Immunosuppression: Concepts and Impacts

Immunosuppression: Concepts and Impacts

Edited by **Jim Wang**

New Jersey

Published by Foster Academics,
61 Van Reypen Street,
Jersey City, NJ 07306, USA
www.fosteracademics.com

Immunosuppression: Concepts and Impacts
Edited by Jim Wang

International Standard Book Number: 978-1-63242-241-5 (Hardback)

Printed in the United States of America.

Contents

Preface

Any act which weakens the efficiency of immune system is classified under Immunosuppression. This book talks about immunology in scientific and curative aspects. The book is rather precise and comprises of matters very relevant to the topic of human immune system and its role in health and diseases. Therapeutic immunosuppression has uses in scientific medicine, which vary from prevention and therapy of organ/bone marrow transplant rejection to organization of autoimmune and inflammatory disorders. This book brings forward significant growth in the area of molecular mechanisms and active therapeutic aspects used for immunosuppression in different human disease situations. This book combines all the important information from different parts of the world, which had been earlier dispersed in different biomedical literature. This text is highly useful to practitioners, doctors, surgeons and biomedical researchers, because it sheds light on different aspects of transplantations and novel therapies.

The researches compiled throughout the book are authentic and of high quality, combining several disciplines and from very diverse regions from around the world. Drawing on the contributions of many researchers from diverse countries, the book's objective is to provide the readers with the latest achievements in the area of research. This book will surely be a source of knowledge to all interested and researching the field.

In the end, I would like to express my deep sense of gratitude to all the authors for meeting the set deadlines in completing and submitting their research chapters. I would also like to thank the publisher for the support offered to us throughout the course of the book. Finally, I extend my sincere thanks to my family for being a constant source of inspiration and encouragement.

Editor

Transplantation and Novel Therapies

Cellular Therapies for Immunosuppression

Nathalie Cools, Viggo F. I. Van Tendeloo and Zwi N. Berneman
Laboratory of Experimental Hematology, Vaccine & Infectious Disease Institute,
University of Antwerp
Belgium

1. Introduction

Almost all current therapeutic approaches to inhibit destructive immune responses in autoimmunity are based on antigen non-specific agents, such as cyclosporine A, which systemically suppress the function of virtually all immune effector cells. This indiscriminate immunosuppression, however, often causes serious and sometimes life-threatening side-effects. Indeed, long-term use of immunosuppressive drugs leads to nephrotoxicity and metabolic disorders, as well as manifestations of hyperimmunosuppression such as opportunistic infections and cancer. It is evident, that treatment would be greatly improved by targeting the fundamental cause of pathogenic immune responses in autoimmunity, i.e. loss of tolerance to self-antigens. For this, manipulation of the immune system in autoimmune diseases should ideally arise in specific tolerance for the self-antigens that stimulate chronic activation of the immune system resulting in long term remissions.

New – more antigen-specific and targeted - therapies are intensively being investigated for the treatment of human diseases (Sabatos-Peyton et al., 2010; Dazzi et al., 2007; Miller et al., 2007). In this context, a variety of cellular therapies have been designed to elicit or amplify immune responses. These cell-based activation immunotherapies have proven to be effective for cancer and infectious diseases. Although still in its infancy, the use of well specified and functionally characterized cellular products as treatment modality for autoimmune disorders and in transplantation tolerance is gaining interest. Indeed, experiences with hematopoietic stem cells and cell types with regulatory properties support the concept of resetting immune tolerance and have made cell-based therapies for autoimmune diseases a realistic alternative. At this point however, it is not yet clear which cell type among a broad arsenal of different tolerogenic entities is best with regard to safety, efficacy and related costs.

This review will explore the molecular and cellular mechanisms underlying T cell tolerance and will focus on emerging cell-based therapies pertaining to reduce, suppress or redirect existing immune responses to self-antigens in human diseases.

2. Control and regulation of immune responses

2.1 Tolerance induction
Immune tolerance is the process by which the body naturally does not launch an immune system attack against its own tissues. A variety of tolerance mechanisms have been

described to exist naturally and to be responsible for protection of the body's own tissue from immune injuries, while effectively fighting pathogens. Central tolerance to self-antigens results primarily from apoptotic deletion of autoreactive T cells during intrathymic T cell development (Burnet, 1959a; Burnet, 1959b). However, some limitations of this process have been observed resulting in escape of potentially autoreactive T cells (Steinman & Nussenzweig, 2002). Therefore additional mechanisms to induce tolerance occur in the periphery. These include (i) T cell anergy (i.e. the induction of functional hyporesponsiveness to antigens) (Schwartz, 2003), (ii) T cell deletion (i.e. the elimination of autoreactive T cells by apoptosis) (Kurts et al., 1998) and (iii) active suppression of the immune response by regulatory T cells (Cools et al., 2007a). Collectively these mechanisms are known as peripheral tolerance. Despite these mechanisms, some autoreactive T cells may escape and be present in the periphery. Their activation may lead to autoimmune disease. These diseases result in cell and tissue destruction by autoreactive T cells or autoantibodies and the accompanying inflammatory processes. Common autoimmune diseases include rheumatoid arthritis (RA), systemic lupus erythematosis (SLE), type 1 diabetes, multiple sclerosis (MS), Sjogren's syndrome, and inflammatory bowel disease (IBD).

2.2 T cell activation

The current paradigm is that the outcome of the immune response is determined by the relative balance between cells that are capable of causing tissue damage, such as T helper type 1 (Th1), type 2 (Th2) and type 17 (Th17) cells versus cells that are designed to suppress immune responses and limit damage, such as regulatory T cells (Treg). It is generally accepted that antigen-presenting cells (APC), particularly dendritic cells (DC), play a central role in the control and maintenance of this delicate balance depending on the level of inflammation in the microenvironment in which T cell activation takes place (Cools et al., 2007b).

(Auto)immune reactions are set in motion with the uptake, processing and presentation of self-antigens through APC. Nevertheless, it is commonly believed now that generation of T cell-mediated (auto)immunity requires a 3-signal T cell activation process (Curtsinger et al., 1999; Curtsinger et al., 2003) (Figure 1). The first signal is provided by the presentation of (self-)antigens by major histocompatibility complex (MHC) molecules on the APC to the T cell receptor (TCR) on the T cell. At this site, antigen recognition will take place which will create an immune synapse determining subsequent T cell fate. Next, interaction of costimulatory molecules on APC and T cells ensures appropriate activation of naïve T cells (Greenfield et al., 1998). For instance, the costimulatory factors CD80 and CD86 bind to CD28 on naïve T cells resulting in activation and proliferation of T cells. Absence of the second signal results in T cell anergy. Besides effector T cell activation, costimulation is also required for the activation and expansion of different regulatory T cell subsets (Salomon et al., 2000). Currently, it is generally accepted that (an) additional signal(s) (i.e. "signal 3"), such as CD40 ligation and/or the production of pro- or anti-inflammatory cytokines are involved in APC-driven polarization of naïve T cells into effector T cell populations. Indeed depending on the cytokines present upon T cell activation, naïve CD4+ T helper cells can acquire a variety of immune effector phenotypes (Strom & Koulmanda, 2009; Zhou et al., 2009). In brief, when CD4+ T cells are activated in the presence of interleukin (IL)-12, they become IFN-γ-producing Th1 cells; while CD4+ T cells that are activated in the presence of

IL-4 will differentiate into Th2 cells producing IL-4, IL-5 and IL-13. Expression of the transcription factor FOXP3 and subsequent generation of Treg is induced by transforming growth factor (TGF)-β, in the absence of additional pro-inflammatory cytokines. In contrast, expression of TGF-β in concert with IL-6 and IL-21 induces IL-17-producing T cells (Th17) (Bettelli et al., 2007; Weaver & Hatton, 2009; Jäger & Kuchroo, 2010).

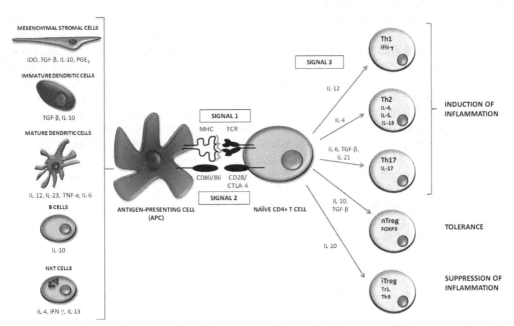

Fig. 1. Molecular mechanisms of T cell activation. Currently, it is accepted that generation of T cell-mediated immunity requires at least 3 signals. In brief, antigen presentation (= "signal 1"), costimulation (= "signal 2"), and the production of immunoregulatory cytokines (= "signal 3") are required for the activation and expansion of different effector and regulatory T cell subsets

It might be evident that the immunological basis of the therapeutic effect of a variety of biological agents used for the induction of immunosuppression lies in the interaction with one, or more, of the above molecular signals. Therefore, immunosuppressants developed for their ability to alter T cell function can generally be divided into 3 categories: (i) TCR-directed agents, (ii) costimulatory antagonists, and (iii) antagonists of cytokines and cytokine receptors. First, Fc receptor (FcR)-non-binding CD3-specific antibodies carrying mutations of the IgG1 Fc chain with elimination of glycosylation sites, are minimally depleting and result in T cell apoptosis and anergy by altering the TCR-CD3 complex and/or induction of Treg. The early results from clinical trials using anti-CD3 antibodies, i.e. Otelixizumab (ChAgly CD3), Tepilizumab [hOKT3γ1(Ala-Ala)], and Visilizumab, in a variety of autoimmune disorders are encouraging (Keymeulen et al., 2005; Bisikirsha et al., 2005; Plevy et al., 2007). Second, agents that block T cell costimulation are currently being tested as maintenance drug in transplant patients. In this context, Abatacept (CTLA4-Ig) blocks the interaction between CD28 expressed on the surface of T cells and CD80/CD86 on the surface of APC. Additionally, Alefacept interferes with the activation of T cells by preventing the interaction between CD2 on T cells and LFA-3 on APC (Vincenti & Luggen, 2007). Furthermore, cytokine– and/or cytokine receptor–directed therapies are also in development in order to promote immunosuppression. Indeed, TNF-α blockers have been extensively used and validated as an efficacious treatment for RA, Crohn's disease and psoriasis (Feldman et al., 1998; Victor et al., 2003). This approach clearly represents one of the greatest successes in biological response–modifying therapies. In addition, the therapeutic efficacy of an anti-IL-12/IL-23 (p40) monoclonal antibody (i.e. Ustekinumab) has been demonstrated in patients with active Crohn's disease (Mannon et al., 2004) and psoriasis (Krueger et al., 2007; Leonardi et al., 2008), but not in MS patients (Segal et al., 2008). For completeness, also biologicals that interfere with lymphocyte trafficking have been approved for the treatment of autoimmune disease. Thus far, the most successfull drug in this class is Natalizumab, a monoclonal antibody to α4-integrin (Yednock et al., 1992; Stüve et al., 2006) blocking the entry of leukocytes into the central nervous system. In addition, Fingolimod (FTY-720) holds promise as a new treatment for MS by promoting tissue retention (O'Connor et al., 2009). In fact, lymphocytes are trapped in the lymph nodes, which reduces peripheral lymphocyte counts and the recirculation of lymphocytes to the inflamed tissues (Mandala et al., 2002; Mehling et al., 2008).

Unlike conventional immunosuppressants for the treatment of patients with autoimmune diseases, biologicals only bind to immune cells or to products secreted by immune cells, thereby reducing or preventing toxicity to non-immune system tissues.

3. Cell therapy approaches aiming at minimizing T cell activation

At present, existing immunomodulatory drugs do not specifically target pathogenic autoreactive T lymphocytes. It is therefore evident, that the "holy grail" for the treatment of autoimmune disease is the development of treatment strategies in which only the pathogenic autoreactive T cells are safely inactivated in an antigen-specific manner, while leaving the remainder of the immune system undisturbed. Therefore, strong efforts are currently undertaken to circumvent various systemic side effects that may occur after overall modulation of protective immunity by harnessing peripheral regulatory mechanisms. Indeed, the anticipated induction of antigen-specific immunosuppression may operate via a number of cell-intrinsic (e.g. anergy) and/or cell-extrinsic (e.g. Treg) mechanisms. Potential candidate cell populations that bear immunomodulating and regulatory properties comprise stem cells of various origins, as well as immune cells such as Treg, DC, NKT and B cells.

3.1 Stem cells
3.1.1 Hematopoietic stem cells (HSC)
Hematopoietic stem cells (HSC) are cells capable of self-renewal and reconstitute all types of blood cells. For this, research on HSC is now providing new approaches to remove autoreactive immune cells and to subsequently generate a new, properly functioning immune system. Although the approach to use high dose myeloablative therapy combined with subsequent hematopoietic stem cell transplantation (HSCT) was first described more than 50 years ago for the treatment of malignant conditions, this principle was adopted in recent years for treatment of various autoimmune diseases. It is evident that complete

immunoablation is a drastic way to achieve maximal treatment efficiency in autoimmune diseases (Teng et al., 2005), with potentially lethal complications such as cardiotoxicity or overt opportunistic infections. For this, HSCT is only considered in patients suffering from severe and progressive autoimmune disease and refractory to conventional immunosuppressants. In contrast to complete ablation of autoreactive T cells, recent immune reconstituting data suggest that non-myeloablative or reduced intensity conditioning protocols could also allow the normal immune-regulatory mechanisms to recontrol the system (Muraro et al., 2005).

To obtain cells for autologous HSCT, stem cells are mobilized from the bone marrow to the peripheral blood, before patient conditioning, using various protocols [e.g. granulocyte colony-stimulating factor (G-CSF)]. Subsequently, the autologous HSC are collected through leukapheresis. After this, the patient is prepared for the transplant by potent immunosuppressive treatment, usually by chemotherapy and/or radiotherapy, in order to eliminate autoreactive T cells. Thereafter, peripheral blood cells or bone marrow cells enriched for HSC or previously purified CD34+ HSC are re-injected and newly developing B and T cells are introduced to self-antigens and controlled by the natural tolerance mechanisms. In most trials, the patient's own stem cells have been used (i.e. autologous HSCT), however small series and case reports of allogeneic HSCT have been reported (Oyama et al., 2001; Burt et al., 2004). Although the advantage of allogeneic HSCT is clear, namely introducing a "healthy" immune system, limited experience is available with regard to this approach for treatment of autoimmune disease. Indeed, the increased toxicity and potential risk of graft-versus-host disease (GVHD) is associated with significant morbidity and mortality of allogeneic HSCT (Griffith et al., 2006).

Several mechanisms may apply for correction of autoimmunity by HSCT. As mentioned above, potent immunosuppressive treatment attributes to the elimination of autoreactive T and B cells. However, incomplete immunoablation may account for the suboptimal responses and high risk rates of early relapse seen in some clinical trials of autologous HSCT. Although HSCT targets a wide array of immune effector cells non-specifically, it has become evident that the therapeutic efficacy of HSCT cannot merely be the consequence of the profound immunosuppression. In contrast, resetting of the abnormal immune regulation underlying the autoimmune conditions most likely attributes to the success of this therapeutic approach. This was well illustrated by Traynor and colleagues who found that following HSCT the deregulated T cell receptor repertoires were restored to those of healthy individuals (Traynor et al., 2000). From this, it can be postulated that re-establishing tolerance in T cells contributes to the beneficial effect of HSCT and thereby decreases the likelihood of disease re-occurrence. Besides the risk associated with allogeneic HSCT, this approach is associated with durable and complete remission in a small number of patients. It is postulated that elimination of autoreactive host lymphocytes by allogeneic donor T cells contributes to this beneficial effect, known as graft–versus–autoimmunity (GVA) effect. However, as stated above, this benefit comes with the associated risk of GVHD. Furthermore tolerance to self-antigens, after allogeneic HSCT, may also be achieved by mixed hematopoietic chimerism, i.e. a state in which HSC of the recipient and donor co-exist and thus also multi-lineage hematopoietic populations. When both donor and host cells contribute to hematopoiesis, the new T cell repertoire in the recipient thymus is rendered tolerant to antigens expressed by hematopoietic cells of both origins.

According to the EBMT/EULAR database (Daikeler et al., 2011), MS is the most frequent diagnosis for which HSCT is being used. Other indications are scleroderma, RA, juvenile idiopathic arthritis (JIA), SLE, Crohn's disease, ulcerative colitis, and vasculitis (Burt et al., 2003; Popat & Krance, 2004; Hough et al., 2005; Tyndall & Saccardi, 2005). Today, HSCT can induce long-term remission lasting for more than six years without any treatment and with a significant decrease in the risks of HSCT, in particular for patients with severe autoimmune disease refractory to conventional treatment. Nonetheless, the major limitation of HSCT in autoimmune patients remains that a considerable amount of treatment-related complications have been reported (e.g. infections, graft failure and malignant relapses), which accounted for the majority of the transplant-related mortality. Currently, several phase III clinical trials are ongoing to evaluate the prospects of autologous HSCT as a cellular treatment strategy for severe autoimmune disease.

3.1.2 Mesenchymal stromal cells (MSC)

Recently another cell, the mesenchymal stromal cell (MSC), has generated great interest for its ability to induce immunosuppression. In pioneering studies, Friedenstein et al. reported more than 30 years ago fibroblast-like cells that could be isolated from bone marrow via their inherent adherence to plastic in culture (Friedenstein et al., 1974). MSC are now known as cells of stromal origin that have the ability of self-renewal and multipotency, which allows their differentiation into various tissues of mesodermal origin (osteocytes, chondrocytes and adipocytes) and other embryonic lineages, and may be isolated from bone marrow, skeletal muscle, adipose tissue, synovial membranes and other connective tissues, and blood. Although still subject of debate, MSC are defined by using a combination of phenotypic markers and functional properties. A generally accepted phenotypic profile of human MSC includes the expression of CD73, CD105 and CD90 as well as the absence of expression of hematopoietic (CD45) and vascular (CD31) markers (Pittenger et al., 1999; Dominici et al., 2006).

MSC are relatively non-immunogenic, i.e. they do not normally express MHC or costimulatory molecules such as CD80 and CD86. Moreover, MSC exert a profound immunosuppressive and anti-inflammatory effect *in vitro* and *in vivo*, which has made these cells of particular interest for therapeutic application (Marigo & Dazzi, 2011). The mechanisms underlying the immunosuppressive effect of MSC remain to be clarified. However, it has been demonstrated that preliminary "licensing" of MSC by inflammatory environmental conditions, such as IFN-γ, is needed to acquire their immunosuppressive properties (Jones et al., 2007). In turn, MSC skew the inflammatory environment into an anti-inflammatory environment both directly, through mechanisms mediated by soluble factors [TGF-β (Di Nicola et al., 2002), indoleamine 2,3-dioxygenase (IDO) (Meisel et al., 2004), hepatocyte growth factor (HGF) (Di Nicola et al., 2002), nitric oxide (Sato et al., 2007), IL-10 (Batten et al., 2006) and prostaglandin E2 (Aggarwal & Pittenger, 2005)] and cell contact [e.g. via the inhibitory molecule programmed death 1 (PD-1) (Augello et al., 2005)], and indirectly via the recruitment of other regulatory networks that involve APC (Beyth et al., 2005) and Treg (Prevosto et al., 2007). Although MSC-induced unresponsiveness lacks any selectivity, its effect is directed mainly at the level of T cell proliferation, as evidenced by cell cycle arrest of MSC-induced anergic T cells. Additionally, recent studies suggest that MSC may induce a cytokine profile shift in the Th1/Th2 balance towards the anti-inflammatory Th2 phenotype (Haniffa et al., 2007; Zhou et al., 2008). Indeed, MSC have been shown to decrease the production of IFN-γ, IL-2 and TNF-α, whilst they increase IL-4 secretion (Aggarwal & Pittenger, 2005). Furthermore, MSC suppress the cytolytic effects of cytotoxic T cells (Rasmusson et al., 2003). However, the effects of MSC on immune responses are not confined to T cells. Indeed, it has been demonstrated that MSC are also capable of inhibiting proliferation of IL-2- and IL-15-stimulated natural killer (NK) cells (Sotiropoulou et al., 2006; Spaggiari et al., 2006), as well as alter the function of B cells and APC. Indeed, MSC affect terminal differentiation of B cells demonstrated by an altered release of humoral factors. Moreover, they increase B cell viability, while inhibiting B cell proliferation through cell cycle arrest of B lymphocytes in the G0/G1 phase (Tabera et al., 2008; Asari et al., 2009). In addition, MSC-derived prostaglandin E2 was shown to act on macrophages by stimulating the production of IL-10 (Németh et al., 2009) and on monocytes by blocking their differentiation towards DC as well as on dendritic cell maturation and function, as demonstrated by a decreased cell-surface expression of MHC class II and costimulatory molecules, and a decreased production of IL-12 and TNF-α (Spaggiari et al., 2009; Jiang et al., 2005; Nauta et al., 2006). Finally, MSC have been reported to promote both *in vitro* and *in vivo*, the formation of potent CD4+CD25+ as well as CD8+ Treg (Prevosto et al., 2007; Maccario et al., 2005), although the precise mode of action is still subject of active research.

Although better understanding of the underlying mechanisms is still required, accumulating evidence with regard to their immunomodulatory properties suggests that MSC have great potential to suppress immune responses in various clinical settings. While MSC represent only a rare fraction in bone marrow and other tissues (i.e. 0.001-0.01% of the total nucleated cells), they can be expanded *ex vivo*, under clinical-grade conditions, to significant numbers from a small bone marrow aspirate in 8 to 10 weeks (DiGirolamo et al., 1999; Sekiya et al., 2002). Treatment of several auto-immune diseases, such as type 1 diabetes, RA, MS (Zappia et al., 2005), and GVHD (Le Blanc et al., 2004; Le Blanc et al., 2008; Lazarus et al., 2005) was performed with administration of MSC derived from allogeneic donors. Several phase I and II clinical trials have been conducted, and encouraging results have been generated from these studies. For example, it has recently been demonstrated that MSC may promote reconstitution of the bone marrow stroma after chemotherapy and enhance HSC engraftment. Indeed, sustained hematopoietic engraftment in pediatric patients was shown after co-transplantation of donor MSC with allogeneic HSC (Ball et al., 2007). In addition, MSC infusion has resulted in striking improvement of therapy-resistant, acute GVHD, as demonstrated by a complete response of 30 out of 55 patients in a multi-center phase II clinical trial (LeBlanc et al., 2008). Although clinical results obtained so far confirm feasibility and safety of the *in vivo* application of MSC without major adverse events, another report has shown an increased risk of relapse in leukemia patients who were co-transplanted with MSC in order to prevent acute GVHD after allogeneic HSCT (Ning et al., 2008), as compared with patients receiving standard HSCT.

3.2 Dendritic cells

A major therapeutic goal in autoimmune diseases is to provide inhibitory mechanisms with the capacity to suppress inappropriate immune activation in an antigen-specific manner with minimal risk and damage to the host. In this perspective, we discuss the role of dendritic cells (DC) and regulatory T cells (Treg) in the design of new cell-based and antigen-specific therapeutic strategies to suppress autoreactive immune responses.

DC are a highly specialized population of white blood cells that are capable of orchestrating the adaptive immune responses (Cools et al., 2007b). In their immature state, DC reside in the peripheral tissues (skin, airways and intestine) where they function as the "sentinels" of the immune system, i.e. they patrol the body to capture antigens, including self-antigens, invading pathogens and certain malignant cells. In the classical view, antigen-loaded DC migrate to the secondary lymphoid organs and the internalized antigen is processed and presented to T cells in a MHC-dependent manner (Trombetta et al., 2005). Depending on the context in which the antigen was captured, DC induce tolerance or immunity. Indeed, in a steady-state condition DC remain immature, expressing only small amounts of MHC and costimulatory molecules, and are believed to induce T cell anergy or regulatory T cells (Lutz & Schuler, 2002). Upon encounter of so-called danger signals, DC undergo a complex maturation process from antigen-capturing cells into antigen-presenting cells, essential for triggering T cell proliferation and differentiation into helper and effector T cells with unique functions and cytokine profiles.

DC are heterogeneous and can be divided into two major subsets: plasmacytoid DC and conventional or myeloid DC, which show several distinct phenotypic and biological features (O'Doherty et al., 1994). Plasmacytoid DC (pDC) originate from a lymphoid progenitor cell in lymphoid organs and are characterized by the production of high amounts of type I interferon in response to viral stimuli (Cella et al., 1999). For this, pDC are believed to be primarily involved in innate immunity (Swiecki & Colonna, 2010; Reizis et al., 2011). On the other hand, a myeloid progenitor cell differentiates towards different DC populations in the bone marrow (Liu, 2001). Subsequently, DC subsets circulate throughout the body: Langerhans cells migrate towards the skin epidermis and interstitial DC migrate towards the skin dermis and various other tissues (airways, liver and intestine). Circulating or migrating DC are found in the blood and in the afferent lymphatics, respectively. In human blood, differences in DC subsets can be identified based on a different expression of Toll-like Receptors (TLR) (Kadowaki et al., 2001), cytokine receptors and cytokines (Kohrgruber et al., 1999), as well as a difference in migratory potential (Penna et al., 2001), indicating a different function in induction and regulation of the immune response by various subtypes [for review on DC subsets see (Ju et al., 2010)].

DC appear to be essential for both central tolerance in the thymus and peripheral tolerance (Liu et al., 2007). Indeed, mature thymic DC present self-antigens to developing T and B cells and subsequently delete lymphocytes with autoreactivity above a certain threshold (Steinman et al., 2003). In addition, DC induce peripheral tolerance through induction of T cell anergy and T cell deletion and through activation of Treg. Antigen presentation in the absence of costimulation can lead to impaired clonal expansion and T cell anergy (Schwartz, 2003). Furthermore, there is increasing evidence that under steady-state conditions antigen presentation by immature DC leads to T cell deletion and peripheral tolerance. In this context, a discrete subset of human DC expressing indoleamine 2,3-dioxygenase (IDO) have been identified (Munn et al., 2002; Mellor & Munn, 2004). IDO is a catabolic enzyme responsible for the degradation of tryptophan, an amino acid essential for T cell proliferation. Additionally, signalling through CD95 (Fas ligation) by DC may be involved in tolerance induction (Süss & Shortman, 1996). Finally, it has also been documented that DC are able to prime Treg in order to maintain tolerance to self-antigens, foreign peptides and allo-antigens (Banerjee et al., 2006; Fehérvári & Sakaguchi, 2004; Kretschmer et al., 2005).

While the pivotal role of DC in immunity is clearly established and results of early studies using DC-based therapeutic vaccines in cancer patients (Van Tendeloo et al., 2011) and HIV-infected individuals (Connolly et al., 2008) are encouraging, the fact that DC are also involved in tolerance induction has provided the prospect for the use of DC to suppress noxious immune responses in allergy, autoimmunity and transplantation (Hilkens et al., 2010). Dendritic cell-based immunotherapeutic strategies for autoimmune and allergic diseases can be developed either by targeting antigen to DC *in vivo* or by culturing the cells *in vitro*, pulsing with antigen and injecting them back into patients. On the one hand, antigens coupled to antibodies specific for DC markers, such as 33D1 or DEC-205, have already been used to deliver antigens to DC *in vivo*, resulting in antigen-specific tolerance which in contrast could not be attained by injection of the same peptide in the Freund's adjuvant (Hawiger et al., 2001; Bonifaz et al., 2002). On the other hand, administration of immature DC has already been shown to induce antigen-specific T cell tolerance. Indeed, when iDC pulsed with influenza matrix protein (IMP) and keyhole limpet hemocyanin (KLH), a general stimulator of CD4+ T cells, were injected, a decline in influenza-specific CD8+ IFN-γ-secreting T cells was observed, while peptide-specific IL-10-secreting T cells appeared (Dhodapkar et al., 2001; Dhodapkar & Steinman, 2002). Aforementioned results suggest that DC can induce antigen-specific T cell tolerance *in vitro* as well as *in vivo*, and have prompted a number of groups to translate these findings into clinical applications. A phase I clinical trial using vitamin D3-treated tolerogenic DC will be started in RA patients at Newcastle University (Harry et al., 2010; Hilkens et al., 2010) (http://clinicaltrials.gov/ct2/show/study/NCT012352858). Furthermore, genetic manipulation of DC by overexpressing immune–regulatory molecules or inhibiting or silencing immune–stimulatory molecules promotes tolerogenic function. In line with this, a first safety study using tolerogenic DC treated with antisense oligonucleotides targeting the primary transcripts of the CD40, CD80, and CD86 costimulatory molecules has recently started at the University of Pittsburg (http://clinicaltrials.gov/ct2/show/study/NCT00445913).

3.3. Regulatory T cells

Different T cell subsets have been identified with the ability to suppress immune responses and are currently subdivided based on expression of cell surface markers, production of cytokines and mechanisms of action. Two broad categories of Treg have been described. The first are naturally-occurring thymic-derived regulatory T cells (nTreg) which constitutively express the IL-2 receptor α chain (CD25), and comprise 1-10% of the CD4+ T cell population in healthy adults. These cells also express the intracellular transcription factor forkhead box P3 (FOXP3) (Ziegler, 2006), which has demonstrated to be critical for the generation of Treg (Gavin et al., 2007; Bacchetta et al., 2006), and its genetic deficiency results in autoimmune and inflammatory diseases (Wildin & Freitas, 2005). Recently, a unique CpG-rich island within an evolutionary conserved region upstream of exon 1, named TSDR (Treg-specific demethylation region), was demonstrated to be unmethylated in nTreg (Lal & Bromberg, 2009a; Lal et al., 2009b). Demethylation of this region resulted in strong and stable induction of FOXP3. In contrast, conventional CD4+ T cells display methylation of the FOXP3 locus. This finding has led to new methods of analysing Treg based on quantitative analysis of methylation patterns of the key transcription factor FOXP3, which may be valuable for quality assessment of *ex vivo* expanded Treg (Wieczorek et al., 2009). There is accumulating evidence that 2 subsets of nTreg exist: a first population that is derived directly from the thymus; the second derives from CD4+CD25- T cell precursors in the periphery. In addition, several other studies have reported the existence of various subsets of (antigen-)induced or adaptive Treg. There are at least two populations of induced Treg (iTreg), subdivided according to different expression of immunosuppressive cytokines: CD4+ regulatory T cells type 1 (Tr1) express high levels of interleukin (IL)-10 (Roncarolo et al., 2006; Battaglia et al., 2004), while T helper 3 (Th3) regulatory T cells secrete large amounts of TGF-β (Faria & Weiner, 2006; Carrier et al., 2007). In addition, we have shown the presence of IL-10/TGF-β double-positive Tr1 cells at the single cell level (Cools et al., 2008). Ultimately, only the demonstration of actual suppressive function confirms the presence of Treg.

Numerous immunosuppressive mechanisms described thus far suggest that multiple, redundant mechanisms are required for optimal Treg function *in vivo*. Indeed Treg mediate suppressive effects by several mechanisms including cell contact-mediated suppression, competition for growth factors and secretion of soluble suppressive factors. Several *in vitro* studies have demonstrated that Treg suppress proliferation and IFN-γ production by effector T cells through a direct cell contact-dependent mechanism between suppressor and effector cells, possibly mediated by the expression of cell surface markers, such as glucocorticoid-induced tumor necrosis factor (TNF) receptor-related protein (GITR), cytotoxic T lymphocyte-associated antigen (CTLA-4) and galectin-1 (Shevach, 2009; Garín et al., 2007). Also, cell surface-bound TGF-β has been reported to mediate cell contact-dependent immunosuppression by Treg (Nakamura et al, 2001). Another mechanism for Treg to affect effector T cell activation can be established by modulating DC function. For example, ligation of CD80/CD86 on DC by CTLA-4 on Treg results in expression and activation of IDO (Fallarino et al., 2003), a catabolic enzyme involved in tryptophan degradation. Furthermore, soluble factors such as the immunosuppressive cytokines IL-10, IL-35 (Collison et al., 2007) and TGF-β have been implicated in the suppressive function of Treg. The roles of these cytokines in immunosuppression include cell cycle arrest and inhibition of proliferation, induction of apoptosis, and suppression of DC maturation and function (Li & Flavell, 2008). Moreover, Treg can express cytotoxic molecules, such as granzyme A, granzyme B and perforin, inducing apoptosis of target cells (Grossman et al., 2004; Gondek et al., 2005). Finally, Treg may also attenuate immune responses by competing with effector cells for essential growth factors, such as IL-2 which has been demonstrated to be essential for both Treg and effector cell function (Busse et al., 2010). It is evident from the studies delineated above that the precise mechanisms of suppression by Treg has yet to be fully elucidated.

Various studies have confirmed the importance and therapeutic potential of Treg. A number of commonly used non-specific therapies have been documented to induce immunomodulatory cytokines and to alter Treg function. For instance, rapamycine (sirolimus), an oral inhibitor of the mammalian target of rapamycin (mTor) pathway, promotes the *de novo* generation and enhances the suppressive capacity of Treg (Gao et al., 2007; Monti et al., 2008). This is in contrast to calcineurin inhibitors which inhibit Treg induction. While the action of these drugs is non-specific, strategies to specifically induce Treg are currently the subject of active investigation. These approaches are based on the fact that exposure to antigen increases Treg frequency and/or potency by either expanding nTreg or inducing the generation of induced Treg from cells that do not originally possess regulatory activity (Long & Wood, 2009). They include adoptive transfer of *ex vivo* generated and/or expanded CD4+CD25+ Treg, and the induction of appropriate Treg populations in patients *in vivo*. Since Treg comprise only a small proportion of peripheral blood CD4+ T cells in human, *ex vivo* expansion of these cells prior to administration to the patient is required. The most commonly used expansion protocol at present is based on stimulation by anti-CD3/anti-CD28 beads in the presence of high doses of recombinant IL-2, supplemented in some protocols with rapamycin (Trzonkowski et al., 2009). This approach is advantageous since the expanded cells can be phenotypically and functionally characterized prior to infusion. Currently, several clinical trials using adoptively transferred Treg are ongoing (Riley et al., 2009). In a phase I/II clinical trial in 28 patients receiving HSCT together with conventional T cells as well as Treg, long-term protection from GVHD and robust immune reconstitution was demonstrated (Di Ianni et al., 2011). In addition, Trzonkowski et al. did not report unexpected adverse effects using *ex vivo* expanded Treg in humans for the treatment of GVHD following HSCT (Trzonkowski et al., 2009). To date, further clinical studies are being planned to test the therapeutic potential of Treg in view of immunosuppression in autoimmunity and in solid organ transplantation.

3.4 Other immune effector cells
3.4.1 B cells

B cells can play a variety of pathogenic roles in human autoimmune diseases. On the one hand, they may serve as potent self-antigen-presenting cells and on the other hand after differentiation into plasma cells they can secrete auto-antibodies that through complexing antigen can promote local inflammatory reactions. Indeed, two major B cell subsets have been demonstrated: (i) early lineage CD20+CD79+CD27+ B cells function primarily as APC expressing MHC and costimulatory antigens that sustain T cell-mediated cellular responses, and (ii) late lineage CD138+ mature plasma cells and CD38+ plasma blasts that relate to the humoral response (Zarkhin et al., 2008; Zarkhin et al., 2010). From these results it is evident that B cells contribute to immunity through production of antibodies, antigen presentation to T cells and secretion of cytokines. The role of B cells as an essential component of the autoimmune reaction that sustains the chronic inflammation has been underlined by successful therapeutic B cell depletion with anti-CD20 monoclonal antibodies. Indeed, rituximab – a chimeric anti-CD20 monoclonal antibody - has been proven to be highly beneficial for patients with certain autoimmune diseases, including RA, MS and type 1 diabetes. However, this treatment also resulted in aggravation of symptoms in a few patients, suggesting that B cells can also protect from autoimmune pathology. In this context, IL-10-producing regulatory CD1d+CD5+ B cells are able to downregulate autoimmune disease initiation, onset, or severity in experimental autoimmune encephalomyelitis (EAE), collagen-induced arthritis, contact hypersensitivity, and inflammatory bowel disease, indicating that B cells can also be essential for immunosuppression of autoreactive T cell responses (Iwata et al., 2011; DiLillo et al., 2010). Therefore, B cell-mediated regulation of the immune system may be of great interest for the development of new cell-based therapies for immunosuppression. Indeed, adoptive transfer of *in vitro* activated B cells isolated from successfully treated mice limited disease severity, suggesting a possible role for regulatory B cells (Yanaba et al., 2008).

3.4.2 Natural killer T cells

A T cell subset with regulatory properties that additionally exhibit natural killer cell characteristics has been identified in mice and humans [extensively reviewed elsewhere (Hegde et al., 2010; Pratschke et al., 2009; Wu & Van Kaer, 2009)]. These natural killer T (NKT) cells are a subset of innate lymphocytes that recognize endogenous or exogenous glycolipids in the context of CD1d molecules expressed by APC, such as monocytes, DC and myeloid suppressor cells. Upon antigenic stimulation NKT cells produce a variety of immunomodulatory cytokines, which endow these cells with potent immunoregulatory properties. Therefore, NKT cells have been tested in animal models of various autoimmune diseases, such as type 1 diabetes, experimental autoimmune encephalomyelitis, arthritis and SLE, but so far only with moderate success.

3.4.3 Peripheral blood mononuclear cells (PBMC)

An alternative approach for effective immunosuppression for treatment of autoimmune disease involves the coupling of self-antigen-derived peptides to cellular vehicles using chemical fixatives (Miller et al., 2007). The induction of immunosuppression by this method is indirect and implies that the fixed cells rapidly undergo apoptotic cell death following fixation and subsequently carry over intact peptides to tolerogenic APC for processing and presentation (Smith & Miller, 2006; Turley & Miller, 2007).

To date, the group of Roland Martin from the University of Hamburg (Germany) has started a phase I/IIa study to evaluate the therapeutic use of autologous peripheral blood mononuclear cells (PBMC) in MRI-proven relapsing-remitting MS patients. These PBMC are coupled with a cocktail of 7 myelin peptides associated with MS pathogenesis against which demonstrable responses can be detected in patient subsets (Lutterotti et al., 2008). This first-in-man exploratory study will provide proof-of-concept of the potential for this cell-based immune-therapeutic approach.

4. Conclusion

Cell-based immunotherapy presents an appealing venue as a substantial component of future individualized treatment modalities for a broad scope of medical fields, including cancer immunotherapies, autoimmune diseases and transplantation tolerance.

Increasing knowledge with regard to the biology, function and mode of immunosuppression of immunoregulatory cell populations opens up new possibilities for antigen-specific manipulation of autoimmunity. Ultimately, this will lead to their clinical application. Nonetheless, the complexity and heterogeneity of autoimmunity, in which multiple dysregulated cell types on various genetic backgrounds are involved, may require integration of several tolerance induction mechanisms to restore tolerance. Therefore, the opportunity to intervene before the appearance of epitope spreading (Miller et al., 2007) using tolerogenic strategies in combination with broader immunosuppressive agents, should be further explored. For instance, induction of immunosuppression may be preceded by treatment with biologicals which can function to reduce the self-antigen-specific T cell frequency to a level that can be effectively and permanently suppressed. Strategies that have shown immunosuppressive effects in animal models include the combination of costimulatory blockade reagents and T cell depletion, as well as adoptively transferred Treg (Chen et al., 2005; Bresson & von Herrath, 2008).

Additionally, also the therapeutic benefit of autologous HSCT could be boosted by the addition of regulatory cell populations, such as tolerogenic DC, Treg, or MSC, which have potent immunosuppressive properties.

Numerous questions still remain in view of the translation of bench findings to the bedside. One challenge for immune tolerance induction is the identification of disease subsets to be considered in evaluating treatment response as well as careful and proper choice of patients to be included for clinical trials evaluating the effects of cellular therapies for immunosuppression. Another quest is how to qualitatively and quantitatively measure immunosuppression in patients. In this context, immunological assays may be used as measures of the effect of immune therapies, although their relationship to the disease process remains speculative. As an example, cellular proliferation assays to islet-specific proteins have distinguished responses in diabetic patients from healthy control subjects (Herold et al., 2009). Ideally, therapies for immunosuppression must also be durable. This means that the ability to regulate the autoimmune response has to be permanent or at least for many years following intervention, for instance via the generation of self-antigen-specific Treg. Nevertheless, major concerns to administer a specified cell product as a tolerizing regimen relates to the risk of *in vivo* re-activation, particularly in response to any underlying inflammatory microenvironment. By means of example, it has indeed been shown that a minority of adoptively transferred Treg lose their FOXP3 expression and can even differentiate into effector T cells (Komatsu et al., 2009). Moreover, a number of groups have identified the ability of Treg to differentiate into proinflammatory Th17 cells (Koenen et al., 2008; Voo et al., 2009). Therefore, such side effects need to be blocked and – in the case of DC – several reports demonstrate that exposure to anti-inflammatory cytokines and immunosuppressive agents can condition DC to a tolerogenic state (Steinman & Banchereau, 2007). Recently, we have shown that *in vitro* exposure of *ex vivo* generated DC from MS patients to IL-10 results in IL-10-, but not IL-12-, secreting DC with low expression levels of CD80/86 and an effective capacity to suppress myelin-specific T cell responses *in vitro* (Cools et al., manuscript submitted for publication). Importantly, further *in vitro* treatment of DC with maturation stimuli did not induce phenotypic changes or modifications in the cytokine secretion profile. Other related safety issues include immunogenicity, carcinogenicity, sensitization to donor HLA, lack of clear mechanistic understanding and cost-benefit relations. In particular the absence of transformation potential of *ex vivo* cultured cells needs to be documented before infusion into (immune-compromised) patients, since failure of immune surveillance mechanisms may favour the development of tumors *in vivo*.

In conclusion, improved understanding of the disease pathogenesis of autoimmunity, the genetic defects underlying different forms of autoimmune diseases, and the mechanisms by which regulatory cell populations suppress autoreactive T and B cells will better define the ultimate role of cellular therapies in the treatment of autoimmune disease.

5. Acknowledgement

This work was supported by grant no. G.0168.09 of the Fund for Scientific Research – Flanders, Belgium (FWO-Vlaanderen), by the grants of the University of Antwerp through the Special Research Fund (BOF), Medical Legacy Fund, and the Methusalem funding program, by a grant of the Hercules Foundation - Belgium, by grants of the Charcot

Foundation - Belgium and of the "Belgische Stichting Roeping" - Belgium. NC is a postdoctoral fellow of the Fund for Scientific Research (FWO)-Flanders.

6. References

Aggarwal S, Pittenger MF. (2005). Human mesenchymal stem cells modulate allogeneic immune cell responses. Blood, 105(4):1815-22.

Asari S, Itakura S, Ferreri K, Liu CP, Kuroda Y, Kandeel F, Mullen Y. (2009). Mesenchymal stem cells suppress B-cell terminal differentiation. Exp Hematol, 37(5):604-15.

Augello A, Tasso R, Negrini SM, Amateis A, Indiveri F, Cancedda R, Pennesi G. (2005). Bone marrow mesenchymal progenitor cells inhibit lymphocyte proliferation by activation of the programmed death 1 pathway. Eur J Immunol, 35(5):1482-90.

Bacchetta R, Passerini L, Gambineri E, Dai M, Allan SE, Perroni L, Dagna-Bricarelli F, Sartirana C, Matthes-Martin S, Lawitschka A, Azzari C, Ziegler SF, Levings MK, Roncarolo MG. (2006). Defective regulatory and effector T cell functions in patients with FOXP3 mutations. J Clin Invest, 116(6):1713-22.

Ball LM, Bernardo ME, Roelofs H, Lankester A, Cometa A, Egeler RM, Locatelli F, Fibbe WE. (2007). Cotransplantation of ex vivo expanded mesenchymal stem cells accelerates lymphocyte recovery and may reduce the risk of graft failure in haploidentical hematopoietic stem-cell transplantation. Blood, 110(7):2764-7.

Banerjee DK, Dhodapkar MV, Matayeva E, Steinman RM, Dhodapkar KM. (2006). Expansion of FOXP3high regulatory T cells by human dendritic cells (DCs) in vitro and after injection of cytokine-matured DCs in myeloma patients. Blood, 108(8):2655-61.

Battaglia M, Gianfrani C, Gregori S, Roncarolo MG. (2004). IL-10-producing T regulatory type 1 cells and oral tolerance. Ann N Y Acad Sci, 1029:142-53.

Batten P, Sarathchandra P, Antoniw JW, Tay SS, Lowdell MW, Taylor PM, Yacoub MH. (2006). Human mesenchymal stem cells induce T cell anergy and downregulate T cell allo-responses via the TH2 pathway: relevance to tissue engineering human heart valves. Tissue Eng, 12(8):2263-73.

Bettelli E, Korn T, Kuchroo VK. (2007). Th17: the third member of the effector T cell trilogy. Curr Opin Immunol, 19(6):652-7.

Beyth S, Borovsky Z, Mevorach D, Liebergall M, Gazit Z, Aslan H, Galun E, Rachmilewitz J. (2005). Human mesenchymal stem cells alter antigen-presenting cell maturation and induce T-cell unresponsiveness. Blood, 105(5):2214-9.

Bisikirska B, Colgan J, Luban J, Bluestone JA, Herold KC. (2005). TCR stimulation with modified anti-CD3 mAb expands CD8+ T cell population and induces CD8+CD25+ Tregs. J Clin Invest. 115(10):2904-13.

Bonifaz L, Bonnyay D, Mahnke K, Rivera M, Nussenzweig MC, Steinman RM. (2002). Efficient targeting of protein antigen to the dendritic cell receptor DEC-205 in the steady state leads to antigen presentation on major histocompatibility complex class I products and peripheral CD8+ T cell tolerance. J Exp Med, 196(12):1627-38.

Bresson D, von Herrath M. (2008). Resuscitating adaptive Tregs with combination therapies? Novartis Found Symp, 292:50-60; discussion 60-7, 122-9, 202-3.

Burnet M. (1959a). Auto-immune disease. I. Modern immunological concepts. Br Med J, 2(5153):645-650.

Burnet M. (1959b). Auto-immune disease. II. Pathology of the immune response. Br Med J, 2(5154):720-725.

Burt RK, Marmont A, Arnold R, Heipe F, Firestein GS, Carrier E, Hahn B, Barr W, Oyama Y, Snowden J, Kalunian K, Traynor A. (2003). Development of a phase III trial of hematopoietic stem cell transplantation for systemic lupus erythematosus. Bone Marrow Transplant, 32 Suppl 1:S49-51.

Burt RK, Oyama Y, Verda L, Quigley K, Brush M, Yaung K, Statkute L, Traynor A, Barr WG. (2004). Induction of remission of severe and refractory rheumatoid arthritis by allogeneic mixed chimerism. Arthritis Rheum, 50(8):2466-70.

Busse D, de la Rosa M, Hobiger K, Thurley K, Flossdorf M, Scheffold A, Höfer T. (2010). Competing feedback loops shape IL-2 signaling between helper and regulatory T lymphocytes in cellular microenvironments. Proc Natl Acad Sci U S A, 107(7):3058-63.

Carrier Y, Yuan J, Kuchroo VK, Weiner HL. (2007). Th3 cells in peripheral tolerance. I. Induction of Foxp3-positive regulatory T cells by Th3 cells derived from TGF-beta T cell-transgenic mice. J Immunol, 178(1):179-85.

Cella M, Jarrossay D, Facchetti F, Alebardi O, Nakajima H, Lanzavecchia A, Colonna M. (1999). Plasmacytoid monocytes migrate to inflamed lymph nodes and produce large amounts of type I interferon. Nat Med, 5(8):919-23.

Chen Z, Benoist C, Mathis D. (2005). How defects in central tolerance impinge on a deficiency in regulatory T cells. Proc Natl Acad Sci U S A, 102(41):14735-40.

Collison LW, Workman CJ, Kuo TT, Boyd K, Wang Y, Vignali KM, Cross R, Sehy D, Blumberg RS, Vignali DA. (2007). The inhibitory cytokine IL-35 contributes to regulatory T-cell function. Nature, 450(7169):566-9.

Connolly NC, Whiteside TL, Wilson C, Kondragunta V, Rinaldo CR, Riddler SA. (2008). Therapeutic immunization with human immunodeficiency virus type 1 (HIV-1) peptide-loaded dendritic cells is safe and induces immunogenicity in HIV-1-infected individuals. Clin Vaccine Immunol, 15(2):284-92.

Cools N, Ponsaerts P, Van Tendeloo VF, Berneman ZN. (2007a). Regulatory T cells and human disease. Clin Dev Immunol, 2007:89195.

Cools N, Ponsaerts P, Van Tendeloo VF, Berneman ZN. (2007b). Balancing between immunity and tolerance: an interplay between dendritic cells, regulatory T cells, and effector T cells. J Leukoc Biol, 82(6):1365-74.

Cools N, Van Tendeloo VF, Smits EL, Lenjou M, Nijs G, Van Bockstaele DR, Berneman ZN, Ponsaerts P. (2008). Immunosuppression induced by immature dendritic cells is mediated by TGF-beta/IL-10 double-positive CD4+ regulatory T cells. J Cell Mol Med, 12(2):690-700.

Curtsinger JM, Lins DC, Mescher MF. (2003). Signal 3 determines tolerance versus full activation of naive CD8 T cells: dissociating proliferation and development of effector function. J Exp Med, 197(9):1141-1151.

Curtsinger JM, Schmidt CS, Mondino A, Lins DC, Kedl RM, Jenkins MK, Mescher MF. (1999). Inflammatory cytokines provide a third signal for activation of naive CD4+ and CD8+ T cells. J Immunol, 162(6):3256-3262.

Daikeler T, Labopin M, Di Gioia M, Abinun M, Alexander T, Miniati I, Gualandi F, Fassas A, Martin T, Schwarze CP, Wulffraat N, Buch M, Sampol A, Carreras E, Dubois B, Gruhn B, Güngör T, Pohlreich D, Schuerwegh A, Snarski E, Snowden J, Veys P,

Fasth A, Lenhoff S, Messina C, Voswinkel J, Badoglio M, Henes J, Launay D, Tyndall A, Gluckman E, Farge D. (2011). Secondary autoimmune diseases occurring after HSCT for an autoimmune disease: a retrospective study of the EBMT Autoimmune Disease Working Party. Blood, Epub ahead of print.

Dazzi F, van Laar JM, Cope A, Tyndall A. (2007). Cell therapy for autoimmune diseases. Arthritis Res Ther, 9(2):206.

Dhodapkar MV, Steinman RM, Krasovsky J, Munz C, Bhardwaj N. (2001). Antigen-specific inhibition of effector T cell function in humans after injection of immature dendritic cells. J Exp Med, 193(2):233-8.

Dhodapkar MV, Steinman RM. (2002). Antigen-bearing immature dendritic cells induce peptide-specific CD8(+) regulatory T cells in vivo in humans. Blood, 100(1):174-7.

Di Ianni M, Falzetti F, Carotti A, Terenzi A, Castellino F, Bonifacio E, Del Papa B, Zei T, Ostini RI, Cecchini D, Aloisi T, Perruccio K, Ruggeri L, Balucani C, Pierini A, Sportoletti P, Aristei C, Falini B, Reisner Y, Velardi A, Aversa F, Martelli MF. (2011). Tregs prevent GVHD and promote immune reconstitution in HLA-haploidentical transplantation. Blood, 117(14):3921-8.

Di Nicola M, Carlo-Stella C, Magni M, Milanesi M, Longoni PD, Matteucci P, Grisanti S, Gianni AM. (2002). Human bone marrow stromal cells suppress T-lymphocyte proliferation induced by cellular or nonspecific mitogenic stimuli. Blood, 99(10):3838-43.

Digirolamo CM, Stokes D, Colter D, Phinney DG, Class R, Prockop DJ. (1999). Propagation and senescence of human marrow stromal cells in culture: a simple colony-forming assay identifies samples with the greatest potential to propagate and differentiate. Br J Haematol, 107(2):275-81.

DiLillo DJ, Matsushita T, Tedder TF. (2010). B10 cells and regulatory B cells balance immune responses during inflammation, autoimmunity, and cancer. Ann N Y Acad Sci, 1183:38-57.

Dominici M, Le Blanc K, Mueller I, Slaper-Cortenbach I, Marini F, Krause D, Deans R, Keating A, Prockop Dj, Horwitz E. (2006). Minimal criteria for defining multipotent mesenchymal stromal cells. The International Society for Cellular Therapy position statement. Cytotherapy, 8(4):315-7.

Fallarino F, Grohmann U, Hwang KW, Orabona C, Vacca C, Bianchi R, Belladonna ML, Fioretti MC, Alegre ML, Puccetti P. (2003). Modulation of tryptophan catabolism by regulatory T cells. Nat Immunol, 4(12):1206-12.

Faria AM, Weiner HL. (2006). Oral tolerance and TGF-beta-producing cells. Inflamm Allergy Drug Targets, 5(3):179-90.

Fehérvári Z, Sakaguchi S. (2004). Control of Foxp3+ CD25+CD4+ regulatory cell activation and function by dendritic cells. Int Immunol, 16(12):1769-80.

Feldman M, Taylor P, Paleolog E, Brennan FM, Maini RN. (1998). Anti-TNF alpha therapy is useful in rheumatoid arthritis and Crohn's disease: analysis of the mechanism of action predicts utility in other diseases. Transplant Proc, 30(8):4126-7.

Friedenstein AJ, Chailakhyan RK, Latsinik NV, Panasyuk AF, Keiliss-Borok IV. (1974). Stromal cells responsible for transferring the microenvironment of the hemopoietic tissues. Cloning in vitro and retransplantation in vivo. Transplantation, 17(4):331-40.

Gao W, Lu Y, El Essawy B, Oukka M, Kuchroo VK, Strom TB. (2007). Contrasting effects of cyclosporine and rapamycin in de novo generation of alloantigen-specific regulatory T cells. Am J Transplant, 7(7):1722-32.

Garín MI, Chu CC, Golshayan D, Cernuda-Morollón E, Wait R, Lechler RI. (2007). Galectin-1: a key effector of regulation mediated by CD4+CD25+ T cells. Blood, 109(5):2058-65.

Gavin MA, Rasmussen JP, Fontenot JD, Vasta V, Manganiello VC, Beavo JA, Rudensky AY. (2007). Foxp3-dependent programme of regulatory T-cell differentiation. Nature, 445(7129):771-5.

Gondek DC, Lu LF, Quezada SA, Sakaguchi S, Noelle RJ. (2005). Cutting edge: contact-mediated suppression by CD4+CD25+ regulatory cells involves a granzyme B-dependent, perforin-independent mechanism. J Immunol, 174(4):1783-6.

Greenfield EA, Nguyen KA, Kuchroo VK. (1998). CD28/B7 costimulation: a review. Crit Rev Immunol, 18(5):389-418.

Griffith LM, Pavletic SZ, Tyndall A, Gratwohl A, Furst DE, Forman SJ, Nash RA. (2006). Target populations in allogeneic hematopoietic cell transplantation for autoimmune diseases--a workshop accompanying: cellular therapy for treatment of autoimmune diseases, basic science and clinical studies, including new developments in hematopoietic and mesenchymal stem cell therapy. Biol Blood Marrow Transplant, 12(6):688-90.

Grossman WJ, Verbsky JW, Barchet W, Colonna M, Atkinson JP, Ley TJ. (2004). Human T regulatory cells can use the perforin pathway to cause autologous target cell death. Immunity, 21(4):589-601.

Haniffa MA, Wang XN, Holtick U, Rae M, Isaacs JD, Dickinson AM, Hilkens CM, Collin MP. (2007). Adult human fibroblasts are potent immunoregulatory cells and functionally equivalent to mesenchymal stem cells. J Immunol, 179(3):1595-604.

Harry RA, Anderson AE, Isaacs JD, Hilkens CM. (2010). Generation and characterisation of therapeutic tolerogenic dendritic cells for rheumatoid arthritis. Ann Rheum Dis, 69(11):2042-50.

Hawiger D, Inaba K, Dorsett Y, Guo M, Mahnke K, Rivera M, Ravetch JV, Steinman RM, Nussenzweig MC. (2001). Dendritic cells induce peripheral T cell unresponsiveness under steady state conditions in vivo. J Exp Med, 194(6):769-79.

Hegde S, Fox L, Wang X, Gumperz JE. (2010). Autoreactive natural killer T cells: promoting immune protection and immune tolerance through varied interactions with myeloid antigen-presenting cells. Immunology, 130(4):471-83.

Herold KC, Brooks-Worrell B, Palmer J, Dosch HM, Peakman M, Gottlieb P, Reijonen H, Arif S, Spain LM, Thompson C, Lachin JM; Type 1 Diabetes TrialNet Research Group. (2009). Validity and reproducibility of measurement of islet autoreactivity by T-cell assays in subjects with early type 1 diabetes. Diabetes, 58(11):2588-95.

Hilkens CM, Isaacs JD, Thomson AW. (2010). Development of dendritic cell-based immunotherapy for autoimmunity. Int Rev Immunol, 29(2):156-83.

Hough RE, Snowden JA, Wulffraat NM. (2005). Haemopoietic stem cell transplantation in autoimmune diseases: a European perspective. Br J Haematol, 128(4):432-59.

Iwata Y, Matsushita T, Horikawa M, Dilillo DJ, Yanaba K, Venturi GM, Szabolcs PM, Bernstein SH, Magro CM, Williams AD, Hall RP, St Clair EW, Tedder TF. (2011).

Characterization of a rare IL-10-competent B-cell subset in humans that parallels mouse regulatory B10 cells. Blood, 117(2):530-41.

Jäger A, Kuchroo VK. (2010). Effector and regulatory T-cell subsets in autoimmunity and tissue inflammation. Scand J Immunol, 72(3):173-84.

Jiang XX, Zhang Y, Liu B, Zhang SX, Wu Y, Yu XD, Mao N. (2005). Human mesenchymal stem cells inhibit differentiation and function of monocyte-derived dendritic cells. Blood, 105(10):4120-6.

Jones S, Horwood N, Cope A, Dazzi F. (2007). The antiproliferative effect of mesenchymal stem cells is a fundamental property shared by all stromal cells. J Immunol, 179(5):2824-31.

Ju X, Clark G, Hart DN. (2010). Review of human DC subtypes. Methods Mol Biol, 595:3-20.

Kadowaki N, Ho S, Antonenko S, Malefyt RW, Kastelein RA, Bazan F, Liu YJ. (2001). Subsets of human dendritic cell precursors express different toll-like receptors and respond to different microbial antigens. J Exp Med, 194(6):863-9.

Keymeulen B, Vandemeulebroucke E, Ziegler AG, Mathieu C, Kaufman L, Hale G, Gorus F, Goldman M, Walter M, Candon S, Schandene L, Crenier L, De Block C, Seigneurin JM, De Pauw P, Pierard D, Weets I, Rebello P, Bird P, Berrie E, Frewin M, Waldmann H, Bach JF, Pipeleers D, Chatenoud L. (2005). Insulin needs after CD3-antibody therapy in new-onset type 1 diabetes. N Engl J Med, 352(25):2598-608.

Koenen HJ, Smeets RL, Vink PM, van Rijssen E, Boots AM, Joosten I. (2008). Human CD25highFoxp3pos regulatory T cells differentiate into IL-17-producing cells. Blood, 112(6):2340-52.

Kohrgruber N, Halanek N, Gröger M, Winter D, Rappersberger K, Schmitt-Egenolf M, Stingl G, Maurer D. (1999). Survival, maturation, and function of CD11c- and CD11c+ peripheral blood dendritic cells are differentially regulated by cytokines. J Immunol, 163(6):3250-9.

Komatsu N, Mariotti-Ferrandiz ME, Wang Y, Malissen B, Waldmann H, Hori S. (2009). Heterogeneity of natural Foxp3+ T cells: a committed regulatory T-cell lineage and an uncommitted minor population retaining plasticity. Proc Natl Acad Sci U S A, 106(6):1903-8.

Kretschmer K, Apostolou I, Hawiger D, Khazaie K, Nussenzweig MC, von Boehmer H. (2005). Inducing and expanding regulatory T cell populations by foreign antigen. Nat Immunol, 6(12):1219-27.

Krueger GG, Langley RG, Leonardi C, Yeilding N, Guzzo C, Wang Y, Dooley LT, Lebwohl M; CNTO 1275 Psoriasis Study Group. (2007). A human interleukin-12/23 monoclonal antibody for the treatment of psoriasis. N Engl J Med, 356(6):580-92.

Kurts C, Heath WR, Kosaka H, Miller JF, Carbone FR. (1998). The peripheral deletion of autoreactive CD8+ T cells induced by cross-presentation of self-antigens involves signaling through CD95 (Fas, Apo-1). J Exp Med, 188(2):415-420.

Lal G, Bromberg JS. (2009a). Epigenetic mechanisms of regulation of Foxp3 expression. Blood, 114(18):3727-35.

Lal G, Zhang N, van der Touw W, Ding Y, Ju W, Bottinger EP, Reid SP, Levy DE, Bromberg JS. (2009b). Epigenetic regulation of Foxp3 expression in regulatory T cells by DNA methylation. J Immunol, 182(1):259-73.

Lazarus HM, Koc ON, Devine SM, Curtin P, Maziarz RT, Holland HK, Shpall EJ, McCarthy P, Atkinson K, Cooper BW, Gerson SL, Laughlin MJ, Loberiza FR Jr, Moseley AB,

Bacigalupo A. (2005). Cotransplantation of HLA-identical sibling culture-expanded mesenchymal stem cells and hematopoietic stem cells in hematologic malignancy patients. Biol Blood Marrow Transplant, 11(5):389-98. PubMed PMID: 15846293.

Le Blanc K, Frassoni F, Ball L, Locatelli F, Roelofs H, Lewis I, Lanino E, Sundberg B, Bernardo ME, Remberger M, Dini G, Egeler RM, Bacigalupo A, Fibbe W, Ringdén O; Developmental Committee of the European Group for Blood and Marrow Transplantation. (2008). Mesenchymal stem cells for treatment of steroid-resistant, severe, acute graft-versus-host disease: a phase II study. Lancet, 371(9624):1579-86.

Le Blanc K, Rasmusson I, Sundberg B, Götherström C, Hassan M, Uzunel M, Ringdén O. (2004). Treatment of severe acute graft-versus-host disease with third party haploidentical mesenchymal stem cells. Lancet, 363(9419):1439-41.

Leonardi CL, Kimball AB, Papp KA, Yeilding N, Guzzo C, Wang Y, Li S, Dooley LT, Gordon KB; PHOENIX 1 study investigators. (2008). Efficacy and safety of ustekinumab, a human interleukin-12/23 monoclonal antibody, in patients with psoriasis: 76-week results from a randomised, double-blind, placebo-controlled trial (PHOENIX 1). Lancet, 371(9625):1665-74.

Li MO, Flavell RA. (2008). Contextual regulation of inflammation: a duet by transforming growth factor-beta and interleukin-10. Immunity, 28(4):468-76.

Liu YJ, Soumelis V, Watanabe N, Ito T, Wang YH, Malefyt Rde W, Omori M, Zhou B, Ziegler SF. (2007). TSLP: an epithelial cell cytokine that regulates T cell differentiation by conditioning dendritic cell maturation. Annu Rev Immunol, 25:193-219.

Liu YJ. (2001). Dendritic cell subsets and lineages, and their functions in innate and adaptive immunity. Cell, 106(3):259-62.

Long E, Wood KJ. (2009). Regulatory T cells in transplantation: transferring mouse studies to the clinic. Transplantation, 88(9):1050-6.

Lutterotti A, Sospedra M, Martin R. (2008). Antigen-specific therapies in MS - Current concepts and novel approaches. J Neurol Sci, 274(1-2):18-22.

Lutz MB, Schuler G. (2002). Immature, semi-mature and fully mature dendritic cells: which signals induce tolerance or immunity? Trends Immunol, 23(9):445-9.

Maccario R, Podestà M, Moretta A, Cometa A, Comoli P, Montagna D, Daudt L, Ibatici A, Piaggio G, Pozzi S, Frassoni F, Locatelli F. (2005). Interaction of human mesenchymal stem cells with cells involved in alloantigen-specific immune response favors the differentiation of CD4+ T-cell subsets expressing a regulatory/suppressive phenotype. Haematologica, 90(4):516-25.

Mandala S, Hajdu R, Bergstrom J, Quackenbush E, Xie J, Milligan J, Thornton R, Shei GJ, Card D, Keohane C, Rosenbach M, Hale J, Lynch CL, Rupprecht K, Parsons W, Rosen H. (2002). Alteration of lymphocyte trafficking by sphingosine-1-phosphate receptor agonists. Science, 296(5566):346-9.

Mannon PJ, Fuss IJ, Mayer L, Elson CO, Sandborn WJ, Present D, Dolin B, Goodman N, Groden C, Hornung RL, Quezado M, Yang Z, Neurath MF, Salfeld J, Veldman GM, Schwertschlag U, Strober W; Anti-IL-12 Crohn's Disease Study Group. (2004). Anti-interleukin-12 antibody for active Crohn's disease. N Engl J Med, 351(20):2069-79.

Marigo I, Dazzi F. (2011). The immunomodulatory properties of mesenchymal stem cells. Semin Immunopathol, Epub ahead of print.

Mehling M, Brinkmann V, Antel J, Bar-Or A, Goebels N, Vedrine C, Kristofic C, Kuhle J, Lindberg RL, Kappos L. (2008). FTY720 therapy exerts differential effects on T cell subsets in multiple sclerosis. Neurology, 71(16):1261-7.

Meisel R, Zibert A, Laryea M, Göbel U, Däubener W, Dilloo D. (2004). Human bone marrow stromal cells inhibit allogeneic T-cell responses by indoleamine 2,3-dioxygenase-mediated tryptophan degradation. Blood, 103(12):4619-21.

Mellor AL, Munn DH. (2004). IDO expression by dendritic cells: tolerance and tryptophan catabolism. Nat Rev Immunol, 4(10):762-74.

Miller SD, Turley DM, Podojil JR. (2007). Antigen-specific tolerance strategies for the prevention and treatment of autoimmune disease. Nat Rev Immunol, 7(9):665-77.

Monti P, Scirpoli M, Maffi P, Piemonti L, Secchi A, Bonifacio E, Roncarolo MG, Battaglia M. (2008). Rapamycin monotherapy in patients with type 1 diabetes modifies CD4+CD25+FOXP3+ regulatory T-cells. Diabetes, 57(9):2341-7.

Munn DH, Sharma MD, Lee JR, Jhaver KG, Johnson TS, Keskin DB, Marshall B, Chandler P, Antonia SJ, Burgess R, Slingluff CL Jr, Mellor AL. (2002). Potential regulatory function of human dendritic cells expressing indoleamine 2,3-dioxygenase. Science, 297(5588):1867-70.

Muraro PA, Douek DC, Packer A, Chung K, Guenaga FJ, Cassiani-Ingoni R, Campbell C, Memon S, Nagle JW, Hakim FT, Gress RE, McFarland HF, Burt RK, Martin R. (2005). Thymic output generates a new and diverse TCR repertoire after autologous stem cell transplantation in multiple sclerosis patients. J Exp Med, 201(5):805-16.

Nakamura K, Kitani A, Strober W. (2001). Cell contact-dependent immunosuppression by CD4(+)CD25(+) regulatory T cells is mediated by cell surface-bound transforming growth factor beta. J Exp Med, 194(5):629-44.

Nauta AJ, Kruisselbrink AB, Lurvink E, Willemze R, Fibbe WE. (2006). Mesenchymal stem cells inhibit generation and function of both CD34+-derived and monocyte-derived dendritic cells. J Immunol, 177(4):2080-7.

Németh K, Leelahavanichkul A, Yuen PS, Mayer B, Parmelee A, Doi K, Robey PG, Leelahavanichkul K, Koller BH, Brown JM, Hu X, Jelinek I, Star RA, Mezey E. (2009). Bone marrow stromal cells attenuate sepsis via prostaglandin E(2)-dependent reprogramming of host macrophages to increase their interleukin-10 production. Nat Med, 15(1):42-9.

Ning H, Yang F, Jiang M, Hu L, Feng K, Zhang J, Yu Z, Li B, Xu C, Li Y, Wang J, Hu J, Lou X, Chen H. (2008). The correlation between cotransplantation of mesenchymal stem cells and higher recurrence rate in hematologic malignancy patients: outcome of a pilot clinical study. Leukemia, 22(3):593-9.

O'Connor P, Comi G, Montalban X, Antel J, Radue EW, de Vera A, Pohlmann H, Kappos L; FTY720 D2201 Study Group. (2009). Oral fingolimod (FTY720) in multiple sclerosis: two-year results of a phase II extension study. Neurology, 72(1):73-9.

O'Doherty U, Peng M, Gezelter S, Swiggard WJ, Betjes M, Bhardwaj N, Steinman RM. (1994). Human blood contains two subsets of dendritic cells, one immunologically mature and the other immature. Immunology, 82(3):487-93.

Oyama Y, Papadopoulos EB, Miranda M, Traynor AE, Burt RK. (2001). Allogeneic stem cell transplantation for Evans syndrome. Bone Marrow Transplant, 28(9):903-5.

Penna G, Sozzani S, Adorini L. (2001). Cutting edge: selective usage of chemokine receptors by plasmacytoid dendritic cells. J Immunol, 167(4):1862-6.

Pittenger MF, Mackay AM, Beck SC, Jaiswal RK, Douglas R, Mosca JD, Moorman MA, Simonetti DW, Craig S, Marshak DR. (1999). Multilineage potential of adult human mesenchymal stem cells. Science, 284(5411):143-7.

Plevy S, Salzberg B, Van Assche G, Regueiro M, Hommes D, Sandborn W, Hanauer S, Targan S, Mayer L, Mahadevan U, Frankel M, Lowder J. (2007). A phase I study of visilizumab, a humanized anti-CD3 monoclonal antibody, in severe steroid-refractory ulcerative colitis. Gastroenterology, 133(5):1414-22.

Popat U, Krance R. (2004). Haematopoietic stem cell transplantation for autoimmune disorders: the American perspective. Br J Haematol, 126(5):637-49.

Pratschke J, Stauch D, Kotsch K. (2009). Role of NK and NKT cells in solid organ transplantation. Transpl Int, 22(9):859-68.

Prevosto C, Zancolli M, Canevali P, Zocchi MR, Poggi A. (2007). Generation of CD4+ or CD8+ regulatory T cells upon mesenchymal stem cell-lymphocyte interaction. Haematologica, 92(7):881-8.

Rasmusson I, Uhlin M, Le Blanc K, Levitsky V. (2007). Mesenchymal stem cells fail to trigger effector functions of cytotoxic T lymphocytes. J Leukoc Biol, 82(4):887-93.

Reizis B, Bunin A, Ghosh HS, Lewis KL, Sisirak V. (2011). Plasmacytoid dendritic cells: recent progress and open questions. Annu Rev Immunol, 29:163-83.

Riley JL, June CH, Blazar BR. (2009). Human T regulatory cell therapy: take a billion or so and call me in the morning. Immunity, 30(5):656-65.

Roncarolo MG, Gregori S, Battaglia M, Bacchetta R, Fleischhauer K, Levings MK. (2006). Interleukin-10-secreting type 1 regulatory T cells in rodents and humans. Immunol Rev, 212:28-50.

Sabatos-Peyton CA, Verhagen J, Wraith DC. (2010). Antigen-specific immunotherapy of autoimmune and allergic diseases. Curr Opin Immunol, 22(5):609-15.

Salomon B, Lenschow DJ, Rhee L, Ashourian N, Singh B, Sharpe A, Bluestone JA. (2000). B7/CD28 costimulation is essential for the homeostasis of the CD4+CD25+ immunoregulatory T cells that control autoimmune diabetes. Immunity, 12(4):431-440.

Sato K, Ozaki K, Oh I, Meguro A, Hatanaka K, Nagai T, Muroi K, Ozawa K. (2007). Nitric oxide plays a critical role in suppression of T-cell proliferation by mesenchymal stem cells. Blood, 109(1):228-34.

Schwartz RH. (2003). T cell anergy. Annu Rev Immunol, 21:305-34.

Segal BM, Constantinescu CS, Raychaudhuri A, Kim L, Fidelus-Gort R, Kasper LH; Ustekinumab MS Investigators. (2008). Repeated subcutaneous injections of IL12/23 p40 neutralising antibody, ustekinumab, in patients with relapsing-remitting multiple sclerosis: a phase II, double-blind, placebo-controlled, randomised, dose-ranging study. Lancet Neurol, 7(9):796-804.

Sekiya I, Larson BL, Smith JR, Pochampally R, Cui JG, Prockop DJ. (2002). Expansion of human adult stem cells from bone marrow stroma: conditions that maximize the yields of early progenitors and evaluate their quality. Stem Cells 20(6):530-41.

Shevach EM. (2009). Mechanisms of foxp3+ T regulatory cell-mediated suppression. Immunity, 30(5):636-45.

Smith CE, Miller SD. (2006). Multi-peptide coupled-cell tolerance ameliorates ongoing relapsing EAE associated with multiple pathogenic autoreactivities. J Autoimmun, 27(4):218-31.

Sotiropoulou PA, Perez SA, Gritzapis AD, Baxevanis CN, Papamichail M. (2006). Interactions between human mesenchymal stem cells and natural killer cells. Stem Cells, 24(1):74-85.

Spaggiari GM, Abdelrazik H, Becchetti F, Moretta L. (2009). MSCs inhibit monocyte-derived DC maturation and function by selectively interfering with the generation of immature DCs: central role of MSC-derived prostaglandin E2. Blood, 113(26):6576-83.

Spaggiari GM, Capobianco A, Becchetti S, Mingari MC, Moretta L. (2006). Mesenchymal stem cell-natural killer cell interactions: evidence that activated NK cells are capable of killing MSCs, whereas MSCs can inhibit IL-2-induced NK-cell proliferation. Blood, 107(4):1484-90.

Steinman RM, Banchereau J. (2007). Taking dendritic cells into medicine. Nature, 449(7161):419-26.

Steinman RM, Hawiger D, Nussenzweig MC. (2003). Tolerogenic dendritic cells. Annu Rev Immunol, 21:685-711.

Steinman RM, Nussenzweig MC. (2002). Avoiding horror autotoxicus: the importance of dendritic cells in peripheral T cell tolerance. Proc Natl Acad Sci U S A, 99(1):351-358.

Strom TB, Koulmanda M. (2009). Recently discovered T cell subsets cannot keep their commitments. J Am Soc Nephrol, 20(8):1677-80.

Stüve O, Marra CM, Jerome KR, Cook L, Cravens PD, Cepok S, Frohman EM, Phillips JT, Arendt G, Hemmer B, Monson NL, Racke MK. (2006). Immune surveillance in multiple sclerosis patients treated with natalizumab. Ann Neurol, 59(5):743-7.

Süss G, Shortman K. (1996). A subclass of dendritic cells kills CD4 T cells via Fas/Fas-ligand-induced apoptosis. J Exp Med, 183(4):1789-96.

Swiecki M, Colonna M. (2010). Unraveling the functions of plasmacytoid dendritic cells during viral infections, autoimmunity, and tolerance. Immunol Rev, 234(1):142-62.

Tabera S, Pérez-Simón JA, Díez-Campelo M, Sánchez-Abarca LI, Blanco B, López A, Benito A, Ocio E, Sánchez-Guijo FM, Cañizo C, San Miguel JF. (2008). The effect of mesenchymal stem cells on the viability, proliferation and differentiation of B-lymphocytes. Haematologica, 93(9):1301-9.

Teng YK, Verburg RJ, Sont JK, van den Hout WB, Breedveld FC, van Laar JM. (2005). Long-term followup of health status in patients with severe rheumatoid arthritis after high-dose chemotherapy followed by autologous hematopoietic stem cell transplantation. Arthritis Rheum, 52(8):2272-6.

Traynor AE, Schroeder J, Rosa RM, Cheng D, Stefka J, Mujais S, Baker S, Burt RK. (2000). Treatment of severe systemic lupus erythematosus with high-dose chemotherapy and haemopoietic stem-cell transplantation: a phase I study. Lancet, 356(9231):701-7.

Trombetta ES, Mellman I. (2005). Cell biology of antigen processing in vitro and in vivo. Annu Rev Immunol, 23:975-1028.

Trzonkowski P, Bieniaszewska M, Juścińska J, Dobyszuk A, Krzystyniak A, Marek N, Myśliwska J, Hellmann A. (2009). First-in-man clinical results of the treatment of patients with graft versus host disease with human ex vivo expanded CD4+CD25+CD127- T regulatory cells. Clin Immunol, 133(1):22-6.

Turley DM, Miller SD. (2007). Peripheral tolerance induction using ethylenecarbodiimide-fixed APCs uses both direct and indirect mechanisms of antigen presentation for prevention of experimental autoimmune encephalomyelitis. J Immunol, 178(4):2212-20.

Tyndall A, Saccardi R. (2005). Haematopoietic stem cell transplantation in the treatment of severe autoimmune disease: results from phase I/II studies, prospective randomized trials and future directions. Clin Exp Immunol, 141(1):1-9.

Van Tendeloo VF, Van de Velde A, Van Driessche A, Cools N, Anguille S, Ladell K, Gostick E, Vermeulen K, Pieters K, Nijs G, Stein B, Smits EL, Schroyens WA, Gadisseur AP, Vrelust I, Jorens PG, Goossens H, de Vries IJ, Price DA, Oji Y, Oka Y, Sugiyama H, Berneman ZN. (2010). Induction of complete and molecular remissions in acute myeloid leukemia by Wilms' tumor 1 antigen-targeted dendritic cell vaccination. Proc Natl Acad Sci U S A, 107(31):13824-9.

Victor FC, Gottlieb AB, Menter A. (2003). Changing paradigms in dermatology: tumor necrosis factor alpha (TNF-alpha) blockade in psoriasis and psoriatic arthritis. Clin Dermatol, 21(5):392-7.

Vincenti F, Luggen M. (2007). T cell costimulation: a rational target in the therapeutic armamentarium for autoimmune diseases and transplantation. Annu Rev Med, 58:347-58.

Voo KS, Wang YH, Santori FR, Boggiano C, Wang YH, Arima K, Bover L, Hanabuchi S, Khalili J, Marinova E, Zheng B, Littman DR, Liu YJ. (2009). Identification of IL-17-producing FOXP3+ regulatory T cells in humans. Proc Natl Acad Sci U S A, 106(12):4793-8.

Weaver CT, Hatton RD. (2009). Interplay between the TH17 and TReg cell lineages: a (co-)evolutionary perspective. Nat Rev Immunol, 9(12):883-9.

Wieczorek G, Asemissen A, Model F, Turbachova I, Floess S, Liebenberg V, Baron U, Stauch D, Kotsch K, Pratschke J, Hamann A, Loddenkemper C, Stein H, Volk HD, Hoffmüller U, Grützkau A, Mustea A, Huehn J, Scheibenbogen C, Olek S. (2009). Quantitative DNA methylation analysis of FOXP3 as a new method for counting regulatory T cells in peripheral blood and solid tissue. Cancer Res, 69(2):599-608.

Wildin RS, Freitas A. (2005). IPEX and FOXP3: clinical and research perspectives. J Autoimmun, 25 Suppl:56-62.

Wu L, Van Kaer L. (2009). Natural killer T cells and autoimmune disease. Curr Mol Med, 9(1):4-14.

Yanaba K, Bouaziz JD, Haas KM, Poe JC, Fujimoto M, Tedder TF. (2008). A regulatory B cell subset with a unique CD1dhiCD5+ phenotype controls T cell-dependent inflammatory responses. Immunity, 28(5):639-50.

Yednock TA, Cannon C, Fritz LC, Sanchez-Madrid F, Steinman L, Karin N. (1992). Prevention of experimental autoimmune encephalomyelitis by antibodies against alpha 4 beta 1 integrin. Nature, 356(6364):63-6.

Zappia E, Casazza S, Pedemonte E, Benvenuto F, Bonanni I, Gerdoni E, Giunti D, Ceravolo A, Cazzanti F, Frassoni F, Mancardi G, Uccelli A. (2005). Mesenchymal stem cells ameliorate experimental autoimmune encephalomyelitis inducing T-cell anergy. Blood, 106(5):1755-61.

Zarkhin V, Chalasani G, Sarwal MM. (2010). The yin and yang of B cells in graft rejection and tolerance. Transplant Rev (Orlando), 24(2):67-78.

Zarkhin V, Kambham N, Li L, Kwok S, Hsieh SC, Salvatierra O, Sarwal MM. (2008). Characterization of intra-graft B cells during renal allograft rejection. Kidney Int, 74(5):664-73.

Zhou H, Jin Z, Liu J, Yu S, Cui Q, Yi D. (2008). Mesenchymal stem cells might be used to induce tolerance in heart transplantation. Med Hypotheses, 70(4):785-7.

Zhou L, Chong MM, Littman DR. (2009). Plasticity of CD4+ T cell lineage differentiation. Immunity, 30(5):646-55.

Ziegler SF. (2006). FOXP3: of mice and men. Annu Rev Immunol, 24:209-26.

2

Current Immunosuppression in Abdominal Organ Transplantation

Raffaele Girlanda, Cal S. Matsumoto,
Keith J. Melancon and Thomas M. Fishbein
Transplant Institute, Georgetown University Hospital, Washington DC
USA

1. Introduction

Organ transplantation has saved the lives of thousands of patients beginning from the mid 1950s. At the end of 2007 the Organ Procurement and Transplantation Network (OPTN) database recorded 183,222 people living with a functioning graft in the United States (Wolfe et al., 2010). Over the last two decades survival rates have continued to improve and currently 81-91% of kidney transplant recipients and 74-79% of liver transplant recipients are alive 5 years post-transplant (Wolfe et al., 2010). This success is a dramatic improvement compared to the early era of transplantation and is the result of advances in organ preservation, surgical technique, intensive care and immunosuppression. Particularly, the development of potent immunosuppressive medications has contributed significantly to the success of organ transplantation by reducing the incidence of rejection and graft loss. In recent large studies the incidence of acute rejection is reported as low as 8-15% 1 year after kidney transplant (Ekberg et al., 2009) and graft loss due to acute rejection has now become very uncommon.

Clinical immunosuppression after organ transplantation has come a long way over the last fifty years. It started with total body irradiation, steroids and azathioprine (see Starzl, 2000 for a review on the history of immunosuppression). The rationale behind total body irradiation was to control the immune response to the allograft by ablation of the bone marrow, a similar principle applied today with the use of depleting agents (see below). Other early attempts at controlling the bone marrow and obtain lymphocyte depletion included splenectomy, thymectomy and thoracic duct drainage, but these had limited success. Instead, anti-lymphocyte globulin (ALG), prepared from the serum of horses or rabbits inoculated with human lymphocytes, was introduced in 1966 with the aim of mitigating cellular immunity using heterologous antibodies. (Starzl et al., 1967)

From the early 1960s to 1980s post-transplant immunosuppression consisted of azathioprine, high dose corticosteroids and antilymphocyte globulin. Cyclosporine was introduced in the early 1980s, followed by monoclonal antibodies, then by tacrolimus in the 1990s and lately by mycophenolic acid and sirolimus (see list below). Immunosuppression regimens have changed since the early era of transplantation as a result of the development of new drugs. Furthermore, the number of available drugs continues to increase. This article will describe the immunosuppressive drugs currently used in clinical transplantation and will focus on recent developments. We will also review current organ-specific IMS protocols for kidney, liver, pancreas and intestine transplant to highlight the differences in abdominal organ transplantation that require specific immunosuppressive strategies (ie immunosuppression in the highly sensitized kidney recipient, prevention of disease recurrence after liver transplant, role of induction in intestinal transplantation). Finally, we will highlight current areas of ongoing research and future developments in clinical immunosuppression.

2. Current immunosuppressive agents

There are several immunosuppressive drugs currently used in different combinations in abdominal organ transplantation (see table 1). Most agents target T cell activation and proliferation, given the central role of T lymphocytes in organ rejection. Indeed, the control of T cell-based mechanisms is key to prevent rejection, especially in the early post-transplant period. However, increasing attention is being given to the role of B cells and to the production of alloantibodies in late graft injury and chronic rejection. In addition, components of the innate immune system (neutrophils, complement) are becoming the target for development of new immunosuppressive agents. Here we discuss the immunosuppressive agents currently used in clinical transplantation and present new drugs being investigated in clinical trials.

Antibodies (monoclonal)
Alemtuzumab
Basiliximab
Daclizumab
Muromonab-CD3 (OKT3)
Rituximab
Antibodies (polyclonal)
ALG
Atgam
Thymoglobulin
Azathioprine
Calcineurin inhibitors
Cyclosporine
Tacrolimus
Corticosteroids
mTOR inhibitors
Everolimus
Sirolimus
Mycophenolic acid
Mycophenolate mofetil
Mycophenolate sodium
Others
Belatacept
Bortezomib

Table 1. Immunosuppressive drugs currently used in clinical transplantation

2.1 Corticosteroids

Corticosteroids (prednisone, prednisolone, methylprednisolone) were the first immunosuppressive drugs to be used in transplantation and remain today first line treatment across organs for both prevention and treatment of rejection. The multiple anti-inflammatory and immunomodulatory effects on a wide variety of cells including lymphocytes, granulocytes, macrophages, monocytes and endothelial cells are well known and the molecular mechanisms of action of steroids have been described extensively (Adcock et al., 2000). Briefly, corticosteroids down regulate cytokine gene expression in lymphocytes, antagonize macrophage differentiation, inhibit neutrophil adhesion to endothelial cells thereby decreasing their extravasation to the site of inflammation, decrease circulating eosinophil and basophil counts, inhibit IgE-dependent release of histamine and leukotriene from basophils and inhibit degranulation of mast cells. Additionally, glucocorticoids downregulate endothelial cell function including expression of class II MHC antigen and expression of adhesion molecules.

Based on these multiple effects on different cellular components of the immune response corticosteroids are very effective in preventing and treating acute allograft rejection. Indeed episodes of acute rejection are routinely treated with pulse steroids with generally good response, although there are instances of steroid-resistant rejection episodes.

The multiple side effects of steroids are also well known and include impaired wound healing, increased risk of infection, hypertension, weight gain, hyperglycemia, osteoporosis, fluid retention, hirsutism, acne and cataracts . Side effects may have an important impact especially in the long term and in children (ie growth pattern), therefore multiple trials of steroid withdrawal and steroid-free regimens have been designed in an attempt to limit the side effects of corticosteroids, with variable results (see below specific organs). In addition, several steroid withdrawal protocols have been associated with increased acute rejection (Knight et al., 2010). Corticosteroids still maintain a central role in the armamentarium of immunosuppressive agents currently available in clinical transplantation.

2.2 Azathioprine

Azathioprine was the main immunosuppressive agent, with steroids, for many years in clinical transplantation. It is a nucleotide analogue originally developed during research on new chemotherapy agents for leukemia. The mechanism of action of azathioprine is to incorporate into and to halt DNA replication thus blocking the *de-novo* purine synthesis in lymphocytes. It was originally tested in experimental kidney transplantation in the 1960s (Calne et al., 1961) and it obtained improved graft survival with less toxicity compared to analogue agents such as 6-mercaptopurine. Azathioprine is now very rarely used and it has been replaced by mycophenolic acid (see below) in many transplant programs.

2.3 Calcineurin inhibitors

Calcineurin inhibitors (CNI) are main immunosuppressive agents in use today in virtually every transplant program. Cyclosporine and tacrolimus are the two CNI currently used in clinical transplantation. Their immunosuppressive effect is to block the production of pro-inflammatory cytokines including IL-2, INF-γ, TNF-α and to inhibit T cell activation and proliferation by inactivating calcineurin, an intracellular calcium/calmodulin phosphatase triggered by the engagement of T cell receptor by donor MHC and responsible for de-phosphorilation of nuclear factor for activated T cells (NF-AT) which promotes the transcription of cytokine genes.

Although CNI remain the cornerstone of current immunosuppressive protocols, increasing attention is being devoted to their long term side effects (ie nephrotoxicity). The impact of these side effects and the concomitant introduction of alternative immunosuppressive agents led to the design of trials to reduce CNI exposure. Strategies to limit CNI exposure include CNI minimization, avoidance, and withdrawal (Flechner SM et al., 2008) However, to date trials incorporating mycophenolate mofetil or mTOR inhibitors showed mixed results because of adverse events or lack of efficacy (Larson et al., 2006, Ekberg et al., 2007).

2.3.1 Cyclosporine

Cyclosporine, a metabolite extracted from the soil fungi *Cylindrocarpon lucidum* and *Trichoderma polysporum*, initially was investigated as an antifungal but was also shown to be immunosuppressive in mice models of skin allotransplantation. Its potent anti-lymphocyte properties prolonged the survival of kidney transplants in the dog. The introduction of cyclosporine in the early 1980s has revolutionized clinical transplantation and has remained the cornerstone of immunosuppression for kidney, liver, heart and other organs for many years. The mechanism of action and the immunologic effects of cyclosporine have been reported above. With cyclosporine a dramatic increase in early graft survival was observed in many centers with some programs reporting almost doubling their 1-year graft survival rate from 50% in the late 1970s to 86% in the 1980s (Merion RM et al, 1984). Since the early 1980s triple immunosuppressive therapy with cyclosporine, azathioprine and steroids has been standard protocol for a long time in many centers and has allowed dramatic growth of transplant programs worldwide.

The main side effects of cyclosporine are nephrotoxicity and hypertension. Other side effects include diabetes and cosmetic changes like gingival hyperplasia and hirsutism. With long-term follow-up, it has become apparent that up to 15% to 20% of patients treated with calcineurin inhibitors experience chronic renal insufficiency requiring dialysis and/or renal transplantation (Ojo et al., 2003). The nephrotoxicity of cyclosporine is thought to result from its vasoconstrictor effects on renal blood vessels. Although early toxicity resulting in renal dysfunction may be reversible, the late stages of cyclosporine nephrotoxicity resulting in advanced tubular interstitial fibrosis and scarring may be irreversible. Now cyclosporine is used less frequently since other potent immunosuppressive drugs became available (see below).

2.3.2 Tacrolimus

The introduction of tacrolimus has further improved the remarkable results previously obtained with cyclosporine by reducing rejection rates and improving long term graft function and survival (Busuttil et al., 2004).

Tacrolimus (FK506) is a metabolite of the fungus *Streptomyces tsukubaensis*. The mechanism of action of tacrolimus is identical to that of cyclosporine. Upon entering the cytoplasm, it binds to an immunophilin referred to as FK-binding protein 12 and inhibits calcineurin, preventing the dephosphorylation of the transcription factor NFAT and inhibiting the transcription of cytokines necessary for rejection. Tacrolimus has gradually replaced cyclosporine in many transplant programs since it was found to be much more potent then cyclosporine. Indeed, its first successful use was reported as rescue therapy for rejected liver grafts failing conventional therapy (Starzl et al., 1989). Subsequently, tacrolimus has gradually been included in routine immunosuppression protocols in liver transplantation. Multicenter trials compared the efficacy and safety of tacrolimus with cyclosporine and showed that tacrolimus was associated with significantly fewer episodes of corticosteroid resistant or refractory rejection, although graft survival and patient survival were not significantly different; additional findings included a lower incidence of chronic rejection and infection. (The U.S. Multicenter FK506 Liver Study Group, 1994; European FK506 Multicentre Liver Study Group, 1994)

Since the early 1990s, an increasing number of patients receiving liver, kidney, heart, and heart-lung has been successfully immunosuppressed with tacrolimus-based regimens rather than cyclosporine. In addition, tacrolimus has made a significant impact on the outcomes of intestinal transplantation (see below). As a result, currently many transplant programs worldwide have adopted tacrolimus-based immunosuppressive regimens. However, like for cyclosporine, the toxicity profile of tacrolimus has become evident with studies showing that the use of tacrolimus is associated with higher risk of diabetes post-transplant and with incidence of nephrotoxicity and neurotoxicity comparable or higher than those of cyclosporine (Ekberg et al., 2007).

Tacrolimus is administered twice daily. To improve compliance with the medication a modified-release once daily dose form of tacrolimus has been developed and shown to have equivalent systemic exposure of conventional twice-daily tacrolimus (Cross et al., 2007) and similar efficacy in preventing kidney (Kramer et al., 2010) and liver (Truneka et al., 2010) transplant rejection.

2.4 Mycophenolic acid

Mycophenolate mofetil and mycophenolate sodium are similar pro-drugs both converted to the active compound mycophenolic acid by liver metabolism and they will be discussed together. Mycophenolic acid emerged as a new immunosuppressive agent in the early 1990s with a mechanism of action different from CNI (Mele et al., 2000) (Stewart et al., 2001). Whereas cyclosporine and tacrolimus both inhibit the enzyme calcineurin and the induction of cytokine synthesis soon after T cell activation, mycophenolic acid has no direct effect on the production of cytokines but prevents T and B cell proliferation by inhibiting a pathway required for cell division. Mycophenolic acid is a selective and noncompetitive inhibitor of inosine monophosphate dehydrogenase, which is an important enzyme in the *de novo* pathway of guanine nucleotide synthesis. This results in the inhibition of DNA synthesis in T and B lymphocytes thereby inhibiting cell proliferation and function. Other cell types can use salvage pathways and are not affected, therefore the effects of mycophenolic acid are largely on the immune cells with few effects on the non-immune system. Clinically, mycophenolate acid has largely replaced azathioprine because of its fewer myelotoxic and hepatotoxic side effects. It is usually combined into a regimen including a calcineurin inhibitor and steroids.

Since the 1990s, when large, double-blind, randomized trials in kidney transplant recipients showed the efficacy of mycophenolate acid in preventing early acute rejection in combination with cyclosporine and prednisone, this drug has been used widely as a part of various combination regimens of immunosuppressive agents. Common mycophenolic acid-related side effects comprise gastrointestinal symptoms such as abdominal pain, diarrhea and nausea, infections (cytomegalovirus) and myelosuppression, namely anemia and leucocytopenia, malignancy (post-transplant lymphoproliferative disorders and non melanoma skin cancer).

Mycophenolate sodium is an enteric-coated preparation that allows delayed release of the active drug in the small intestine rather than the stomach. This may help alleviate some of the gastrointestinal side effects of mycophenolate mofetil. There is no significant difference in rejection and side effects in large randomized trial of mycophenolate mofetil versus mycophenolate sodium (Ciancio et al., 2011). The ability of mycophenolic acid to facilitate sparing of other immunosuppressive agents, particularly cyclosporine and its related nephrotoxicity, is promising. By permitting reduction in cyclosporine doses, mycophenolic acid may stabilize or improve renal graft function in patients with cyclosporine-related nephrotoxicity or chronic allograft nephropathy.

2.5 mTOR inhibitors

The mTOR inhibitors sirolimus and everolimus are among the most recently introduced immunosuppressive agents with a mechanism of action different from CNI and from antimetabolites. Sirolimus (or rapamycin) is a macrolide antibiotic, structurally similar to tacrolimus, isolated from the fungus *Streptomyces hygroscopicus* in 1968 and found to have immunosuppressive properties in the late 1980s. Like the calcineurin inhibitors, sirolimus acts by binding to an intracellular immunophilin FKB12. This complex sirolimus-immunophilin inhibits a protein called mammalian target of rapamycin (*mTOR*). Inhibition of mTOR results in selective inhibition of synthesis of new ribosomal proteins which are essential for progression of the cells from the G1 to the S phase. This results in blockage of T cell activation. In addition, sirolimus has been associated with inhibition of fibroblast growth factors required for tissue repair. This antifibrotic effect has two potentially beneficial effects after transplantation in reducing the progression to fibrosis in post liver transplant hepatitis C recurrence (see below) and in reducing the risk of malignancy in transplant recipients because of its antiangiogenic effects (Geisler et al., 2010).

The half life of sirolimus is 60 hours which allows single daily dose unlike other agents given twice daily and this has an important impact on patient compliance to immunosuppression regimens. Everolimus is a modified form of sirolimus to improve its absoprion. Its half life is shorter and is administred twice daily. Everolimus is currently undergoing clinical trials in liver transplantation. In addition to being used as immunosuppressant, it has been investigated in the treatment of renal cell carcinoma for its proliferation signal inhibition and in drug-coated stents to prevent restenosis of coronary arteries for its antifibrotic effect (Gabardi et al., 2010)

There have been a number of studies investigating the impact of adding sirolimus to low dose CNI regimens in order to reduce nephrotoxicity of CNI after kidney (Schena et al., 2009), liver (Harper et al., 2011) and heart (Raichlin et al., 2007) transplantation. The use of sirolimus with mycophenolate mofetil or azathioprine to avoid *de novo* CNI exposure has improved glomerular filtration rate for at least two years in most studies in kidney transplantation with comparable incidence of rejection, however experience is limited in liver and heart transplantation. However, there have been also reports of an increased risk of nephrotoxicity when combining sirolimus with high doses calcineurin inhibitors (Kahan, 2000)

Sirolimus, unlike calcineurin inhibitors, has been shown to enhance the development and function of regulatory T cells, a subset of CD4(+)CD25(+) lymphocytes with the ability to suppress alloimmune responses in vitro and in vivo. It is therefore being evaluated as a component of strategies to promote tolerance in organ transplant recipients (Knektle 2010).

In intestinal transplant recipients the introduction of sirolimus in tacrolimus-based regimens has significantly delayed the onset and reduced the severity of rejection (see below).

The adverse effects of sirolimus include thrombocytopenia, leukopenia, anemia, arthralgias, hyperlipidemia, pneumonitis, and diarrhea. There have also been reports of wound complications (delayed wound healing, incisional hernia) in the post-transplant period, an affect probably secondary to its antiproliferative effects on fibroblasts. Oral ulcers were seen with the liquid preparation; however, this seems to be less frequent with the use of the pill preparation.

2.6 Antibodies

The use of antibodies as part of the immunosuppression regimen post-transplant dates from the beginning of clinical transplantation when anti-lymphocyte globulin (ALG) prepared from the serum of horses or rabbits inoculated with human lymphocytes was added to azathioprine and steroids. In 1986 muromonab CD3, a monoclonal antibody (mAb) targeting CD3, was first approved for prevention and treatment of renal allograft rejection. Originally, the rationale for the use of antibodies as immunosuppressants was to deplete and block the function of immune competent cells. The purified IgG fraction of polyclonal antibody preparations is directed against cell-surface molecules expressed on T cells, B cells, NK cells and macrophages, causing complement mediated cell lysis, uptake of opsonised cells by the reticulo-endothelial system and modulation of surface receptors of lymphocytes. Infact the administration of polyclonal antibodies results in profound lymphopenia. Polyclonal antibodies are obtained by inoculating rabbits or horses with human lymphocytes or thymocytes. Currently available preparations include Thymoglobulin and Atgam. Monoclonal antibodies are produced in response to a single antigen. These include the mouse monoclonal antibody muromonab (OKT3), which is specific to the CD3 receptor and was the first monoclonal antibody to be used in transplantation to treat acute rejection. Other monoclonal antibodies include the anti-IL-2 receptor antibodies daclizumab and basiliximab, anti CD20 rituximab, antiCD52 alemtuzumab. Other new mAbs are emerging, targeting co-stimulatory signals, cell surface receptors and novel protein constructs.

Antibodies are further classified into lymphocyte-depleting or nondepleting agents (review Klipa et al., 2010) The total lymphocyte counts and CD3 counts are usually measured during therapy to monitor the achievement of effective depletion and to make dose adjustments in case of incomplete depletion.

Currently, antibodies are administered as induction immunosuppression to the majority of kidney, pancreas and intestine transplant recipients in the United States, and less frequently to liver recipients. Induction therapy, as opposed to maintenance immunosuppression, refers to the use of biological agents and high dose steroids to prevent immune engagement and T-cell activation during tissue injury from organ preservation, reperfusion, and alloresponse immediately after transplant. The agents most commonly used are thymoglobulin and alemtuzumab (depleting) and basiliximab, daclizumab and rituximab (non depleting) (review in Aparna et al., 2009).

The benefits of induction therapy include a decreased incidence and delayed onset of acute rejection, and also delayed introduction of or lowering dose of CNI in the early post-transplant period allowing for peri-operative renal dysfunction to recover. Other uses of antibodies are in desensitization protocols in sensitized kidney transplant recipients (see below) and in the treatment of steroid resistant rejection. Rituximab has also been used to treat antibody-mediated rejection in kidney transplant (Kaposztas et al., 2009). In addition to considerable cost, side effects include cytokine release phenomena secondary to cytolysis and characterized by fevers, chills, hypotension. Other side effects are nausea, diarrhea, arthralgias, thrombocytopenia, dyspnea, and seizures. The risk of infection and of posttransplantation lymphoproliferative disease is increased with antibody therapy.

2.7 New immunosuppressive drugs

Different pathways and stages of the immunologic response are the target of strategies to develop new immunosuppressive drugs: cell-surface molecules, signaling mechanisms, T-cell proliferation, cell trafficking and cell recruitment.

New immunosuppressive drugs include mainly proteins targeting T-cell and B-cell surface receptors and non-protein drugs (also called small molecules) targeting intracellular pathways. **Belatacept** is a fusion protein composed of the Fc fragment of a human IgG1 immunoglobulin linked to the extracellular domain of CTLA-4. (review Weclawiak et al., 2010) It represents a new class of immunosuppressants. Unlike calcineurin inhibitors that block or diminish the effects of T-cell activation on allografts, belatacept prevents T-cell activation by selectively blocking T-cell costimulation molecules. In the initial trial in kidney transplant recipients it was as effective as cyclosporine in preventing acute rejection but with better preservation of kidney function and reduction of chronic allograft nephropathy (Vincenti et al., 2005) The stability of graft function and the safety profile of belatacept at 5 years has been reported in a subsequent study (Vincenti et al., 2010).

Memory T cells play a crucial role in acute and chronic rejection and are a potent barrier to transplantation tolerance. **Alefacept**, a fusion protein combining Leukocyte Function associated Antigen-3 (LFA3) with IgG currently approved for psoriasis, binds to CD2 on T cells (Ellis et al, 2001). Unlike belatacept that prevents activation of naïve T cells, alefacept targets memory T cells (Weaver et al., 2008) since CD2 is espressed more on memory than naïve T cells.

Efalizumab (Dedrick et al., 2002) is a humanized antiCD11a (LFA1) monoclonal antibody used in patients with chronic plaque psoriasis (Kuschei et al., 2011). It blocks the binding of LFA1 to intracellular adhesion molecule-1 (ICAM-1) causing loss of activation, adhesion and migration of T-cells. Preliminary experience with efalizumab in kidney transplantation showed efficacy in controlling rejection but raised concern of overimmunosuppression since 8% of patients developed post-transplant lymphoproliferative disease (Vincenti et al., 2007).

New non-protein drugs (also identified as small molecules) target intracellular pathways of the immune response to the allograft, such as Janus kinase proteins (JAK), which mediate signal transmission between cell membrane receptors and the nucleus. The immunosuppressive effect of inhibition of JAK3 results from blocking the signaling of the gamma chain subfamily of cytokines (interleukins 2, 4, 7, 9, 15 and 21). **Tofacitinib**, a Janus kinase 1/3 inhibitor developed for the treatment of rheumatoid arthritis (Flanagan et al., 2010) prolonged kidney allograft survival in cynomolgus monkeys without concomitant use of calcineurin inhibitor (Borie et al., 2005). In clinical kidney transplantation it has been used in a calcineurin inhibitor- free regimen (Busque et al., 2009). This study reported comparable acute rejection rates between tofacitinib and tacrolimus-based immunosuppression but raised concern of overimmunosuppression in the form of increased BK virus infection rates.

Two new other biologic agents being developed are **4D11,** a costimulation blockade agent targeting CD40 (Aoyagi et al., 2009) and **natalizumab,** a humanized IgG4 approved for multiple sclerosis and Crohn's disease targeting alpha4 submunit of integrins thus inhibiting leucocyte adhesion (Hutchinson 2010).

Voclosporine (ISA247) is a novel oral semisynthetic structural analogue of cyclosporine that has been modified at the first amino acid residue of the molecule. This drug has been shown to be more potent than cyclosporine in vitro and in vivo in rat heterotopic heart transplantation. The advantage of this cyclosporine-analogue drug is the lack of nephrotoxicity. There is still limited experience with this drug in clinical transplantation.

Preliminary results show non-inferiority to tacrolimus in preventing rejection (Gaber et al., 2008). More data is needed on the efficacy and safety profile in the long term.

Protein kinases (PKC) play a key role in signaling pathways downstream of the T-cell receptor (signal 1) and CD28 (signal 2) and thereby are involved in early T-cell activation. There are several isoforms of PKC. PKCh is largely restricted toT lymphocytes and mediates activation of the transcription factors activator protein-1 and nuclear factor (NF) jB, leading to downstream IL-2 production. The PKCh knockout mice demonstrate impaired T-cell activation. **Sotrastaurin (AEB071)** is a new oral low molecular weight compound that effectively blocks early T-cell activation by selective inhibition of PKC and therefore has a different mechanism of action from that of the CNIs. (Kovarik et al., 2011)

In kidney transplantation the deleterious effects of the humoral (antibody-mediated) component of acute rejection and their impact on long term graft survival are being increasingly recognized. This has prompted the development of more targeted antihumoral therapies. **Bortezomib** is an antineoplastic agent originally developed for the treatment of multiple myeloma. It is a proteasome inhibitor that induces apoptosis in rapidly dividing cells with active protein synthesis like plasma cells. In kidney transplantation it has been reported to revert antibody-mediated rejection (Perry et al., 2009, Walsh et al., 2010). Early antibody-mediated rejection demonstrated increased response to proteasome inhibitors than late AMR (Walsh et al.,2011)

3. Immunosuppression in kidney transplantation

Kidney transplant is the most frequently performed among abdominal organ transplants and in 2010 16,896 patients received a kidney transplant in the United States, 37% of which were from live donor. (unos) (http://optn.transplant.hrsa.gov/latestData/rptData.asp). The advantages of live-donor versus deceased donor kidney transplant are multiple including shorter time on the waiting list, shorter cold ischemia time (ie the interval between organ procurement and transplantantation), less preservation injury and overall better graft function in the short and long term. However, the immunologic risk in live-donor kidney transplant is not inferior to deceased donor, even in case of live-related donor (ie between non-identical siblings). On the contrary, live donor kidney transplant is becoming a bigger immunological challenge than deceased donor with the increasing number of transplants performed in highly sensitized or ABO incompatible recipients (see below).

There are several immunosuppression protocols currently used in kidney transplantation, but the majority include induction with depleting or non-depleting antibodies and maintenance immunosuppression based on a combination of agents (usually triple therapy) including CNI, mycophenolic acid, sirolimus and steroids.

Current acute rejection rate is 10-15% (Gaston et al., 2009) and usually the function of the graft is maintained after treatment of the rejection episode. Immunosuppression regimens currently available are very effective in treating episodes of acute rejection so that graft loss due to acute rejection has now become a rare event. Instead, chronic rejection (or chronic allograft nephropathy) remains a major cause of graft loss, usually a late event (years) after transplant. The causes of chronic allograft nephropathy and graft loss are multiple including repeated episodes of rejection, disease recurrence, CNI toxicity and others. Indeed, one of the main side effects of CNI is nephrotoxicity, affecting up to 16% of non-renal transplant recipients at 3 years and resulting in end stage kidney disease requiring dialysis in 5-20% of patients 5 years after transplant (Ojo et al.,2003). This prompted the design of several trials of CNI withdrawal, minimization or avoidance in an attempt to limit the impact of CNI nephrotoxicity. However, CNI cannot be avoided completely in kidney transplantation without paying the price of high rejection rate up to 53% within the first year (Vincenti et al., 2001). So another approach would be to reduce CNI (Ekberg et al., 2007).

Increasing attention is being recently devoted to the role of late antibody mediated rejection causing chronic sub-acute immune mediated injury. Chronic antibody mediated injury is being recognized as a cause of late graft loss and is a process that is not controlled by CNI or other current drugs (Colvin 2010, Kirk et al., 2010).

Highly sensitized and ABO-incompatible recipients

Immunologic sensitization in a transplant candidate refers to the presence of pre-formed antibodies and it is measured as PRA (Panel of Reactive Antibodies), which express the percentage of the antigenic repertoire in the general population to which the transplant candidate has developed antibodies (0-100%). The causes of sensitization are multiple and include blood transfusions, previous transplant, pregnancies and infections. Highly sensitized patients have PRA of 80% or higher. These patients are at greater risk of rejection and graft loss than non-sensitized patients. In addition, highly sensitized patients are likely to wait longer for a 0-mismatch kidney graft than non-sensitized patients. This has prompted the development of desensitization protocols to enable highly sensitized patients to receive a successful transplant in a timely manner. The aim of desensitization protocols is to reduce the amount of circulating HLA antibodies and to prevent the formation of new antibodies. Strategies currently adopted to achieve these goals include plasmapheresis to remove HLA antibodies, intravenous immunoglobulins (IvIg) to neutralize circulating antibodies and to inhibit complement activation, rituximab (a chimeric anti CD20 monoclonal antibody) to deplet B cells and, more recently, bortezomib, a proteasome inhibitor that targets plasma cells (see above). The protocol at our Institute also includes mycophenolate sodium started the week before transplant as part of the strategy to control the B cell component of the immune response (Melancon et al., 2011) Current results of desensitization programs demonstrate graft function and graft survival comparable to non-sensitized patients (Montgomery et al., 2010, Melancon et al., 2011, Niederhaus et al., 2011).

Until recently, another barrier to a successful kidney transplant has been ABO-incompatibility between donor and recipient (ie donor blood type is A or B and recipient blood type is O). Over the last decade this barrier has been overcome in some transplant centers by the implementation of programs of paired kidney exchange and antibody reduction therapies in which a number of donor-recipient pairs are entered into a pool and matched according to blood type compatibility (Montgomery et al., 2006) (Melancon et al., 2011). In addition to entering an exchange program, the recipient of an ABO incompatible pair with high isohemoagglutinin titers can also be treated with plasmapheresis and anti-B cell agents to reduce the isohemoagglutinin titer to 1:16 or below, a level considered safe to proceed with ABO incompatible transplant. Since the number of kidneys from deceased donors remains inadequate, living kidney donation has allowed for more patients to be removed from the waiting list. Programs of paired kidney exchange and the implementation of antibody reduction therapies have allowed the use of ABO incompatible donors and also the inclusion of non-directed *good Samaritan* donors, who enter the system with a desire to donate a kidney to someone for purely altruistic purposes. These strategies have all contributed to magnify the opportunities for a successful transplant for patients who otherwise would have had to wait 5-7 years for a matched kidney from deceased donor. In our recent series, all patients received a transplant within 90 days of their initial evaluation for living donor transplantation (Melancon et al., 2011).

4. Immunosuppression in liver transplantation

Liver transplantation has become an established treatment for patients with decompensated cirrhosis and acute liver failure and today the liver is the second most commonly performed abdominal organ transplant. Currently, 6,000 liver transplants are performed in the US yearly (unos). (http://optn.transplant.hrsa.gov/ar2009/Chapter_IV_AR_CD.htm?cp=5#TOC).

In parallel to the success of kidney transplantation, the outcomes of liver transplantation have continued to improve over the last two decades following better surgical techniques and the introduction of more potent immunosuppression. The introduction of cyclosporine first and later tacrolimus has allowed to control the rejection rate and prolong allograft survival ((Starzl et al., 1985, Busuttil et al., 2004). Especially tacrolimus has played an important role in liver transplantation since its introduction by allowing to rescue grafts from cyclosporine resistant rejection (Starzl et al., 1989). As a result, cyclosporine is less commonly used today in liver transplantation and most immunosuppression protocols are based on tacrolimus, associated to mycophenolic acid and steroids (reviewed in Geissler et al., 2009 and Pillai et al., 2009).

Usually liver transplant recipients do not receive antibody-based induction immunosuppression. Rather, high-dose methylprednisolone (500 mg – 1 g) is given intravenously as induction at the time of implantation of the liver and rapidly tapered from the time of surgery to a daily maintenance dose of 5 to 10 mg per day. Many programs taper and discontinue prednisone at 3 to 6 months to avoid the side effects of long-term prednisone use. Prednisone cessation does not seem to have a negative impact on graft function. Indeed, steroid withdrawal trials have demonstrated that corticosteroid-free regimens do not lead to increased rejection rates. However, in patients transplanted for immune-mediated liver disease such as primary biliary cirrhosis, primary sclerosing cholangitis and autoimmune hepatitis it seems prudent to maintain prednisone therapy in the long term, albeit at a low-dose, in order to reduce the risk of disease recurrence.

Corticosteroids are also used in the treatment of episodes of acute cellular rejection: intravenous methylprednisolone is usually given at a dose of 1,000 mg on alternate days for a total of 3 doses, followed by taper.

Acute rejection does not impact on graft function in the long term in the vast majority of cases given the resilience and the regenerative capacity of the liver as opposed to kidney or other solid organs.

An important issue in immunosuppression in liver transplant recipients is the prevention of nephrotoxicity associated with CNI. Chronic renal damage is affecting up to 16% of non-renal transplant recipients treated with CNI (Ojo et al., 2003) and the search for the best renal sparing immunosuppression strategy in liver transplantation is still ongoing. A key factor seems to be the tailoring of the immunosuppression *regimen* to the individual patient. In patients with renal insufficiency at the time of transplant one strategy is to hold calcineurin inhibitors and to use an IL-2 receptor blocker as induction agent. This will obtain effective immunosuppression early post-transplant allowing the introduction of CNI to be delayed until after resolution of peri-operative renal dysfunction. In the event of non-recovery of renal function, the addition of sirolimus may be considered. A number of studies have reported on the use of sirolimus in patients with renal insufficiency after liver transplantation and especially in those with calcineurin inhibitor (CNI)-associated nephrotoxicity. The results of these studies have not been conclusive. A recent meta-analysis showed that conversion to sirolimus from CNIs in LT recipients with renal insufficiency [glomerular filtration rate (GFR) < 60 mL/minute or creatinine level ≥ 1.5 mg/dL] is associated with a non-significant improvement in renal function. In addition, although patient and graft survival were not significantly different, infections, ulcers and discontinuation of therapy were significantly more common in patients treated with sirolimus compared to control (Asrani et al., 2010). This adds to an earlier concern raised by previous randomized studies when sirolimus was first tried in liver transplantation in 1999. One study (Wiesner et al 2002) reported increased risk of hepatic artery thrombosis and death compared to standard immunosuppression. This study was interrupted and led the FDA to issue an alert on the use of sirolimus in liver transplant. (http://www.fda.gov/Drugs/DrugSafety/PostmarketDrugSafetyInformationforPatientsan dProviders/DrugSafetyInformationforHeathcareProfessionals/ucm165015.htm).

However, sirolimus is currently being used by transplant programs in selected patients. A recent single center retrospective study on 148 patients converted to sirolimus at any time post-transplant for renal function impairment or for progression of fibrosis in HCV positive recipients documents that sirolimus was safe and effective with low rejection rates (3.4%) and no cases of hepatic artery thrombosis (Harper et al., 2011). Another large single center retrospective study reported on the safety and efficacy of sirolimus in liver transplant with lower incidence of rejection and similar survival rates compared to other regimens (Campsen et al., 2011).

Finally, other recent studies have reported that the antifibrotic and antiangiogenic effects of sirolimus may have a favorable impact in HCV positive recipients and patients transplanted for hepatocellular carcinoma, respectively (see below).

A special consideration has been given over the last few years to immunosuppression regimens used in HCV positive liver transplant recipients. HCV-related cirrhosis is now the most common indication for liver transplantation in the US and HCV recurrence in the graft is a major risk factor for graft loss. To date there is no single best strategy to successfully prevent HCV recurrence post-transplant, although new antivirals are being developed that may have a positive impact. The management of immunosuppression in HCV liver transplant recipients has been the focus of several studies but consensus on the best immunosuppression regimen in HCV recipients is lacking. However, it seems to be now accepted in many centers that the use of steroids, especially high-dose intravenous boluses to treat acute cellular rejection should be considered very carefully in patients with hepatitis C because of the risk of severe recurrence of hepatitis C. (Berenguer 2011). Therefore, the prevention of rejection by obtaining and maintaining adequate levels of tacrolimus from the very early post-operative period is very important. Cyclosporine has been suggested to be superior to tacrolimus in controlling HCV recurrence post-transplant given the antiviral effects of cyclosporine in vitro but clinical trials failed to confirm this expectation and currently there is no evidence that the choice of CNI (cyclosporine or tacrolimus) makes a significant difference in outcome in HCV recipients (Berenguer et al., 2010). Antiviral therapy with interferon and ribavirin is an option in selected transplant recipients with recurrent HCV: progression to cirrhosis is slower, risk of graft decompensation is lower and patient survival is longer in responders to antiviral treatment compared to non-responders (Berenguer et al., 2008). However, the pro-inflammatory effects of interferon increase the risk of acute rejection, chronic rejection and de-novo autoimmune hepatitis post-transplant

(Nazia et al., 2011). Pre-transplant antiviral treatment is poorly tolerated in Child C patients (Melero et al., 2009).

The antifibrotic effect of sirolimus has been considered to have a potential impact on slowing down fibrosis progression in HCV-positive recipients (Wagner et al., 2010). A recent study on 88 patients treated with sirolimus-based immunosuppression reports that, although timing or severity of post-transplant HCV recurrence were not affected, hepatitis activity and fibrosis scores were lower on serial biopsy compared to conventional immunosuppression regimens (Asthana et al., 2011). Further studies will have to confirm the role of sirolimus in HCV-infected grafts.

Liver transplantation is the most radical and successful treatment for selected patients with hepatocellular carcinoma (HCC) who fulfill transplant criteria. Tumor recurrence affects 10-20% of patients within 2 years after transplant and is a major determinant of patient survival. Multiple factors determine the risk of recurrence of HCC after liver transplant, including staging and biologic aggressivity of HCC. Post-transplant immunosuppression increases the risk of tumor recurrence and the choice of the immunosuppression regimen may have an impact on outcomes. Drugs like mTOR inhibitors (sirolimus, see above) effectively reduce cell growth and angiogenesis in animal models of hepatocellular cancer (review in Treiber 2009) and may have a role in reducing the risk of recurrence in patients transplanted for HCC. In a recent study patients transplanted for HCC and treated with sirolimus had lower recurrence rates than patients treated with tacrolimus (Chinnakotla et al., 2009); a subsequent study on registry data confirmed better survival rates in sirolimus patients compared to non-sirolimus (Toso et al., 2010).

New drugs are being developed for the treatment of HCC. Sorafenib is a tyrosine kinase inhibitor shown to increase survival in patients with advanced HCC (Llovet et al., 2008). Trials are ongoing on the use of sorafenib to prevent recurrence after transplant (Villanueva et al., 2011).

Currently, antibodies are not commonly used in liver transplantation. OKT3 has been in the past the most commonly used monoclonal antibody in liver transplantation. It was originally introduced in 1987 for prophylaxis of acute cellular rejection but now it is mainly used in patients with steroid-resistant cellular rejection. The use of OKT3 and of other depleting agents is associated with early and severe recurrences of hepatitis C and must be used with caution in this cohort of patients. (Rosen et al., 1997, Eghtesad et al., 2005)

Two non-depleting IL-2 receptor antibodies, daclizumab and basiliximab, are being used in liver transplantation for induction immunosuppression in patients with renal failure to allow a delayed introduction of CNI (Verna et al., 2011).

Alemtuzumab has been used in tolerance inducing protocols in liver transplantation but is not currently used outside research protocols (Weissenbacher et al., 2010).

5. Immunosuppression in pancreas transplantation

Currently about 1,100 patients receive a pancreas transplant in the US per year. The main indication is to restore normoglycemia in patients with type I diabetes on high insulin regimens to improve or at least to arrest the progression of diabetic nephropathy, retinopathy and neuropathy. The advantages of pancreas transplant versus insulin therapy in obtaining normoglycemia have been well documented (Gremizzi et al., 2010). Hypoglycemia unawareness, a complication of insulin therapy, is also an indication for pancreas transplant. Since the year 2000 islet cell transplant has been introduced as an alternative less invasive treatment for diabetes (Shapiro et al., 2000) with reports of variable success over the years (review in (de Kort et al., 2011)). The long term function of transplanted islets remains an unresolved issue. Recent studies report that pancreas transplant obtains higher rates of and longer lasting insulin independence compared to islet cell transplant, but with higher risk of surgical complications (Vardanyan et al., 2010, Maffi et al., 2011). The immunological aspects and immunosuppression regimens specific to islet transplant have been extensively reviewed (Azzi et al., 2010) and will not be discussed here. The pancreas is transplanted either simultaneously with the kidney for patients with renal failure due to type 1 diabetes mellitus or as isolated pancreas. In addition, the pancreas is included in the multivisceral graft for selected patients transplanted for intestinal failure (see below). Advances in surgical techniques and immunosuppression management have obtained current pancreas graft survival rates of 86% at 1 year, between 60 and 80% at 3 years and 53% at 10 years, respectively (Gruessner et al., 2010).

Most pancreas transplant recipients receive induction therapy with T-cell-depleting agents thymoglobulin or alemtuzumab and maintenance immunosuppression with a combination of CNI (mostly tacrolimus), mycophenolate mofetil, sirolimus and rapid steroid withdrawal (review in Heilman et al., 2010). The incidence of acute rejection after pancreas transplant is reported between 20 and 35% at 3 years (Farney et al., 2009). Like in kidney transplant, the combination of sirolimus with full dose CNI may accentuate nephrotoxicity. There have been trials of elimination of CNI to avoid nephrotoxicity with similar patient and graft survival at 6 months compared to tacrolimus based regimens, but with higher rates of acute rejection (Gruessner et al 2005). Over the last years, more and more maintenance protocols have avoided the use of steroids (Knight et al., 2010).

6. Immunosuppression in intestinal transplantation

Intestinal transplantation is the newest and most recently developed among abdominal organ transplants. Although it has been attempted experimentally for decades since the pioneering work of Lillehei (Lillehei et al 1959), the first successful intestinal transplant in humans was reported in 1990 (Grant et al., 1990). Over the last decade intestinal transplantation has become clinically established as an effective treatment for patients with intestinal failure and life-threatening complications of parenteral nutrition (Fishbein 2009). In recent years 150-180 intestinal transplants are performed in US per year. (unos) http://optn.transplant.hrsa.gov/latestData/rptData.asp

Rejection has been a formidable obstacle to successful intestinal transplantation. The development of effective immunosuppression together with advanced surgical techniques and improved patient management have significantly contributed to the success of intestinal transplantation. Although initially rejection and mortality rates were high, the outcomes of intestinal transplantation have markedly improved over the last decade and now survival rates are close to other solid organ transplants. However, still transplantation of the intestine remains a greater immunologic challenge compared to other solid organs. The high immunogenicity of the intestinal graft is related to its rich composition in lymphoid tissue (80% of the body immune cells reside in the gut) and also to the presence of a complex innate immune system continuously exposed to intraluminal foreign antigens and microbes. A delicate and fine balance between absorption of nutrients and defense from infection is regulated at the level of the intestinal surface and the interplay between innate and acquired components of the immune response at the level of the intestinal mucosa is being better understood in recent years (see below).

The introduction of tacrolimus in the early 1990 and induction immunotherapy (Reyes et al 2005) have decreased the rejection rate from historical rates of 80 or more to 20-40% in most recent series. Episodes of acute rejection are treated with intravenous pulse steroids and/or thymoglobulin, depending on severity. The severity of rejection episodes has been better controlled with the introduction of sirolimus in addition to tacrolimus-based maintenance immunosuppression (Fishbein et al., 2002, Gupta et al., 2005). Infliximab, an anti-tumor necrosis factor alpha antibody used for Crohn's disease, has been successful in isolated cases as salvage therapy in patients with thymoglobulin resistant rejection (De Greef et al., 2011). Immunosuppression protocols continue to evolve (Abu-Elmagd et al., 2009, Pirenne et al., 2009) and different drug combinations are used with the cornerstone for maintenance immunosuppression being tacrolimus.

New insight in intestine transplant function and on new strategies to control allograft rejection comes from studies on gut microflora and innate immunity. The normal intestinal flora is dominated by anaerobic species Bacteroides and Clostridia. Post-transplant the composition of the gut microflora changes and the microbial community is dominated by Lactobacilli and Enterobacteria, which are facultative anaerobes (Hartman et al., 2009). This represents an inversion of the normal flora. After surgical closure of the ileostomy, which is usually undertaken three months post-transplant, the microbial community reverts to the normal flora. Therefore, the transplanted intestine can function with either of two alternate microbial populations. As in patients with inflammatory bowel disease, the functional impact of alterations in the gut microflora is only recently being recognized and may have implications for the management of intestinal transplant rejection.

The nucleotide-binding oligomerization domain 2 (NOD2) is an intracellular sensor for pathogen/microbe associated molecular patterns that recognizes a component of the bacterial cell wall. NOD2 protein is a critical regulator of bacterial immunity in the intestine and is required for the expression of intestinal anti-microbial peptides. Mutations of NOD2 are highly correlated with Crohn's disease. We found that 35% of intestinal transplant recipients have NOD2 mutations associated with Crohn's disease and that the risk severe rejection and of graft failure were significantly greater in the NOD2 mutant recipients compared with the NOD2 wild-type recipients (Fishbein et al 2008). The presence of a NOD2 polymorphism in the recipient may influence the viability of the allograft by interrupting NOD2- dependent circuits required to maintain intestinal homeostasis with respect to commensal flora: a recipient lacking a functional intestinal microbial-sensing system may be more exposed to allograft damage secondary to rejection than a recipient with an intact system.

7. Future perspectives

Renal function impairment, opportunistic infections (Cytomegalovirus, Epstein-Barr related post-transplant lymphoproliferative disease and others) and metabolic disorders (diabetes and others) are frequent complications of prolonged immunosuppression and remain a major challenge to improve the long term outcomes of transplant recipients. Future strategies to limit the impact of these complications include the development of new non-nephrotoxic agents, the individualization of organ-specific immunosuppression regimens tailored to patient needs and the design of protocols of minimization of immunosuppression and tolerance induction. Studies on gene expression profiling and other methods derived from the –omics approach will further contribute to characterize the rejection process and to monitor the immune response.

The role of B cells and antibodies is increasingly being investigated and recognized as a target for treatment. The presence and persistence of donor-specific antibodies in the long term follow-up of kidney transplant recipients led to the recognition that chronic antibody mediated injury may be responsible for late graft loss. (Colvin 2010). This has prompted interest in new **B-cell** based therapeutic strategies and trials are under way involving agents to control humoral immunity.

The contribution of memory T cells (Lo et al., 2011) and of systemic complement activation (Damman et al., 2011) to the rejection process will also be better characterized by ongoing trials.

8. References

Abu-Elmagd KM, Costa G, Bond GJ, Wu T, Murase N, Zeevi A, et al. (2009). Evolution of the immunosuppressive strategies for the intestinal and multivisceral recipients with special reference to allograft immunity and achievement of partial tolerance. *Transplant International* 22 :96–109.

Adcock IM, Ito K. (2000).Molecular mechanisms of corticosteroid actions. *Monaldi Arch Chest Dis* 55(3):256–66.

Aoyagi T, Yamashita K, Suzuki T, Uno M, Goto R, Taniguchi M, et al. (2009). A human anti-CD40 monoclonal antibody, 4D11, for kidney transplantation in cynomolgus monkeys: induction and maintenance therapy. *Am J Transplant*. 9(8):1732-41.

Aparna P, Augustine JJ, Hricik DE. (2009).Induction Antibody Therapy in Kidney Transplantation. *Am J Kidney Dis* 54:935-944.

Asrani SK, Leise MD, West CP, Murad MH, Pedersen RA, Erwin PJ, Tian J, Wiesner RH, Kim WR (2010). Use of sirolimus in liver transplant recipients with renal insufficiency: a systematic review and meta-analysis. *Hepatology*. 52(4):1360-70.

Asthana S, Toso C, Meeberg G (2011). The impact of sirolimus on hepatitis C recurrence after liver transplantation. *Can J Gastroenterol*, 25(1):28-34.

Azzi J, Geara AS, El-Sayegh S, Abdi R. (2010).Immunological aspects of pancreatic islet cell transplantation. *Expert Rev Clin Immunol*. 6(1):111-24.

Berenguer M, Palau A, Aguilera V, Rayón JM, Juan FS, Prieto M. (2008).Clinical benefits of antiviral therapy in patients with recurrent hepatitis C following liver transplantation. *Am J Transplant*. 8(3):679-87.

Berenguer M, Aguilera V, San Juan F, Benlloch S, Rubin A, López-Andujar R, Moya A, Pareja E, Montalva E, Yago M, de Juan M, Mir J, Prieto M. (2010). Effect of calcineurin inhibitors in the outcome of liver transplantation in hepatitis C virus-positive recipients. *Transplantation*. 90(11):1204-9.

Berenguer M. (2011).Hot topic debate on HCV: The type of immunosuppression does not matter. *Liver Transpl*. Jun 1. doi: 10.1002/lt.22347. [Epub ahead of print]

Borie DC, Changelian PS, Larson MJ et al.(2005). Immunosuppression by the JAK3 inhibitor CP-690,550 delays rejection and significantly prolongs kidney allograft survival in nonhuman primates. *Transplantation* 79: 791–801

Busque S, Leventhal J, Brennan DC, Steinberg S, Klintmalm G, Shah T, Mulgaonkar S, Bromberg JS, Vincenti F, Hariharan S, Slakey D, Peddi VR, Fisher RA, Lawendy N, Wang C, Chan G.(2009). Calcineurin-inhibitor-free immunosuppression based on the JAK inhibitor CP-690,550: a pilot study in de novo kidney allograft recipients. *Am J Transplant*. 9(8):1936-45

Busuttil RW, Lake JR.(2004). Role of tacrolimus in the evolution of liver transplantation. *Transplantation*. 77(9 Suppl):S44-51.

Calne RY (1961) Inhibition of the rejection of renal homografts in dogs by purine analogues. *Transpl Bull* 28(2):445-461

Campsen J, Zimmerman MA, Mandell S, Kaplan M, Kam I. (2011). A Decade of Experience Using mTor Inhibitors in Liver Transplantation. *J Transplant*. 2011;2011:913094. Epub 2011 Mar 15.

Chinnakotla S, Davis GL, Vasani S.(2009). Impact of sirolimus on the recurrence of hepatocellular carcinoma after liver transplantation. *Liver Transpl*, 15(12): 1834-42.

Ciancio G, Gaynor JJ, Zarak A, Sageshima J, Guerra G, Roth D, Brown R, Kupin W, Chen L, Tueros L, Hanson L, Ruiz P, Burke GW 3rd.(2011) Randomized trial of mycophenolate mofetil versus enteric-coated mycophenolate sodium in primary renal transplantation with tacrolimus and steroid avoidance: four-year analysis. *Transplantation*. 91(11):1198-1205.

Colvin RB, Hirohashi T, Farris AB, Minnei F, Collins AB, Smith RN. (2010). Emerging role of B cells in chronic allograft dysfunction. *Kidney Int Suppl*. 119:S13-7.

Colvin RB. (2010). Dimensions of antibody-mediated rejection. *Am J Transplant*. 10(7):1509-10.

Cross SA, Perry CM. (2007).Tacrolimus once-daily formulation in the prophylaxis of transplant rejection in renal or liver allograft recipients. *Drugs*. 67(13):1931-43.

Damman J, Seelen MA, Moers C, Daha MR, Rahmel A, Leuvenink HG, Paul A, Pirenne J, Ploeg RJ. (2011) Systemic Complement Activation in Deceased Donors Is Associated With Acute Rejection After Renal Transplantation in the Recipient. *Transplantation*. 92(2):163-169.

Dedrick RL, Walickeb P, Garovoya M. (2002). Anti-adhesion antibodies. Efalizumab, a humanized anti-CD11a monoclonal antibody. *Transplant Immunology* 9: 181–186.

De Greef E, Avitzur Y, Grant D, De-Angelis M, Ng V, Jones N, Ngan B, Shapiro R, Steinberg R, Gana JC. (2011). The Successful Use of Infliximab as Salvage Therapy in Pediatric Intestinal Transplant Patients with Steroid and Thymoglobulin Resistant Late Acute Rejection. *J Pediatr Gastroenterol Nutr*. [Epub ahead of print]

de Kort H, de Koning EJ, Rabelink TJ, Bruijn JA, Bajema IM (2011). Islet transplantation in type 1 diabetes. *BMJ*.;342:d217. doi: 10.1136/bmj.d217.

Eghtesad B, Fung JJ, Demetris AJ, Murase N, Ness R, Bass DC, Gray EA, Shakil O, Flynn B, Marcos A, Starzl TE (2005). Immunosuppression for liver transplantation in HCV-infected patients: mechanism-based principles. *Liver Transpl*. 11(11):1343-52.

Ellis CN, Krueger GG; Alefacept Clinical Study Group.(2001).Treatment of chronic plaque psoriasis by selective targeting of memory effector T lymphocytes. *N Engl J Med*. 345(4):248-55

Ekberg H, Tedesco-Silva H, Demirbas A, Vítko S, Nashan B, Gürkan A, Margreiter R, Hugo C, Grinyó JM, Frei U, Vanrenterghem Y, Daloze P, Halloran PF; ELITE-Symphony Study. (2007) Reduced exposure to calcineurin inhibitors in renal transplantation. *N Engl J Med*. 357(25):2562-75

Ekberg H, Grinyó J, Nashan B, Vanrenterghem Y, Vincenti F, Voulgari A, Truman M, Nasmyth-Miller C, Rashford M. (2007) Cyclosporine sparing with mycophenolate mofetil, daclizumab and corticosteroids in renal allograft recipients: the CAESAR Study. *Am J Transplant*. 7(3):560-70.

Ekberg H, Bernasconi C, Tedesco-Silva H, Vítko S, Hugo C, Demirbas A, Acevedo RR, Grinyó J, Frei U, Vanrenterghem Y, Daloze P, Halloran P. (2009). Calcineurin inhibitor minimization in the Symphony study: observational results 3 years after transplantation. *Am J Transplant.* 9(8):1876-85.

European FK506 Multicentre Liver Study Group.(1994) Randomised trial comparing tacrolimus (FK506) and cyclosporin in prevention of liver allograft rejection. *Lancet.* 344(8920):423-8

Farney AC, Doares W, Rogers J, Singh R, Hartmann E, Hart L, Ashcraft E, Reeves-Daniels A, Gautreaux M, Iskandar SS, Moore P, Adams PL, and Stratta RJ.(2009) A Randomized Trial of Alemtuzumab Versus Antithymocyte Globulin Induction in Renal and Pancreas Transplantation.*Transplantation* 88: 810–819.

Fishbein TM, Florman S, Gondolesi G, Schiano T, LeLeiko N, Tschernia A, Kaufman S. (2002). Intestinal transplantation before and after the introduction of sirolimus. *Transplantation.* 73(10):1538-42

Fishbein T, Novitskiy G, Mishra L, Matsumoto C, Kaufman S, Goyal S, Shetty K, Johnson L, Lu A, Wang A, Hu F, Kallakury B, Lough D, Zasloff M (2008). NOD2-expressing bone marrow-derived cells appear to regulate epithelial innate immunity of the transplanted human small intestine. *Gut.* 57(3):323-30.

Fishbein TM.(2009) Intestinal transplantation. *N Engl J Med.* 361(10):998-1008.

Flanagan ME, Blumenkopf TA,Brissette WH,Brown MF, Casavant JM, Shang-Poa C, Doty JL,Elliott EA, Fisher MB, Hines M, Kent C,Kudlacz EM, Lillie BM, Magnuson KS, McCurdy SP,Munchhof MJ,Perry BD, Sawyer PS, Strelevitz TJ, Subramanyam C,Sun J,Whipple DA, Changelian PS (2010). Discovery of CP-690,550: A Potent and Selective Janus Kinase (JAK) Inhibitor for the Treatment of Autoimmune Diseases and Organ Transplant Rejection *J. Med. Chem.* 53: 8468–8484.

Flechner SM, Kobashigawa J, Klintmalm G.(2008) Calcineurin inhibitor-sparing regimens in solid organ transplantation: focus on improving renal function and nephrotoxicity. *Clin Transplant.* 22(1):1-15.

Gabardi S, Baroletti SA. (2010) Everolimus: a proliferation signal inhibitor with clinical applications in organ transplantation, oncology, and cardiology. *Pharmacotherapy.* 30(10):1044-56.

Gaber AO, Busque S, Mulgaonkar S, Gaston R, Jevnikar A,Meier-Kriesche H-U. (2008) ISA247: A phase IIB multicenter, open label,concentration-controlled trial in de novo renal transplantation. *Am J Transplant* 8(Suppl 2): 336.

Gaston RS, Kaplan B, Shah T, Cibrik D, Shaw LM, Angelis M, Mulgaonkar S, Meier-Kriesche HU, Patel D, Bloom RD. (2009) Fixed- or controlled-dose mycophenolate mofetil with standard- or reduced-dose calcineurin inhibitors: the Opticept trial. *Am J Transplant.*9(7):1607-19.

Geissler EK, Schlitt HJ.(2009) Immunosuppression for liver transplantation. *Gut* 58: 452-463

Geissler EK, Schlitt HJ.(2010) The potential benefits of rapamycin on renal function, tolerance, fibrosis, and malignancy following transplantation. *Kidney Int.* 78(11):1075-9.

Grant D, Wall W, Mimeault R, Zhong R, Ghent C, Garcia B, (1990) Successful small-bowel/liver transplantation. *Lancet* 335(8683):181-4.

Gremizzi C, Vergani A, Paloschi V, Secchi A.(2010) Impact of pancreas transplantation on type 1 diabetes-related complications. *Curr Opin Organ Transplant.* 15(1):119-23.

Gruessner RW, Kandaswamy R, Humar A, Gruessner AC, Sutherland DE.(2005) Calcineurin inhibitor- and steroid-free immunosuppression in pancreas-kidney and solitary pancreas transplantation. *Transplantation* 79:1184–1189.

Gruessner AC, Sutherland DE, Gruessner RW (2010) Pancreas transplantation in the United States: a review. *Curr Opin Organ Transplant.* 15(1):93-101.

Gupta P, Kaufman S, Fishbein TM.(2005) Sirolimus for solid organ transplantation in children. *Pediatr Transplant.* 9(3):269-76

Harper SJ, Gelson W, Harper IG, Alexander GJ, Gibbs P.(2011) Switching to sirolimus-based immune suppression after liver transplantation is safe and effective: a single-center experience. *Transplantation.* 91(1):128-32.

Hartman A, Denver ML, Barupal DK, Fiehn O, Fishbein T, Zasloff M and Eisen JA (2009) Human gut microbiome adopts an alternative state following small bowel transplantation *PNAS* 106(40):17187–17192

Heilman RL, Mazur MJ, Reddy KS. (2010) Immunosuppression in Simultaneous Pancreas-Kidney Transplantation. Progress to Date . *Drugs* 70 (7): 793-804

(http://optn.transplant.hrsa.gov/ar2009/Chapter_III_AR_CD.htm?cp=4#1)

Hutchinson M (2010) Natalizumab therapy of multiple sclerosis. *J Interferon Cytokine Res.* 30(10):787-9.

Kahan BD.(2000) Efficacy of sirolimus compared with azathioprine for reduction of acute renal allograft rejection: a randomized multicentre study. The Rapamune US Study Group. *Lancet* 356(15):194.

Kaposztas Z, Podder H, Mauiyyedi S, Illoh O, Kerman R, Reyes M, Pollard V, Kahan BD.(2009) Impact of rituximab therapy for treatment of acute humoral rejection. *Clin Transplant.* 23(1):63-73.

Kirk AD, Turgeon NA, Iwakoshi NN (2010). B cells and transplantation tolerance. *Nat Rev Nephrol.* 6(10):584-93.

Klipa D, Mahmud N, Ahsan N.(2010) Antibody immunosuppressive therapy in solid organ transplant: Part II. *MAbs.* 2(6):607-12.

Knechtle SJ. (2010) Immunoregulation and tolerance. *Transplant Proc.* 42(9 Suppl):S13-5.

Knight RJ, Podder H, Kerman RH, Lawless A, Katz SM,Van Buren CT, Gaber AO, Kahan BD.(2010) Comparing an early corticosteroid/late calcineurin-free immunosuppression protocol to a sirolimus-, cyclosporine A-, and prednisone based regimen for pancreas-kidney transplantation. *Transplantation* 89:727–732.

Kovarik JM, Steiger JU, Grinyo JM, Rostaing L, Arns W, Dantal J, Proot P, Budde K, Sotrastaurin Renal Transplant Study Group (2011). Pharmacokinetics of sotrastaurin combined with tacrolimus or mycophenolic acid in de novo kidney transplant recipients. *Transplantation.* 91(3):317-22.

Krämer BK, Charpentier B, Bäckman L, Silva HT Jr, Mondragon-Ramirez G, Cassuto-Viguier E, Mourad G, Sola R, Rigotti P, Mirete JO; Tacrolimus Prolonged Release Renal Study Group.(2010) Tacrolimus once daily (ADVAGRAF) versus twice daily (PROGRAF) in de novo renal transplantation: a randomized phase III study. *Am J Transplant.* 10(12):2632-43.

Kuschei WM, Leitner J, Majdic O, Pickl WF, Zlabinger GJ, Grabmeier-Pfistershammer K, Steinberger P.(2011) Costimulatory signals potently modulate the T cell inhibitory capacity of the therapeutic CD11a antibody Efalizumab. *Clin Immunol.* 139(2):199-207.

Larson TS, Dean PG, Stegall MD, Griffin MD, Textor SC, Schwab TR, Gloor TM, Cosio FG, Lund WJ, Kremers WK, Nyberg SL, Ishitani MB, Prieto M, Velosa JA

(2006).Complete Avoidance of Calcineurin Inhibitors in Renal Transplantation: A Randomized Trial Comparing Sirolimus and Tacrolimus. *Am J Transpl* 6:514–522

Lillehei RC, Goot B, Miller FA.(1959) The physiological response of the small bowel of the dog to ischemia including prolonged in vitro preservation of the bowel with successful replacement and survival. *Ann Surg* 150(4): 543-560

Llovet JM, Ricci S, Mazzaferro V(2008). Sorafenib in advanced hepatocellular carcinoma. *N Engl J Med* 359(8):378–390.

Lo DJ, Weaver TA, Stempora L, Mehta AK, Ford ML, Larsen CP, Kirk AD (2011). Selective targeting of human alloresponsive CD8+ effector memory T cells based on CD2 expression. *Am J Transplant.* 11(1):22-33.

Maffi P, Scavini M, Socci C, Piemonti L, Caldara R, Gremizzi C, Melzi R, Nano R, Orsenigo E, Venturini M, Staudacher C, Del Maschio A, Secchi A. (2011). Risks and benefits of transplantation in the cure of type 1 diabetes: whole pancreas versus islet transplantation. A single center study. *Rev Diabet Stud.* 8(1):44-50.

Melancon JK, Cummings LS, Graham J, Rosen-Bronson S, Light J, Desai CS, Girlanda R, Ghasemian S, Africa J, Johnson LB.(2011). Paired kidney donor exchanges and antibody reduction therapy: novel methods to ameliorate disparate access to living donor kidney transplantation in ethnic minorities. *J Am Coll Surg.* 212(4):740-5.

Mele TS, Halloran PF.(2000) The use of mycophenolate mofetil in transplant recipients. *Immunopharmacology* 47:215–245.

Melero J, Berenguer M. (2009).Antiviral therapy in patients with HCV-cirrhosis. *Ann Hepatol.* 8(4):292-7.

Merion RM, White DJ, Thiru S, Evans DB, Calne RY.(1984). Cyclosporine: five years' experience in cadaveric renal transplantation. *N Engl J Med.* 310(3):148-54

Montgomery RA, Gentry SE,Marks WH. (2006). Domino paired kidney donation: a strategy to make best use of live non-directed donation. *Lancet* 368:419–421.

Montgomery RA. (2010) Renal transplantation across HLA and ABO antibody barriers: integrating paired donation into desensitization protocols. *Am J Transplant* 10:449–457.

Nazia S, Guindi M, Renner EL, Berenguer M. (2011). Immune-mediated complications of the graft in interferon-treated hepatitis C positive liver transplant recipients. *J of Hepatol* 55: 207–217

Niederhaus SV, Muth B, Lorentzen DF, Wai P, Pirsch JD, Samaniego-Picota M, Leverson GE, D'alessandro AM, Sollinger HW, Djamali A. (2011) Luminex-based desensitization protocols: the university of wisconsin initial experience. *Transplantation.* 92(1):12-7.

Ojo AO, Held PJ, Port FK, Wolfe RA, Leichtman AB, Young EW, Arndorfer J, Christensen L, Merion RM.(2003) Chronic renal failure after transplantation of a nonrenal organ. *N Engl J Med.* 349(10):931-40

Perry DK, Burns JM, Pollinger HS, Amiot BP, Gloor JM, Gores GJ, Stegall MD. (2009). Proteasome Inhibition Causes Apoptosis of Normal Human Plasma Cells Preventing Alloantibody Production. *Am J Transpl* 9(1) 201-209.

Pillai AA, Levitsky J.(2009) Overview of immunosuppression in liver transplantation. *World J Gastroenterol.* 15(34):4225-33.

Pirenne J, Kawai M.(2009). Intestinal transplantation: evolution in immunosuppression protocols. *Current Opinion in Organ Transplantation* 14:250–255

Raichlin E, Khalpey Z, Kremers W, Frantz RP, Rodeheffer RJ, Clavell AL, Edwards BS, Kushwaha SS. (2007). Replacement of calcineurin-inhibitors with sirolimus as primary immunosuppression in stable cardiac transplant recipients.*Transplantation*. 84(4):467-74.

Reyes J, Mazariegos GV, Abu-Elmagd K, Macedo C, Bond GJ, Murase N, Peters J, Sindhi R, Starzl TE. (2005). Intestinal transplantation under tacrolimus monotherapy after perioperative lymphoid depletion with rabbit anti-thymocyte globulin (thymoglobulin). *Am J Transplant*. 5(6):1430-6.

Rosen HR, Shackleton CR, Higa L, Gralnek IM, Farmer DA, McDiarmid SV, Holt C, Lewin KJ, Busuttil RW, Martin P.(1997) Use of OKT3 is associated with early and severe recurrence of hepatitis C after liver transplantation. *Am J Gastroenterol*. 92(9):1453-7

Schena FP, Pascoe MD, Alberu J, del Carmen Rial M, Oberbauer R, Brennan DC, Campistol JM, Racusen L, Polinsky MS, Goldberg-Alberts R.(2009). Conversion from calcineurin inhibitors to sirolimus maintenance therapy in renal allograft recipients: 24-month efficacy and safety results from the CONVERT trial. *Transplantation*. 87(2):233-42.

Shapiro AMJ, Lakey JRT, Ryan EA, Korbutt GS, Toth E, Warnock GL.(2000) Islet transplantation in seven patients with type 1 diabetes mellitus using a glucocorticoid-free immunosuppressive regimen. *N Engl J Med* 343:230-8.

Starzl TE, Marchioro TL, Hutchinson DE, Porter KA, Cerilli GJ, Brettschneider L.(1967) The clinical use of antilymphocyte globulin in renal homotransplantation. *Transplantation*. 5(4):Suppl:1100-5.

Starzl TE.(2000) History of clinical transplantation. *World J Surg*. 24(7):759-82.

Starzl TE, Iwatsuki S, Shaw BW Jr, Gordon RD, Esquivel CO (1985) Immunosuppression and other nonsurgical factors in the improved results of liver transplantation. *Semin Liver Dis*. 5(4):334-43.

Starzl TE, Todo S, Fung J, Demetris AJ, Venkataramman R, Jain A (1989). FK 506 for liver, kidney, and pancreas transplantation. *Lancet*. 8670 (2):1000-4.

Stewart SF, Hudson M, Talbot D, Manas D, Day CP.(2001) Mycophenolate mofetil monotherapy in liver transplantation. *Lancet* 357: 609-610

The U.S. Multicenter FK506 Liver Study Group.(1994) A comparison of tacrolimus (FK 506) and cyclosporine for immunosuppression in liver transplantation. *N Engl J Med*. 331(17):1110-5.

Toso C, Merani S, Bigam DL.(2010). Sirolimus-based immunosuppression is associated with increased survival after liver transplantation for hepatocellular carcinoma. *Hepatology*, 51(4): 1237-43.

Treiber G.(2009) mTOR inhibitors for hepatocellular cancer: a forward-moving target. *Expert Rev Anticancer Ther*. 9(2):247-61.

Trunečka P, Boillot O, Seehofer D, Pinna AD, Fischer L, Ericzon BG, Troisi RI, Baccarani U, Ortiz de Urbina J, Wall W.(2010). Once-daily prolonged-release tacrolimus (ADVAGRAF) versus twice-daily tacrolimus (PROGRAF) in liver transplantation. Tacrolimus Prolonged Release Liver Study Group. *Am J Transplant*. 10(10):2313-23.

Vardanyan M, Parkin E, Gruessner C, Rodriguez Rilo HL. (2010) Pancreas vs. islet transplantation: a call on the future. *Curr Opin Organ Transplant*. 15(1):124-30.

Verna EC, Farrand ED, Elnaggar AS, Pichardo EM, Balducci A, Emond JC, Guarrera JV,Brown RS (2011). Basiliximab Induction and Delayed Calcineurin Inhibitor Initiation in Liver Transplant Recipients With Renal Insufficiency. *Transplantation* 91: 1254–1260.

Villanueva A, Llovet JM.(2011) Targeted therapies for hepatocellular carcinoma. *Gastroenterology*. 140(5):1410-26.

Vincenti F, Ramos E, Brattstrom C, Cho S, Ekberg H, Grinyo J, Johnson R, Kuypers D, Stuart F, Khanna A, Navarro M, Nashan B.(2001) Multicenter trial exploring calcineurin inhibitors avoidance in renal transplantation.*Transplantation*. 71(9):1282-7.

Vincenti F, Larsen C, Durrbach A, Wekerle T, Nashan B, Blancho G, Lang P, Grinyo J, Halloran PF, Solez K, Hagerty D, Levy E, Zhou W, Natarajan K, Charpentier B for the Belatacept Study Group (2005). Costimulation Blockade with Belatacept in Renal Transplantation. *N Engl J Med* 353:770-781

Vincenti F, Mendez R, Pescovitz M, Rajagopalan PR, Wilkinson AH, Butt K, Laskow D, Slakey DP, Lorber MI, Garg JP, Garovoy M (2007) A phase I/II randomized open-label multicenter trial of efalizumab, a humanized anti-CD11a, anti-LFA-1 in renal transplantation. *Am J Transplant*. 7(7):1770-7.

Vincenti F, Blancho G, Durrbach A, Friend P, Grinyo J, Halloran PF, Klempnauer J, Lang P, Larsen CP, Mühlbacher F, Nashan B, Soulillou JP, Vanrenterghem Y, Wekerle T, Agarwal M, Gujrathi S, Shen J, Shi R, Townsend R, Charpentier B. (2010). Five-year safety and efficacy of belatacept in renal transplantation. *J Am Soc Nephrol*. 21(9):1587-96.

Wagner D, Kniepeiss D, Schaffellner S. (2010). Sirolimus has a potential to influent viral recurrence in HCV positive liver transplant candidates. *Int Immunopharmacol*, 10(8):990-3.

Walsh RC, Everly JJ, Brailey P, Rike AH, Arend LJ, Mogilishetty G, Govil A, Roy-Chaudhury P, Alloway RR, Woodle ES. (2010). Proteasome inhibitor-based primary therapy for antibody-mediated renal allograft rejection. *Transplantation*. 89(3):277-84.

Walsh RC, Brailey P, Girnita A, Alloway RR, Shields AR, Wall GE, Sadaka BH, Cardi M, Tevar A, Govil A, Mogilishetty G, Roy-Chaudhury P, Woodle ES.(2011). Early and late acute antibody-mediated rejection differ immunologically and in response to proteasome inhibition. *Transplantation*. 91(11):1218-26

Weaver TA, Charafeddine AH, Agarwal A,1 Leopardi F, Kampen R, Starost MF,Larsen CP, Kirk AD.(2008) Targeting of Costimulation Blockade Resistant T Effector Memory (TEM) Cells in Non-Human Primate Renal Transplantation withLFA-3-Ig (Alefacept) Prolongs Allograft Survival. *Am J Transpl* 8(suppl2):204

Wéclawiak H, Kamar N, Ould-Mohamed A, Cardeau-Desangles I, Rostaing L.(2010) Biological agents in kidney transplantation: belatacept is entering the field. *Expert Opin Biol Ther*. 10(10):1501-8.

Weissenbacher A, Boesmueller C, Brandacher G, Oellinger R, Pratschke J, Schneeberger S.(2010) Alemtuzumab in solid organ transplantation and in composite tissue allotransplantation. *Immunotherapy*. 2(6):783-90.

Wiesner, R, for the Rapamune Liver Transplant Study Group (2002) The safety and efficacy of sirolimus and low-dose tacrolimus vs. tacrolimus in de novo orthotopic liver transplant recipients: results from a pilot study. *Hepatology*, 36: 208A.

Wolfe RA, Roys EC, Merion RM. (2010) Trends in organ donation and transplantation in the United States, 1999-2008. *Am J Transplant*. 10(4 Pt 2):961-72.

3

Spleen Tyrosine Kinase: A Novel Target in Autoimmunity

Stephen P. McAdoo and Frederick W. K. Tam
Imperial College Kidney and Transplant Institute, London
United Kingdom

1. Introduction

Spleen tyrosine kinase (Syk) is a non-receptor tyrosine kinase that is highly expressed in cells of haematopoietic lineage, where it has an important role in the intra-cellular signalling cascades for various immunoreceptors, such as the B cell receptor and the Fc receptor. As such, it is a potential target in allergic and autoimmune diseases. Emerging evidence also suggests that Syk may have additional roles beyond its well defined functions in classical immunoreceptor signalling, which may have implications, potentially useful or harmful, for therapies directed at this protein. Given these diverse functions in numerous cell types, it is unsurprising that Syk has been the subject of hundreds of original research articles, as well as several excellent reviews in recent years (Sada, Takano et al. 2001; Ruzza, Biondi et al. 2009; Mocsai, Ruland et al. 2010; Riccaboni, Bianchi et al. 2010). In this chapter we aim to summarise current understanding of the basic structure and function for Syk, before developing a rationale for targeting Syk in autoimmune disease. We will then review progress towards Syk-directed therapies in clinical practice, and finally we shall consider the emerging functions of Syk beyond the adaptive immune response, and what implications these may have for therapy.

2. Discovery

Syk was identified in the early 1990s in the cytostolic fractions of lysates from porcine spleen and bovine thymus as a 40kDa protein with intrinsic kinase activity. This 40kDa protein was subsequently shown to be a fragment, containing only the catalytic domain, of a larger 72kDa protein that was identified from a porcine spleen cDNA library (from whence it gained its name) using oligonucleotides designed according to the partial sequence of the purified 40kDa fragment (Taniguchi, Kobayashi et al. 1991). The *Syk* gene was subsequently mapped to chromosome 9q22 in humans (Ku, Malissen et al. 1994).

3. Basic structure and function

The Syk molecule has a multi-domain structure (Figure 1a) containing two N-terminal tandem Src Homology 2 (SH2) domains and a C-terminal kinase domain (Sada, Takano et al. 2001). Interdomains A and B connect the SH2-SH2 and SH2-kinase domains, respectively. At least 10 major phosphorylation sites have been identified within the molecule (Furlong,

Mahrenholz et al. 1997) – one located in interdomain A, five within interdomain B, two within the kinase domain, and two near the extreme C-terminus. An alternatively spliced form of Syk - SykB – lacks a 23 amino acid sequence in interdomain B, and in this respect is similar to ZAP-70, the only other member of the Syk family of kinases. ZAP-70 has approximately 60% overall homology to Syk and its expression appears to be more restricted, in particular to T lymphocytes and natural killer (NK) cells (Au-Yeung, Deindl et al. 2009).

In the resting state, it is thought that Syk assumes a closed, auto-inhibited structure (Figure 1b), wherein interdomain A and interdomain B bind to the C-terminal kinase domain, preventing its interaction with potential substrates, in what is termed a 'linker-kinase sandwich' (Deindl, Kadlecek et al. 2007; Kulathu, Grothe et al. 2009). Upon activation, structural changes within the molecule result in an open conformation that allows the exposed catalytic kinase domain to interact with downstream targets.

The canonical mechanism of Syk activation is via its interaction with immunoreceptor tyrosine-based activation motifs (ITAMs) (Turner, Schweighoffer et al. 2000). ITAMs are short peptide sequences characterised by a consensus sequence that contains two tyrosine residues 6-12 amino acids apart. As their name suggests, they are found in association with the cytoplasmic components of classical immunoreceptors, including the T-cell receptor (TCR), B-cell receptor (BCR) and Fc-receptor (FcR) for immunoglobulins, either as an associated adapter protein, or within the cytoplasmic region of the receptor itself.

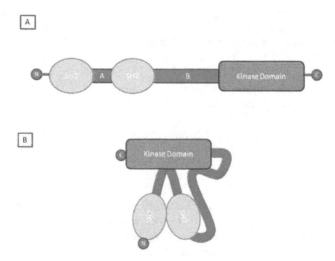

Fig. 1. a. Schematic diagram showing the multi-domain structure of Syk, including two N-terminal SH2-domains, C-terminal kinase domain, and interdomains A and B. Figure 1b: Schematic diagram of the 'linker-kinase sandwich' conformation that has been suggested for resting Syk (see text for details)

Upon receptor engagement, the tyrosine residues on ITAMs are rapidly phosphorylated, primarily by Lyn and other members of the Src family of kinases (Figure 2). The phosphorylated ITAM can now act as a docking site for the SH2 domains of Syk, resulting in conformational changes, exposure of the kinase domain, autophosphorylation and propagation of downstream signalling. In addition, disruption of the 'linker-kinase sandwich' may occur upon phosphorylation of tyrosine residues alone, particularly those within interdomain B. This may occur by autophosphorylation following ITAM-mediated activation, or by transphosphorylation by other kinases, such as Lyn or other Src family kinases that are often co-localised with ITAMs at the cell membrane. As a consequence, positive feedback and sustained Syk activity is possible in the absence of phosphorylated ITAMs. This 'dual' mechanism of activation has recently lead to the proposal of Syk as an 'OR' gate in signalling pathways (Tsang, Giannetti et al. 2008; Bradshaw 2010).

In addition to releasing the enzymatic domain of the protein from the 'linker-kinase sandwich', these changes in structure and phosphorylation, particularly within the tyrosine-rich interdomain B, create docking sites for downstream targets of Syk, for which it can perform both enzymatic and adapter functions (Kulathu, Grothe et al. 2009). These downstream targets include a host of adapter proteins and other enzyme targets (including LAT, SLP76, Vav1, PLC-γ, PI3K and MAP kinases) that are then able to effect complex cellular responses including proliferation, differentiation, phagocytosis and cytokine production (Mocsai, Ruland et al. 2010).

Two groups simultaneously reported the effects of targeted disruption of the *Syk* gene in mice in the mid-90s (Cheng, Rowley et al. 1995; Turner, Mee et al. 1995). *Syk* knockout resulted in perinatal death with a severe haemorrhagic phenotype. This was subsequently shown to be due to a failure of communication between developing vasculature and lymphatics during embryogenesis (Abtahian, Guerriero et al. 2003). Analysis of Syk-deficient lymphoid cells derived from these knock-out animals was critical in developing our early understanding of the functional role of Syk in immunoreceptor signalling in various cell types.

Bone marrow chimera animals, reconstituted with haematopoietic stem cells from Syk-deficient mice, showed no reduction in the numbers of circulating erythrocytes, platelets and total leucocytes. These animals had relatively normal reconstitution of T cells, however detailed analysis revealed impaired differentiation of the B cell lineage, with development arrested at the pro-B to pre-B cell stage, consistent with a role for Syk in pre-BCR signalling (Cheng, Rowley et al. 1995; Turner, Mee et al. 1995). Subsequent *in vitro* work, using a variety of cell lines and cell-based reconstitution systems, has defined a clear role for Syk in initiating downstream signalling following engagement of the BCR (Geahlen 2009), and indeed it was study in this area that was responsible for much of our understanding of the basic structure and function of Syk. The functional role of Syk in mature B cells (such as on antibody production by plasma cells) *in vivo*, however, is less well defined and future studies using small molecule inhibitors, or potentially conditional knockout in this cellular compartment, will be informative.

Analysis of myeloid cells, such as macrophages and neutrophils, from *Syk* knockout bone marrow chimeras showed ablation of FcR-mediated responses including phagocytosis and the generation of reactive oxygen intermediates (Crowley, Costello et al. 1997; Kiefer, Brumell et al. 1998). The role of Syk in signal transduction for activatory FcR in these and a variety of other cell types is now well established, including mast cells bearing FcεR (de Castro 2011). A critical role for Syk in FcγR-mediated antigen internalisation and maturation by dendritic cells has also been described (Sedlik, Orbach et al. 2003), and is notable given the important role of dendritic cells in initiating adaptive immune responses.

In addition to FcR-mediated responses, Syk has been implicated in integrin signalling in myeloid cells (Mocsai, Zhou et al. 2002; Mocsai, Abram et al. 2006). Integrins are transmembrane receptors that have a critical role in cell adhesion and migration, via their interaction with adhesion molecules expressed on other cells, particularly the vascular endothelium. Syk deficient myeloid cells show impaired integrin-mediated responses, thought to be dependent on the association of integrins with ITAM-containing adapter proteins such as FcRγ-chain and DAP12, as myeloid cells deficient in these adapter proteins show similar defects.

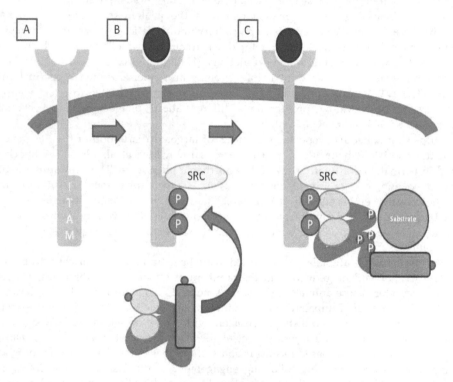

Fig. 2. Simplified schematic showing activation of Syk by interaction with ITAM.
2a: Unengaged receptor bearing non-phosphorylated ITAM motif within its cytoplasmic tail.
2b: Upon receptor engagement Src family kinases (SRC) phosphorylate (P) tyrosine residues within the ITAM motif. 2c: Phosphorylated ITAM motif acts as a docking site for the SH2 domains of Syk, resulting in conformational changes, auto- and transphosphorylation of tyrosines within Syk, thus resulting in activation and phosphorylation of downstream targets

4. Syk in autoimmunity

Given our understanding of its role in BCR- and FcR-mediated signalling, the rationale for targeting Syk in autoimmunity is clear. The presence of autoantibodies is the hallmark of many autoimmune diseases. Whilst not universally pathogenic, these antibodies often contribute to disease via their interaction with FcR expressed on many immune effector cells (and other mechanisms including complement activation). Notably, FcR-deficient mice are resistant to a variety of animal models of autoimmunity, and FcR polymorphisms have been shown to be important determinants of human autoimmune disease (Takai 2002; Nimmerjahn 2006). Syk inhibition may, therefore, have the desirable double effect of preventing the production of pathogenic autoantibodies, via inhibiting B cell activation via the BCR, and simultaneously inhibiting their downstream effects via disrupting signalling from their receptors.

It is encouraging that other therapeutic approaches that target B-cells have recently shown efficacy in clinical practice (Townsend, Monroe et al. 2010). Interestingly, however, clinical benefit cannot always be attributed to eradication of circulating autoantibody, and it is probable that effects on other B cell functions, such as antigen presentation, cytokine production, and provision of co-stimulation to other immune cells, contribute to the benefit seen. Disruption of Syk-dependent BCR signalling may provide similar benefits.

In addition, Syk inhibition may have the additional effect of inhibiting migration and recruitment of immune effector cells to sites of tissue inflammation, via inhibited integrin signalling.

Therapeutic strategies to target Syk, therefore, are desirable and can be broadly classified into two main approaches: pharmacological inhibition of Syk activity, and gene-based therapies aiming to silence Syk expression (Ruzza, Biondi et al. 2009). Whilst the application of the latter has yet to advance to clinical studies, we shall briefly review their future potential, before focusing on the progress of Syk inhibition therapies.

5. Gene-based therapies targeting Syk

5.1 Antisense oligonucleotides (ASO)

ASO are short, single stranded nucleic acid sequences that bind sense mRNA via complementary base-pairing, and thus inhibit the translation of the relevant protein. ASO directed against Syk have shown activity in a variety of cell types *in vitro*, including inhibitory effects of FcγR-mediated signalling in monocytes (Matsuda, Park et al. 1996). Published *in vivo* studies using Syk ASO are limited to animal models of allergic inflammation (Stenton, Kim et al. 2000; Stenton, Ulanova et al. 2002). These have shown that aerosolized Syk ASO, delivered in a liposomal complex, suppress Syk expression in, and inflammatory mediator release from, alveolar macrophages. In addition, markers of pulmonary inflammation were reduced in two distinct animal models. Whilst there have been no *in vivo* studies in autoimmune models, the proposed mechanism of action in these allergic models is via inhibition of activatory FcR-mediated responses, suggesting similar approaches my be effective in autoimmune disease. However, progress in the clinical use of ASO based therapy has been frustratingly slow since the introduction of Fomivirsen, the first antisense therapy to be licensed by the Food and Drug Administration (FDA), being approved for use in AIDS-related cytomegalovirus (CMV) retinitis over 10 years ago. This is due, in part, to the difficulty of producing reliable delivery systems to target the cells, tissues or organs of choice (White, Anastasopoulos et al. 2009) – a not insignificant problem given the multi-system nature of many autoimmune diseases.

5.2 RNA interference (RNAi)

RNAi is an innate cellular process that is thought to regulate endogenous gene expression and protect against viral infection. A variety of small RNA molecules, such as endogenous, genetically encoded microRNA (miRNA) or exogenous small interfering RNA (siRNA), may bind target mRNA via Watson-Crick complementary base pairing, and then direct this target mRNA into an RNA-induced silencing complex (RISC), a natural degradation pathway, thus effecting gene silencing prior to translation. Since this first description of RNAi in 1998, advance in the field has been rapid, and there have been promising early phase clinical studies in a number of conditions, including retinal diseases, malignancies and viral infections. The most commonly used technique to harness RNAi for therapy has been to transfect siRNA into target cells. siRNA specific to Syk, for example, have been shown to inhibit antibody-mediated phagocytosis by human macrophages (Lu, Wang et al. 2011). Again, *in vivo* studies in this field are limited to models of allergic inflammation, and to date are only reported in international patent applications. Aerosolised delivery of Syk siRNA, using similar methods as used for ASO delivery, resulted in decreased pulmonary inflammation, as determined by recruitment of cells to bronchoalveolar lavage fluid, in a rat model of ovalbumin-induced asthma. Again, these findings augur well for the translation and use of RNAi in autoimmune disease. As with antisense therapy, outstanding challenges for harnessing RNAi include the development of effective delivery systems, escape of the innate 'interferon' response directed against foreign nucleic acids, and avoidance of 'off-target' gene silencing (Davidson and McCray 2011).

6. Pharmacological inhibition

A number of biotechnology and pharmaceutical companies are working to develop compounds to inhibit Syk (Ruzza, Biondi et al. 2009; Riccaboni, Bianchi et al. 2010). To date, two such inhibitors, both identified by Rigel Pharmaceuticals, and now in development by AstraZeneca, have progressed to clinical trials – initially R112, and more recently the related compound, R406 (and its respective prodrug, R788).

6.1 Preclinical studies with small molecule inhibitors

Cell based high-throughput screening of small molecules identified R112 as a potent inhibitor of Syk activity, as assayed by production and release of inflammatory mediators following FcRε crosslinking by anti-IgE (Rossi, Herlaar et al. 2006). Subsequent characterization showed that R112 is an ATP-competitive inhibitor of Syk activity, as demonstrated by *in vitro* kinase assays (IC_{50} = 226 nmol/l). These assays also showed activity against other kinases such as Lyn (IC_{50} = 300nmol/l) and Lck (IC_{50} =645 nmol/l). However, when tested in cell-based assays, R112 was shown to be relatively selective for Syk as determined by phosphorylation of target proteins, despite the similar IC_{50} values in the *in vitro* assays.

Rigel subsequently developed the related compound R406, another potent competitive ATP inhibitor for Syk (*in vitro* IC_{50} = 41 nmol/l) (Braselmann, Taylor et al. 2006). Again, selectivity assessments using over 90 *in vitro* kinase assays showed an inhibitory effect on other kinases, although cell based assays confirmed selectivity for Syk – FLT3 was the next most potently inhibited kinase, though at 5-fold less activity. R406 has been shown to inhibit FcR-mediated responses in a variety of cell types *in vitro*, including mast cells, macrophages, neutrophils and dendritic cells (Braselmann, Taylor et al. 2006; Matsubara, Koya et al. 2006). In addition, activity against BCR-mediated responses has been shown in primary human B cells *in vitro*. Notably, R406 did not show significant activity in Syk-independent pathways (such as following lipopolysaccharide stimulation) at the concentrations necessary to inhibit

FcR- and BCR-mediated pathways, in keeping with the selectivity for Syk seen in the cell based phosphorylation assays. R788, or fostamatinib disodium (see McAdoo and Tam 2011 for review) was then developed as the methylene phosphate prodrug of R406, to improve its solubility and potential for oral dosing.

The efficacy of R406/R788 has been studied in numerous animal models of autoimmunity. In a murine model of immune cytopenias, for example, treatment with R788 prevented haemolysis and the development of thrombocytopenia following the administration of anti-red blood cell and anti-platelet antibodies respectively (Podolanczuk, Lazarus et al. 2009). Treatment with R406/R788 reduced clinical, histological and radiographic evidence of joint inflammation following the induction of collagen-induced arthritis, a rodent model of rheumatoid arthritis (Pine, Chang et al. 2007). R788 has shown efficacy in three animal models of SLE (Bahjat, Pine et al. 2008; Deng, Liu et al. 2010). Treatment of the lupus-prone NZB/NZW mouse strain reduced kidney disease, as determined by proteinuria and renal histology, and improved platelet counts and survival. In the BAK/BAX knockout mouse, treatment with R788 reduced lupus-like skin disease and lymphadenopathy. Similarly, in the MRL/lpr strain, treatment improved renal and skin disease, in addition to reducing lymphadenopathy. In a rodent model of antibody-mediated glomerulonephritis, treatment with R788 prevented the induction of disease (Smith, McDaid et al. 2010). In addition, treatment had a profound effect on established disease, reversing the histological features of crescentic glomerulonephritis even when initiated after the induction of disease. Finally, in an autoimmune diabetes model, R788 delayed the onset of insulinitis and spontaneous diabetes in NOD mice (Colonna, Catalano et al. 2010). Again, significant effects were seen even when treatment was initiated after the onset of glucose intolerance. Though not strictly a model of autoimmunity, treatment with R788 reduced local and remote inflammation in mesenteric ischaemia-reperfusion in mice (Pamuk, Lapchak et al. 2010), suggesting effects independent of the FcR and BCR, such as inhibition of leucocyte migration.

The safety of R788/R406 has also been assessed in detailed rodent toxicity and immunotoxicology studies (Zhu, Herlaar et al. 2007). At high doses, R406 was associated with a reduction in circulating lymphocyte count, bone marrow cellularity, and thymic and spleen weight. These changes generally resolved during a drug-withdrawal recovery period. In murine host resistance models, treatment with R788 did not significantly impair clearance of influenza, Listeria or streptococcal infection.

Other pharmaceutical companies have developed a number of other small molecule inhibitors. The majority of these, like R112 and R406, are competitive inhibitors for the ATP binding site of the catalytic domain. Bayer, for example, has developed the imidazopyrimidine analogue BAY 61-3606, which inhibits Syk-mediated responses *in vitro* and has demonstrated efficacy in animal models of allergy *in vivo* (*Yamamoto, Takeshita et al. 2003*). However, the published selectivity profile is limited to only 6 other kinases, and comparison with genetic knockdown suggests that BAY 61-3606 may have significant off-target effects (Lin, Huang et al. 2010).

Other groups have chosen to target the non-kinase domains of the Syk molecule. By inhibiting the interaction of the SH2-domains with their docking proteins, it has been proposed that Syk inhibition may be achieved whilst avoiding off-target effects on other kinases, and one such approach has been shown to inhibit IgE-mediated responses *in vitro* and *in vivo* (*Mazuc, Villoutreix et al. 2008*). Whilst the precise molecular mechanism of the inhibitory effects of this molecule are yet to be definitively described, it should be noted that the SH2-domain is a highly conserved motif found in a large number of proteins involved in signal transduction, and targeting this domain may in turn have diverse off target effects.

6.2 Clinical studies

R112 was the first Syk inhibitor treatment to be assessed in clinical studies, where it showed benefit in relieving symptoms of allergic rhinitis when delivered as an intranasal preparation (Meltzer, Berkowitz et al. 2005). Subsequent work focused on R406/R788, with early phase clinical studies confirming that R406/788 is highly bioavailable following oral administration, rapidly absorbed systemically, and well tolerated at doses needed to achieve biological effects such as inhibition of basophil activation in response to anti-IgE *ex vivo* (IC$_{50}$ 1.06 microM) (Braselmann, Taylor et al. 2006; Sweeny, Li et al. 2010).

To date, the results of five phase II studies with R788 (fostamatinib) have been published. Three of these investigated the effects of fostamatinib in rheumatoid arthritis (RA) (Table 1). The first recruited almost 200 patients with active disease despite standard therapy with methotrexate (Weinblatt, Kavanaugh et al. 2008). Clinical responses were seen as early as one week following the initiation of treatment, and sustained at three months, with significant improvements in disease activity scores in the treatment groups versus placebo. The second study enrolled over 450 patients with active disease despite long-term methotrexate therapy, and this confirmed benefit at six months, with improved American College of Rheumatology 20% improvement criteria (ACR20), ACR50, ACR70 and DAS28 scores (Weinblatt, Kavanaugh et al. 2010). Notably, both these studies included a significant proportion of patients who had failed biological therapy with anti-TNF or anti-CD20 agents, and benefit with fostamatinib was seen in these subgroups (although overall response rates were lower than for the whole study population). A subsequent trial designed specifically to examine the efficacy of fostamatinib in this group of patients failing biologic therapy, however, did not achieve its primary endpoint of improved ACR20 in the treatment group (Genovese, Kavanaugh et al. 2011). There were, however, significant improvements in radiographic and biochemical markers of inflammation.

A small open label study in immune thrombocytopenic purpura (ITP) has also shown promising results (Podolanczuk, Lazarus et al. 2009). Although the numbers are small (n=16), the majority of patients had refractory disease with multiple previous ITP treatments (commonly steroids, intravenous immunoglobulin, rituximab and splenectomy). As such, the sustained (50%) and transient (25%) response rates seen during the average follow up time of 36 weeks represent encouraging results and further studies are planned.

In addition to these studies in autoimmune disease, a fifth phase II study examined the effects of fostamatinib in haematological malignancy (Friedberg, Sharman et al. 2010), the rationale for which is discussed below. Again, in a study population that included a significant proportion of patients with heavily pre-treated, relapsed or refractory disease, fostamatinib showed modest but significant clinical activity and a manageable side-effect profile.

The most frequent adverse event seen in these clinical studies was gastrointestinal toxicity, a common side effect of many kinase inhibitors. Symptoms were dose-related, and seen at rates of up to 45% in groups receiving the highest doses of fostamatinib, and this was the most common reason for patient withdrawal from the RA trials.

REF	N	ENTRY CRITERIA	FOLLOW UP	ENDPOINT	OUTCOMES	COMMENTS
Weinblatt, Kavanaugh et al. 2008)	189	Active RA (≥12 months from diagnosis) despite ≥ 6 months methotrexate therapy	12 weeks	ACR20 response rate (ACR50, ACR70, DAS28 response rates)	Significant benefits in all disease activity scores in patients treated with fostamatinib 100-150mg bd. Clinical responses notes as early as one week after initiation of treatment.	Approximately 1/3 of patients continued to receive other DMARDs during the study; Approximately 20% had received prior biologic therapy (with appropriate washout period before entering study).
Weinblatt, Kavanaugh et al. 2010)	457	Active RA (≥ 6 months from diagnosis) despite ≥ 3 months methotrexate therapy	6 months	ACR20 response rate (ACR50, ACR70, DAS28 response rates)	Significant benefits in all disease activity scores in patients treated with fostamatinib 100-150mg bd. Again, responses noted as early as one week.	15% of patients in this study had received prior biologic therapy. Although overall response rates were lower in this subgroup, still significantly more patients demonstrated responses than the equivalent placebo group.
Genovese, Kavanaugh et al. 2011)	229	Active RA (≥ 12 months from diagnosis) with disease unresponsive to current or previous biologic therapy	3 months	ACR20 response rate (ACR50, ACR70, DAS28 response rates; synovitis scores on MRI)	No difference in disease activity scores across treatment and placebo groups. Significant improvements in circulating inflammatory markers and synovitis scores on MRI noted in treatment groups.	Despite randomisation, baseline differences in steroid dose, previous biologic exposure and synovitis scores were noted between groups, which authors suggest may account for lack of efficacy.

Table 1. Summary of Phase II trials with fostamatinib in patients with rheumatoid arthritis (RA). ACR20/50/70, American College of Rheumatology 20/50/70% improvement criteria; DAS28, disease activity score using 28 joint counts; MRI, magnetic resonance imaging; DMARD, disease modifying anti-rheumatic drug

Neutropenia occurred in up to 30% of patients receiving fostamatinib in the RA trials. Again, this finding appeared to be dose-related and responded to dose reduction or temporary withdrawal of the drug. Although no direct pharmacokinetic interaction has been detected between fostamatinib and methotrexate (Baluom, Samara et al. 2011), synergistic effects on haematopoiesis beyond individual pharmacokinetic parameters (along with underlying bone marrow disease or other concomitant immunosuppressant therapy) may have contributed to this phenomenon, as neutropenia was not reported in the ITP trial. An increased rate of uncomplicated upper respiratory tract infections was seen in the treatment group of the largest RA trial. However, this was not associated with neutropenia. In addition, no opportunistic or atypical infections were reported in any of the clinical trials.

7. Beyond adaptive immunity: problems and potential for Syk-directed therapy

Recently, Syk has been implicated in a number of signalling pathways beyond the adaptive immune response that may have implications for Syk-directed therapy in clinical practice. These include the aforementioned role in cell adhesion, as well as possible roles in innate immunity, platelet function, bone metabolism and tumorigenesis (Mocsai, Ruland et al. 2010). Disruption of these functions may lead to significant toxicity, or alternatively open novel therapeutic avenues, in targeting Syk. The basic mechanism of these functions has been reviewed in detail elsewhere (Mocsai, Ruland et al. 2010); we shall here consider the potential clinical implications.

7.1 Innate Immunity and Infection

Given its diverse effects on adaptive immune responses, coupled to a role in inflammatory cell adhesion and migration, the preeminent concern with Syk directed therapies must be of over-immunosuppression and the associated risk of infection. It is also notable that Syk has recently been associated with a variety of pathogen recognition receptors (PRRs), important components of the innate immune response that recognise pathogen-associated molecular patterns (PAMPs). C-type Lectins, one such class of PRR, play an important role in antifungal immunity in particular, and Syk has been implicated in the intracellular signalling cascades for these receptors (Drummond, Saijo et al. 2011). Some, such as Dectin-1, contain an ITAM motif on their cytoplasmic domain, and others may associate with ITAM containing adaptor proteins such as FcRγ chain or DAP12. As such, Syk inhibition may potentially lead to excessive downregulation of multiple inflammatory, innate and adaptive immune responses, resulting in risk of overwhelming infection. The results of the preclinical toxicity assessments and host resistance models are reassuring in this respect (although a host resistance model of fungal infection has not been studied), as is the absence of severe, atypical or opportunistic infection in the clinical studies thus far. Larger and longer clinical studies are, however, needed to establish the long term and cumulative effects of Syk inhibition on innate immune responses and infection risk, particularly in patient groups who have had extensive treatment histories with other immunosuppressant agents.

7.2 Platelet function

Syk has been shown to be involved in a number of platelet activation pathways, including via the glycoprotein GPVI receptor (an FcRγ chain-associated receptor that bears an ITAM motif), integrin αIIbβ3, and C-type Lectin 2 (CLEC-2; a type II membrane protein containing a single tyrosine-based motif in its cytoplasmic tail that has been termed a hemITAM) (Watson, Auger et al. 2005; Watson, Herbert et al. 2010). In addition, R406 has demonstrated inhibitory activity in these pathways (Spalton, Mori et al. 2009). Notably, however, very high dose exposure to R406 did not prolong bleeding time in mice, and in phase I human studies, R406 did not inhibit collagen or ADP-induced platelet aggregation *ex vivo (Braselmann, Taylor et al. 2006)*, perhaps suggesting redundancy of Syk dependent pathways *in vivo*. Based on these observations, it would appear that targeting Syk in isolation would not be an effective anti-thrombotic therapy. However, synergistic effects, potentially both therapeutic and harmful, with other anti-platelet agents have not been explored in clinical studies.

7.3 Bone metabolism

Syk has been shown to regulate osteoclastic bone resorption, via its association with integrin $\alpha v\beta 3$ and ITAM bearing proteins, such as DAP12 and FcRγ chain, expressed at the osteoclast cell surface (Zou, Kitaura et al. 2007). In addition, Syk has recently been implicated in the suppression of osteoblast differentiation (Yoshida, Higuchi et al. 2011). Thus, Syk may represent a therapeutic target in disorders of bone metabolism such as osteoporosis, although potential effects of Syk inhibition on normal bone, such as osteosclerosis and increased fragility and fracture risk, have yet to be investigated *in vivo* or in clinical studies.

7.4 Tumorigenesis

It has been suggested that Syk is a negative regulator of progression in various types of malignancy (including breast, gastric and melanoma) based on the observation of decreased Syk expression in these tumour types and experimental studies where Syk transfection and re-expression in tumour cell lines suggested a tumour- and metastasis- suppressive effect (Coopman and Mueller 2006). The molecular mechanism of this suppressive role has yet to be established. Conversely, fostamatinib has shown activity in NCI-60 (a panel of 60 diverse human cancer cell lines), although this may be due to off-target effects, rather than Syk inhibition specifically. On this basis, however, a broad multi-histology Phase II study is currently recruiting (NCT00923481).

Syk signalling through the BCR has also been implicated as an important survival signal in various lymphoid malignancies, and R406 has shown antiproliferative and proapoptotic activity in B cell lymphoma and CLL lines *in vitro* (Chen, Monti et al. 2008; Buchner, Fuchs et al. 2009; Quiroga, Balakrishnan et al. 2009). Furthermore, R788 is highly active in animal models of non-Hodgkin's lymphoma (NHL) and chronic lymphocytic leukaemia (CLL) (Young, Hardy et al. 2009; Suljagic, Longo et al. 2010), and in a Phase II clinical trial, fostamatinib showed significant clinical activity in a heterogeneous group of NHL and CLL (Friedberg, Sharman et al. 2010). Based on these findings, larger Phase II trials in haematological malignancy are ongoing (NCT00446095, NCT00798096). Interestingly, some oncogenic viruses have been shown to encode ITAM-containing proteins – for example, Epstein Barr virus (EBV) latent membrane protein 2A (LMP2A) contains an ITAM motif, and has been shown to promote B cell development and survival (Caldwell, Wilson et al. 1998).

7.5 Cardiovascular risk

Hypertension was a commonly reported adverse event in clinical studies with fostamatinib. It is unclear whether this was due to Syk inhibition *per se*, or potentially due to off-target effects on other kinases – the vascular endothelial growth factor receptor 2 being a putative candidate. Whilst usually mild, and responsive to dose reduction of fostamatinib or augmented antihypertensive therapy, the long-term effects of even small increases in blood pressure in patients with autoimmune rheumatic diseases such as RA and lupus, who already have dramatically increased cardiovascular risk, need to be considered. Interestingly, administration of fostamatinib was recently shown to attenuate plaque development in a rodent model of atherosclerosis, an effect thought to be mediated by impaired recruitment of inflammatory cells, suggesting that Syk inhibition is a potential target in atherosclerotic cardiovascular disease (Hilgendorf, Eisele et al. 2011). Syk has also been implicated in the mechanism of high-glucose induced NF-κB activation in glomerular endothelial cells, suggesting a potential role of Syk inhibition in preventing end-organ complications of diabetes mellitus (Yang, Seo et al. 2008).

8. Conclusions

The rationale, the experimental data, and the clinical experience to date augur well for the efficacy of Syk inhibition in autoimmune disease. Several large phase II-III trials in RA are currently in progress (NCT01242514, NCT01264770, NCT01197521, NCT01197534, NCT01197755) and it is hoped that if successful, efficacy could translate to a wide range of organ-specific and systemic autoimmune diseases. Indeed, it is tempting to propose that Syk-directed therapy, with its proven clinical efficacy in early trials, along with potential benefits in cardiovascular disease, hyperglycaemia, bone metabolism and malignancy (particularly those related to oncogenic viruses) is the proverbial 'Holy Grail' of immunosuppressant therapy following 40 years of steroid- and cytotoxic-based regimes complicated by hypertension, diabetes, osteoporosis and lymphoproliferative disease. However, the widespread role of Syk in numerous immune functions raises serious concerns regarding the risk of opportunistic infection, and some questions about the oncogenic potential of Syk disruption in certain cell types remain unanswered. In addition, it is disappointing that Syk inhibition with fostamatinib, the drug furthest through clinical development, showed only improvement by objective assessment using MRI or biochemical markers, rather than clinical benefit in patients who had not responded to biologic therapy. Future clinical studies will need to establish both the long-term safety and superiority of Syk inhibition in practice.

9. Acknowledgements

S.P.M. is in receipt on an MRC Research Training Fellowship
F.W.K.T. has been supported by the Diamond Fund from Imperial College Healthcare Charity, MRC and the Wellcome Trust. F.W.K.T. has received research project grants from Roche Palo Alto, AstraZeneca Limited and Baxter Biosciences.

10. References

Abtahian, F., A. Guerriero, et al. (2003). Regulation of blood and lymphatic vascular separation by signaling proteins SLP-76 and Syk. *Science* 299(5604): 247-251.
Au-Yeung, B. B., S. Deindl, et al. (2009). The structure, regulation, and function of ZAP-70. *Immunol Rev* 228(1): 41-57.

Bahjat, F. R., P. R. Pine, et al. (2008). An orally bioavailable spleen tyrosine kinase inhibitor delays disease progression and prolongs survival in murine lupus. *Arthritis Rheum* 58(5): 1433-1444.

Baluom, M., E. Samara, et al. (2011). Fostamatinib, a syk-kinase inhibitor, does not affect methotrexate pharmacokinetics in patients with rheumatoid arthritis. *J Clin Pharmacol* 51(9): 1310-1318.

Bradshaw, J. M. (2010). The Src, Syk, and Tec family kinases: distinct types of molecular switches. *Cell Signal* 22(8): 1175-1184.

Braselmann, S., V. Taylor, et al. (2006). R406, an orally available spleen tyrosine kinase inhibitor blocks fc receptor signaling and reduces immune complex-mediated inflammation. *J Pharmacol Exp Ther* 319(3): 998-1008.

Buchner, M., S. Fuchs, et al. (2009). Spleen tyrosine kinase is overexpressed and represents a potential therapeutic target in chronic lymphocytic leukemia. *Cancer Res* 69(13): 5424-5432.

Caldwell, R. G., J. B. Wilson, et al. (1998). Epstein-Barr virus LMP2A drives B cell development and survival in the absence of normal B cell receptor signals. *Immunity* 9(3): 405-411.

Chen, L., S. Monti, et al. (2008). SYK-dependent tonic B-cell receptor signaling is a rational treatment target in diffuse large B-cell lymphoma. *Blood* 111(4): 2230-2237.

Cheng, A. M., B. Rowley, et al. (1995). Syk tyrosine kinase required for mouse viability and B-cell development. *Nature* 378(6554): 303-306.

Colonna, L., G. Catalano, et al. (2010). Therapeutic targeting of Syk in autoimmune diabetes. *J Immunol* 185(3): 1532-1543.

Coopman, P. J. and S. C. Mueller (2006). The Syk tyrosine kinase: a new negative regulator in tumor growth and progression. *Cancer Lett* 241(2): 159-173.

Crowley, M. T., P. S. Costello, et al. (1997). A critical role for Syk in signal transduction and phagocytosis mediated by Fcgamma receptors on macrophages. *J Exp Med* 186(7): 1027-1039.

Davidson, B. L. and P. B. McCray, Jr. (2011). Current prospects for RNA interference-based therapies. *Nat Rev Genet* 12(5): 329-340.

de Castro, R. O. (2011). Regulation and function of syk tyrosine kinase in mast cell signaling and beyond. *J Signal Transduct* 2011: 507291.

Deindl, S., T. A. Kadlecek, et al. (2007). Structural basis for the inhibition of tyrosine kinase activity of ZAP-70. *Cell* 129(4): 735-746.

Deng, G. M., L. Liu, et al. (2010). Suppression of skin and kidney disease by inhibition of spleen tyrosine kinase in lupus-prone mice. *Arthritis Rheum* 62(7): 2086-2092.

Drummond, R. A., S. Saijo, et al. (2011). The role of Syk/CARD9 coupled C-type lectins in antifungal immunity. *Eur J Immunol* 41(2): 276-281.

Friedberg, J. W., J. Sharman, et al. (2010). Inhibition of Syk with fostamatinib disodium has significant clinical activity in non-Hodgkin lymphoma and chronic lymphocytic leukemia. *Blood* 115(13): 2578-2585.

Furlong, M. T., A. M. Mahrenholz, et al. (1997). Identification of the major sites of autophosphorylation of the murine protein-tyrosine kinase *Syk*. *Biochim Biophys Acta* 1355(2): 177-190.

Geahlen, R. L. (2009). Syk and pTyr'd: Signaling through the B cell antigen receptor. *Biochim Biophys Acta* 1793(7): 1115-1127.

Genovese, M. C., A. Kavanaugh, et al. (2011). An oral Syk kinase inhibitor in the treatment of rheumatoid arthritis: a three-month randomized, placebo-controlled, phase II study in patients with active rheumatoid arthritis that did not respond to biologic agents. *Arthritis Rheum* 63(2): 337-345.

Hilgendorf, I., S. Eisele, et al. (2011). The Oral Spleen Tyrosine Kinase Inhibitor Fostamatinib Attenuates Inflammation and Atherogenesis in Low-Density Lipoprotein Receptor-Deficient Mice. *Arterioscler Thromb Vasc Biol.*

Kiefer, F., J. Brumell, et al. (1998). The Syk protein tyrosine kinase is essential for Fcgamma receptor signaling in macrophages and neutrophils. *Mol Cell Biol* 18(7): 4209-4220.

Ku, G., B. Malissen, et al. (1994). Chromosomal location of the Syk and ZAP-70 tyrosine kinase genes in mice and humans. *Immunogenetics* 40(4): 300-302.

Kulathu, Y., G. Grothe, et al. (2009). Autoinhibition and adapter function of Syk. *Immunol Rev* 232(1): 286-299.

Lin, Y. C., D. Y. Huang, et al. (2010). Anti-inflammatory actions of Syk inhibitors in macrophages involve non-specific inhibition of toll-like receptors-mediated JNK signaling pathway. *Mol Immunol* 47(7-8): 1569-1578.

Lu, Y., W. Wang, et al. (2011). Antibody-mediated platelet phagocytosis by human macrophages is inhibited by siRNA specific for sequences in the SH2 tyrosine kinase, *Syk. Cell Immunol* 268(1): 1-3.

Matsubara, S., T. Koya, et al. (2006). Syk activation in dendritic cells is essential for airway hyperresponsiveness and inflammation. *Am J Respir Cell Mol Biol* 34(4): 426-433.

Matsuda, M., J. G. Park, et al. (1996). Abrogation of the Fc gamma receptor IIA-mediated phagocytic signal by stem-loop Syk antisense oligonucleotides. *Mol Biol Cell* 7(7): 1095-1106.

Mazuc, E., B. O. Villoutreix, et al. (2008). A novel druglike spleen tyrosine kinase binder prevents anaphylactic shock when administered orally. *J Allergy Clin Immunol* 122(1): 188-194, 194 e181-183.

McAdoo, S. P. and F. W. K. Tam (2011). FOSTAMATINIB DISODIUM Tyrosine-Protein Kinase SYK/FLT3 Inhibitor Treatment of Rheumatoid Arthritis Oncolytic. *Drugs of the Future* 36(4): 273-280.

Meltzer, E. O., R. B. Berkowitz, et al. (2005). An intranasal Syk-kinase inhibitor (R112) improves the symptoms of seasonal allergic rhinitis in a park environment. *J Allergy Clin Immunol* 115(4): 791-796.

Mocsai, A., C. L. Abram, et al. (2006). Integrin signaling in neutrophils and macrophages uses adaptors containing immunoreceptor tyrosine-based activation motifs. *Nat Immunol* 7(12): 1326-1333.

Mocsai, A., J. Ruland, et al. (2010). The SYK tyrosine kinase: a crucial player in diverse biological functions. *Nat Rev Immunol* 10(6): 387-402.

Mocsai, A., M. Zhou, et al. (2002). Syk is required for integrin signaling in neutrophils. *Immunity* 16(4): 547-558.

Nimmerjahn, F. (2006). Activating and inhibitory FcgammaRs in autoimmune disorders. *Springer Semin Immunopathol* 28(4): 305-319.

Pamuk, O. N., P. H. Lapchak, et al. (2010). Spleen tyrosine kinase inhibition prevents tissue damage after ischemia-reperfusion. *Am J Physiol Gastrointest Liver Physiol* 299(2): G391-399.

Pine, P. R., B. Chang, et al. (2007). Inflammation and bone erosion are suppressed in models of rheumatoid arthritis following treatment with a novel Syk inhibitor. *Clin Immunol* 124(3): 244-257.

Podolanczuk, A., A. H. Lazarus, et al. (2009). Of mice and men: an open-label pilot study for treatment of immune thrombocytopenic purpura by an inhibitor of Syk. *Blood* 113(14): 3154-3160.

Quiroga, M. P., K. Balakrishnan, et al. (2009). B-cell antigen receptor signaling enhances chronic lymphocytic leukemia cell migration and survival: specific targeting with a novel spleen tyrosine kinase inhibitor, R406. *Blood* 114(5): 1029-1037.

Riccaboni, M., I. Bianchi, et al. (2010). Spleen tyrosine kinases: biology, therapeutic targets and drugs. *Drug Discov Today* 15(13-14): 517-530.

Rossi, A. B., E. Herlaar, et al. (2006). Identification of the Syk kinase inhibitor R112 by a human mast cell screen. *J Allergy Clin Immunol* 118(3): 749-755.

Ruzza, P., B. Biondi, et al. (2009). Therapeutic prospect of Syk inhibitors. *Expert Opin Ther Pat* 19(10): 1361-1376.

Sada, K., T. Takano, et al. (2001). Structure and function of Syk protein-tyrosine kinase. *J Biochem* 130(2): 177-186.

Sedlik, C., D. Orbach, et al. (2003). A critical role for Syk protein tyrosine kinase in Fc receptor-mediated antigen presentation and induction of dendritic cell maturation. *J Immunol* 170(2): 846-852.

Smith, J., J. P. McDaid, et al. (2010). A spleen tyrosine kinase inhibitor reduces the severity of established glomerulonephritis. *J Am Soc Nephrol* 21(2): 231-236.

Spalton, J. C., J. Mori, et al. (2009). The novel Syk inhibitor R406 reveals mechanistic differences in the initiation of GPVI and CLEC-2 signaling in platelets. *J Thromb Haemost* 7(7): 1192-1199.

Stenton, G. R., M. K. Kim, et al. (2000). Aerosolized Syk antisense suppresses Syk expression, mediator release from macrophages, and pulmonary inflammation. *J Immunol* 164(7): 3790-3797.

Stenton, G. R., M. Ulanova, et al. (2002). Inhibition of allergic inflammation in the airways using aerosolized antisense to Syk kinase. *J Immunol* 169(2): 1028-1036.

Suljagic, M., P. G. Longo, et al. (2010). The Syk inhibitor fostamatinib disodium (R788) inhibits tumor growth in the Emu- TCL1 transgenic mouse model of CLL by blocking antigen-dependent B-cell receptor signaling. *Blood* 116(23): 4894-4905.

Sweeny, D. J., W. Li, et al. (2010). Metabolism of fostamatinib, the oral methylene phosphate prodrug of the spleen tyrosine kinase inhibitor R406 in humans: contribution of hepatic and gut bacterial processes to the overall biotransformation. *Drug Metab Dispos* 38(7): 1166-1176.

Takai, T. (2002). Roles of Fc receptors in autoimmunity. *Nat Rev Immunol* 2(8): 580-592.

Taniguchi, T., T. Kobayashi, et al. (1991). Molecular cloning of a porcine gene syk that encodes a 72-kDa protein-tyrosine kinase showing high susceptibility to proteolysis. *J Biol Chem* 266(24): 15790-15796.

Townsend, M. J., J. G. Monroe, et al. (2010). B-cell targeted therapies in human autoimmune diseases: an updated perspective. *Immunol Rev* 237(1): 264-283.

Tsang, E., A. M. Giannetti, et al. (2008). Molecular mechanism of the Syk activation switch. *J Biol Chem* 283(47): 32650-32659.

Turner, M., P. J. Mee, et al. (1995). Perinatal lethality and blocked B-cell development in mice lacking the tyrosine kinase Syk. *Nature* 378(6554): 298-302.

Turner, M., E. Schweighoffer, et al. (2000). Tyrosine kinase SYK: essential functions for immunoreceptor signalling. *Immunol Today* 21(3): 148-154.

Watson, S. P., J. M. Auger, et al. (2005). GPVI and integrin alphaIIb beta3 signaling in platelets. *J Thromb Haemost* 3(8): 1752-1762.

Watson, S. P., J. M. Herbert, et al. (2010). GPVI and CLEC-2 in hemostasis and vascular integrity. *J Thromb Haemost* 8(7): 1456-1467.

Weinblatt, M. E., A. Kavanaugh, et al. (2008). Treatment of rheumatoid arthritis with a Syk kinase inhibitor: a twelve-week, randomized, placebo-controlled trial. *Arthritis Rheum* 58(11): 3309-3318.

Weinblatt, M. E., A. Kavanaugh, et al. (2010). An oral spleen tyrosine kinase (Syk) inhibitor for rheumatoid arthritis. *N Engl J Med* 363(14): 1303-1312.

White, P. J., F. Anastasopoulos, et al. (2009). Overcoming biological barriers to in vivo efficacy of antisense oligonucleotides. *Expert Rev Mol Med* 11: e10.

Yamamoto, N., K. Takeshita, et al. (2003). The orally available spleen tyrosine kinase inhibitor 2-[7-(3,4-dimethoxyphenyl)-imidazo[1,2-c]pyrimidin-5-ylamino]nicotinamide dihydrochloride (BAY 61-3606) blocks antigen-induced airway inflammation in rodents. *J Pharmacol Exp Ther* 306(3): 1174-1181.

Yang, W. S., J. W. Seo, et al. (2008). High glucose-induced NF-kappaB activation occurs via tyrosine phosphorylation of IkappaBalpha in human glomerular endothelial cells: involvement of Syk tyrosine kinase. *Am J Physiol Renal Physiol* 294(5): F1065-1075.

Yoshida, K., C. Higuchi, et al. (2011). Spleen tyrosine kinase suppresses osteoblastic differentiation through MAPK and PKCalpha. *Biochem Biophys Res Commun*.

Young, R. M., I. R. Hardy, et al. (2009). Mouse models of non-Hodgkin lymphoma reveal Syk as an important therapeutic target. *Blood* 113(11): 2508-2516.

Zhu, Y., E. Herlaar, et al. (2007). Immunotoxicity assessment for the novel Spleen tyrosine kinase inhibitor R406. *Toxicol Appl Pharmacol* 221(3): 268-277.

Zou, W., H. Kitaura, et al. (2007). Syk, c-Src, the alphavbeta3 integrin, and ITAM immunoreceptors, in concert, regulate osteoclastic bone resorption. *J Cell Biol* 176(6): 877-888.

4

Low Immunogenic Potential
of Human Neural Stem Cells

L. De Filippis[1], L. Rota Nodari[1] and Maurizio Gelati[2]
[1]Department of Biotechnologies and Biosciences, Università Milano Bicocca, Milan,
[2]Laboratorio Cellule Staminali, Cell Factory e Biobanca,
Azienda Ospedaliera "Santa Maria", Terni
Italy

1. Introduction

Grafting of neural stem cells into the mammalian central nervous system (CNS) has been performed for some decades now, both in basic research and clinical applications for neurological disorders such as Parkinson's and Huntington's disease, stroke, and spinal cord injuries. Albeit the "proof of principle" status that neural grafts can reinstate functional deficits and rebuild damaged neuronal circuitries, many critical roadblocks have still to be overcome to reach clinical applications. Among these are the manifold immunological aspects that are encountered during the graft–host interaction in vivo. In this chapter we will elucidate different aspects of cellular therapy, particularly using CNS derived stem cells and their ability to modulate immune system in order to avoid rejection and/or affect inflammatory reactions related to neurodegenerative diseases.

2. Neural transplantation for the therapy of neurodegenerative diseases

2.1 NSCs: Use into humans and animal models

Grafting of neural stem cells (NSCs) into the mammalian central nervous system in association with their ability to induce active neurogenesis in the adult CNS has fostered a flurry of studies to investigate the exploitation of NSC for the therapy of neurodegenerative disorders including both genetic diseases like Metachromatic Leukodystrophy (MLD), Huntington's Disease (HD), Alzheimer's Disease (AD) (sporadic) and idiopathic diseases like Parkinson's Disease (PD), AD, Multiple Sclerosis (MS), Amyotrophyc Lateral Sclerosis (ALS), stroke.

Regenerative medicine strongly relies on the capacity of intrinsic subsets of cells to replenish the damaged ones. Although for a long time the CNS was thought to be a "perennial", i.e. post-mitotic tissue, the discovery of active neurogenesis in the adult mammalian brain has debunked this dogma and spurred ongoing research efforts to focus on stem/ precursor cell therapy to treat neurodegeneration and neurotrauma.

Given the intrinsic resilience of NSC to fast proliferation and prompt expansion in vivo, the spontaneous recovery of most CNS injuries remains limited and a feasible strategy to support the endogenous NSC-mediated therapy would be the autologous transplantation of adult stem cells from various tissue compartments than the CNS. Different sources of stem cells have been proposed, but they mostly generate a restricted range of cell phenotypes.

Induced pluripotent stem cells (iPS) have been recently proposed for autologous transplantation, but a major drawback of these genetically manipulated cells is the high risk of cancer formation, mainly due to the uncontrolled integration of retroviral vectors and recombination events.

Therefore, the most feasible candidates to clinical neurological applications are currently the embryonic stem cells (ESCs) and adult somatic stem cells, particularly NSCs.

ESCs are the most primitive type of stem cells properly belonging to the human body and are pluripotent, meaning that they are able to generate all the types of cells present in the human body. As such and thanks to their easy handling and proliferation ex vivo, they would represent ideal candidates to provide a wide array of cell types for the therapy of different disorders. Alas, the limited availability of primary tissue due to ethical concerns and their remarkable teratogenic potential in vivo has strongly discouraged their application in clinical trials. On the contrary, NSC are mostly considered as the optimal cell type for cell-mediated therapy of neural disorders because they share the same tissue origin of the damaged cells they are meant to replenish and are amenable to local environmental cues able to commit their differentiation choice (Cao et al. 2001;Shihabuddin et al. 2000;Suhonen et al. 1996). Accordingly, NSC have been shown to exert multiple therapeutic effects, such as secretion of neurotrophic factors and cytokines, scavenging of toxic molecules, immunomodulation of inflammatory milieu, where neural cell replacement plays only a minor role in the recovery of CNS damage (Bacigaluppi et al. 2009;Behrstock et al. 2006;Ebert et al. 2008;Lindvall and Kokaia 2010). The major roadblock to their procurement from an autologous tissue source can be currently circumvented by their derivation from the fetal human brain, while the requirement for immunosuppression to prevent transplant rejection remains object of conflicting debates.

Above all the disavantages of using immunosuppressive treatment during stem cells therapies include an increased risk for opportunistic infections (Garrido et al. 2006), toxic side effects (Rezzani 2006) and potential negative effects on donor cells as recently described (Guo et al. 2007) for cyclosporin treatment able to reduce cell proliferation and affect differentiation of rat NSCs in vitro.

In this manuscript we will discuss about NSC immunogenic potential and the exploitation of –mild- and/or transient immune suppressive protocols after NSC transplantation.

3. Neural stem cells

Somatic adult NSCs are undifferentiated cells that reside in specialized regions, namely the niche, of the fetal and adult CNS; they possess life-long self-renewal ability and a multipotent differentiation potential, given their ability to generate neurons, astrocytes and oligodendrocytes. Reynolds and Weiss (Reynolds and Weiss 1992) have first demonstrated a stem cell niche in the CNS. In particular, the finding of adult neurogenesis in the SVZ, which leads to the generation of neural progenitors migrating to the olfactory bulbs and to the cortex, has favoured the idea that newborn neurons might subserve cognitive functions and contribute to the homeostasis of the telencephalic-diencephalic area.

Therefore, NSCs maintain the functional and structural integrity of the brain in physiological conditions, thus contributing to tissue homeostasis and repair throughout adulthood (Gage et al. 1998;Reynolds and Weiss 1992;Temple and Alvarez-Buylla 1999). Alas, given the inherent resilience of NSC to rapidly expand into the adult CNS, there is limited spontaneous recovery after brain damage (Popa-Wagner et al. 2009;Romanko et al.

2004), so the integration of new functional neurons following injury can be achieved by transplanting exogenous cells. In vitro, NSCs can be propagated as free-floating aggregates called neurospheres or as a cell monolayer (on adhesion) and demonstrate the same characteristics of self-renewal and potential to differentiate into functionally mature neural cells. The establishment of protocols to isolate and culture NSC as stable cell lines able to maintain unaltered their functional properties over passaging ex vivo, has allowed to set up important model systems for studying neurogenic processes during development and neurobiological mechanisms for maintaining cellular complexity and plasticity. Moreover, compelling evidence from transplantation experiments in animal models suggested the potential use of NSC lines in novel cell-based therapies for brain injury and neurodegenerative disease. Interesting, functional recovery by NSC transplantation was mostly reached through alternative mechanisms rather than cell replacement (Pluchino et al. 2005). These mechanisms include neuroprotection and reduction of host cell death (Chu et al. 2004), enhancement of endogenous angiogenesis after stroke (Jiang et al. 2005), immunomodulatory effects on inflammatory damage (Pluchino, et al. 2005;Rota Nodari et al. 2010;Ziv et al. 2006a) and scavenging of neurotoxic molecules (Emsley et al. 2004).

Thus far, cells with stem-like properties have been identified in the mammalian CNS, including that of humans, throughout development and adulthood (Alvarez-Buylla et al. 2001;Gage 2000;Temple 2001). In particular, NSCs have been derived from germinative zones of the brain such as the hippocampal dentate gyrus, olfactory bulb, subventricular zone, subcallosal zone and spinal cord of embryonic, neonatal, and adult rodents (Gritti et al. 1996;Reynolds and Weiss 1992;Weiss et al. 1996). The SVZ has the greatest potential for neurogenesis and is one of the best characterized niches in the adult brain (Doetsch 2003). It consists of a cell layer adjacent to the ependymal layer which lines the lateral ventricles and contains three major cell types. The stem-like cells (type B cells) have an astroglial phenotype express the glial-fibrillary acidic protein (GFAP), are slow-proliferating but endowed of long-term self-renewal ability (Alvarez-Buylla and Garcia-Verdugo 2002). They give rise to transiently amplifying progenitor cells (type C cells) which are typically GFAP- and express at meaning levels distal-less homeobox 2 (Dlx2) and Epidermal Growth Factor Receptor (EGFR) genes (Pastrana et al. 2009). These type C cells can, in turn, originate migrating neuroblasts (type A cells) which acquire the expression of polisyalylated form of neural cell adhesion molecule (PSA-NCAM) and of doublecortin (Dcx) and migrate to the olfactory bulbs through the a physiological pathway named -rostral migratory stream- (RMS). Altogether these cell characteristics suggest that NSCs are the best candidate in advanced therapies on neurodegenerative/inflammatory diseases. Indeed in the last decade NSC were used to putative treatment in a number of different diseases.

4. Therapeutic potential of NSC

4.1 NSCs: Therapy, proof of concept

Experimentation with intracerebral transplantation of NSCs into animal models has helped to individuate strategies to develop pharmacological and cell replacement therapies for different neurodegenerative pathologies (Anderson et al. 2001), including both genetic diseases like metachromatic leukodystrophy, Huntington's disease and sporadic Alzheimer's disease (AD), and idiopathic diseases like Parkinson's disease (PD), multiple sclerosis (MS), amyotrophic lateral sclerosis (ALS), and stroke (Kim and de Vellis 2009).

In particular, Pluchino et al. recently showed that following intravenous or intracerebral injection in mice affected by an experimental form of MS (EAE), fetal hNSCs can selectively reach brain and spinal cord areas affected by the demyelinating-inflammatory process and contribute to myelin restoration and reduction of astrogliosis in those damaged areas (Pluchino et al. 2009;Pluchino et al. 2003). However, a crucial step toward successful clinical application of NSC-mediated therapy is to unravel how immunocompetent *in vitro* expanded hNSCs are, whether they are amenable to host rejection following transplantation, and whether they present immunomodulatory besides neuroprotective effects after nervous system lesions. The major disadvantage of immune suppression is to excessively undermine the immunity of the patient and the ensuing enhancement of sensitiveness to multiple infections. For a long time a widely held view was that whatever immune activity in the brain was detrimental to the neuronal tissue. However recent studies have elucidated a neuroprotectant role of immune response on neural repair, which basically relies on the mutual interaction between infiltrating blood-immune cells, microglia and neuronal cells, namely a cross-play of regenerative signals generated by the "neurovascular niche" (Madri 2009). Indeed it has been recently shown that both traumatic injury and chronic neurodegeneration induce the activation of resident microglia and infiltration of T-cells and macrophages from the blood vessels, which can exert evident beneficial besides detrimental effects on the surrounding neural tissue (Beers et al. 2006;Glezer et al. 2007;Neumann et al. 2006;Schwartz and Moalem 2001;Ziv, et al. 2006a;Ziv et al. 2006b). These results in combination with unsuccessful clinical studies (in some cases leading to an exacerbation of the disease) radically revised the theory of immune suppression as a therapeutic approach for neurodegenerative disorders. Moreover, the use of immune suppression in order to prevent the rejection of donor NSC transplants can block the immune mediated guidance cues required for the "homing" of NSC to the lesion sites (Ben-Hur 2008). In particular, Fibroblast Growth Factor 2 (FGF2) (Craig et al. 1996;Kuhn et al. 1997), tumor necrosis factor-a (TNF-α) and Interferon-γ (IFN-γ) have been shown to induce cell mobilization (Ben-Hur et al. 2003), while other cytokines drive NSC migration to the lesion through specific physiological pathways, such as the monocyte chemoattractant protein-1 (MCP-1) (Belmadani et al. 2006), hepatocyte growth factor (HGF) (Lalive et al. 2005), Epidermal Growth Factor (EGF), platelet Growth Factor (PDGF) (Armstrong et al. 1990), and stromal derived growth factor (SDF-1 or CXCL12) (Imitola et al. 2004b).

Interestingly, the majority of hNSC lines expanded *in vitro* display low dissimilarities in the major histocompatibility complex (MHC) expression pattern, most likely owing to different culture conditions and to the origin of the primary tissue.

The presence of MHC class I and II molecules on human NSC isolated by our group (Figure 1), or described by Akesson and colleagues (Akesson et al. 2009) would presumably predict a risk for rejection after transplantation. However, Akesson demonstrated that neither NSCs nor differentiated cells were recognized by alloreactive lymphocytes.. Indeed, human NSCs and newly formed astrocytes, but not neurons, suppressed lymphocyte stimulation to alloantigens, suggesting low risk for alloreaction and a role as immunomodulators. Despite these results, in accordance with providing evidence of NSCs low immunogenicity (Odeberg et al. 2005) and ability to produce TGF-β cytokine with a potent bystander effect on limpho/monocytes (Ubiali et al. 2007), the presence of MHC class I and II molecules on hNSCs implies a risk for recognition by alloreactive T cells after transplantation, thus indicating a potential risk for immunological rejection due to MHC incompatibility and subsequent requirement of immunosuppressive treatment to avoid rejection.

The disadvantages of using immunosuppressive treatment include an increased risk for opportunistic infections, toxic side effects and potential negative effects on donor cells.

Notwithstanding several clinical trials harnessing various sources of neural stem cells such as ESC-derived progenitors, spinal cord NSC and fetal NSC are currently ongoing (www.clinicaltrials.org).

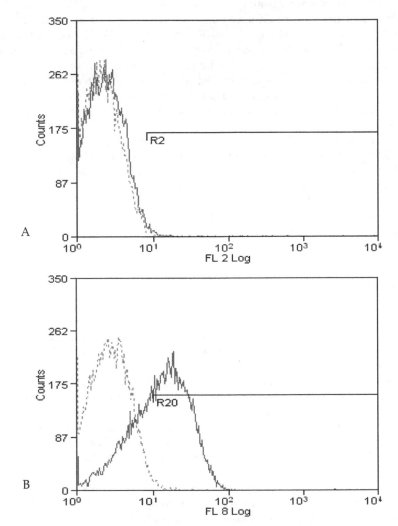

Fig. 1. Cytofluorimetric analysis of HLA class I and II on cultured human neural stem cells (hNSC). A) absence of HLA DR (Class II) on hNSC cell surface. B) Expression of HLA ABC (Class I) on hNSC cell surface

5. Establishment of human NSC lines for clinical application

5.1 NSCs: Cells "clinical grade" produced under GMPs guidelines

Our hNSCs have now been serially expanded under chemically defined conditions and are being cryopreserved, establishing a Good Manufacturing Practice (GMP)-grade, hNSCs bank. In order to certify these cells by the GMP standard, a panel of cellular, functional and biochemical criteria must be met prior to cell release, which include, but are not limited to, karyotype analysis, stable differentiation and growth capacity, and lack of biological contamination by adventitious agents.

In our GMP facility designed to produce human neural stem cells for advanced therapies, quality control is only part of overall quality assurance for cell lines which includes: evaluation and quality control measures for cells and critical reagents coming into the laboratory, control of the laboratory environment, equipment and procedures, control of data arising from cell culture, control of the delivery of research materials, including cells, to other laboratories and traceability of raw material, especially tissue from donors.

Four critical characteristics of cell cultures are fundamental to assure the quality of cell culture work:

1. Identity, i.e., the cells need to possess a specific behaviour:
   i. Self Renewal: growth kinetic stable for a elevated number of passages in vitro
   ii. Multipotency: NSCs are able to differentiate into 3 neural lineages (Astrocytes, Neuron and oligodendrocytes) after growth factors (EGF and bFGF) removal
2. Purity, i.e., freedom from microbiological contamination (all the assays need to be performed according to official Europeian Pharmacopeia, current edition)
   i. Sterility (Bacteria and fungi)
   ii. Mycoplasma
   iii. Bacterial Endotoxins
   iv. Viral contamination
   v. BSE (at least a risk analysis)
3. Maintenance of stable functional properties over passaging *in vitro*
   i. Growth curve: constant positive slope over passages
   ii. Constant ratio neurons/astrocytes/oligodendrocytes upon differentiation assay
   iii. Karyology (healthy karyotype asset and deeper analysis like SKY or comparative genomic hybridisation)
4. Tumorigenicity, i.e., Cell lines not toxic or tumorigenic
   i. Growth factor dependence: the cells died into a few passages after EGF and bFGF removal from culture medium.
   ii. No tumor signs after transplantation into the brain of Nude mice (Figure 2). The cells are able to migrate, differentiate and integrate into host tissue.

Because all of the characteristics above mentioned, raw material (media, cell culture plastic disposable, etc.) were obtained from GMP certified suppliers. Human Neural Stem Cells were produced into controlled environment (class A surrounded by Class B) according to Annex I Vol.4 European GMP Guidelines. Tissue samples were obtained from screened donors according to European Guidelines on "Certain technical requirements for the donation, procurement and testing of human tissues and cell" (Implementing Directive 2004/23/EC of the European Parliament and of the Council).

6. Current immunosuppression in transplant

6.1 Immunosuppressive drugs in cells transplant

Immunosuppression after transplantations is complex and improved therapeutic strategies have contributed to ameliorate the quality of the patient's life and to enhance the survival of the graft; however, the adverse effects associated with immunosuppressive compounds and

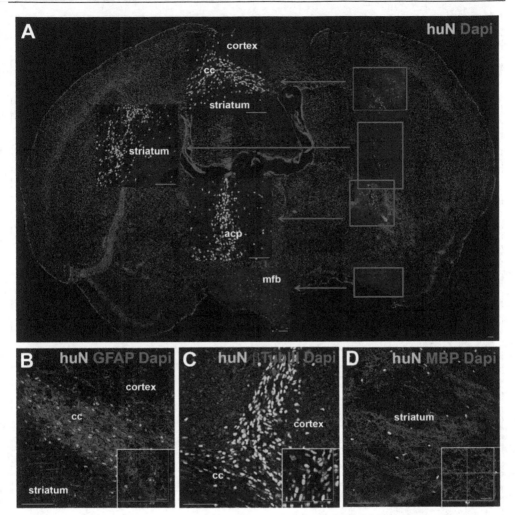

Fig. 2. Panel A-D) Nude mice were injected in striatum with hNSCs. Six months after transplantation mice with hNSCs were sacrificed and immunohistochemistry analysis showed that hNSCs engraft efficiently and migrate throughout the injected hemisphere. (A) Brain map showing the localization of huN+ cells the cells colonized cortex, cc, striatum, acp and mfb. B-D Confocal microscopy analysis showing integration and differentiation of hNSC at 6 months from transplantation into the striatum of nude mice. A) migration of gfp-Transduced hNSC along the corpus callosum and to the striatum of the ipsilateral emisphere. B-D) expression of differentiation and proliferation markers by hNSC identified as human-Nuclei (huN)-immunoreactive cells. Immunostaining with the astroglial marker Glial Fibrillary Acidic Protein (GFAP, B), the neuronal protein β-TubulinIII (C) and the late oligodendroglial marker Myelin Basic Protein (MBP, D). Insets show huN+/MBP colocalization. Nuclei are shown by dapi staining (blue). Scale bars: in A=100μm; in B-D=75μm inset scale bar: B-D=12-17μm. apc: posterior part of anterior commissure; cc: corpus callosum; mfb = medial forebrain bundle

DRUG		MECHANISM OF ACTION	EFFECTS	ADVERSE EFFECTS
Cyclosporine	Calcineurin inhibitor	Binding to the cytosolic protein cyclophilin of immunocompetent lymphocytes and preventing the production of IL-2.	Induction and maintenance of immunosuppression	Nephrotoxicity, hypertension, hyperkalemia, hypomagnesemia, nausea, intestinal diseases, hypertrichosis, gingival hyperplasia, hyperlipidemia, infection, malignancy
Tacrolimus (FK-506)	Macrolide antibiotic (calcineurin inhibitor)	Reducing peptidyl-prolyl isomerase activity by binding to the immunophilin FKBP12 and creating a new complex FKBP12-FK506 which inhibits both T-lymphocyte signal transduction and IL-2 transcription.	Maintenance immunosuppression and for rescue therapy in patients with refractory rejection under cyclosporine based therapy	Infection, cardiac damage, hypertension, liver and kidney problems, hyperkalemia, hypomagnesemia, hyperglycemia, diabetes mellitus, itching, lung damage, neurological problems,
Sirolimus (Rapamycin)	Macrolide	Binding the cytosolic protein FK-binding protein 12 and inhibiting the response to IL-2 and the activation of T and B-cells.	Maintenance immunosuppression and protection from chronic rejection	Hyperkalemia, hypomagnesemia, hyperlipidemia, leukopenia, anemia, healing and joint pain
Mycophenolate mofetil (MMF)	Prodrug of Mycophenolic Acid	Inhibiting inosine monophoshate dehydrogenase impairing B and T-cells proliferation.	Maintenance immunosuppression and protection from chronic rejection	Nausea, vomiting, diarrhea, leukopenia, anemia and thrombocytopenia
Azathioprine	Purine analogue	Decreasing DNA and RNA synthesis and inhibiting the proliferation of fast-growing lymphocytes (T and B-cells particulary)	Maintenance immunosuppression	Leukopenia, thrombocytopenia, hepatitis, cholestasis, alopecia
Corticosteroids	Steroids hormones	Preventing interleukin IL-1 and IL-6 production by macrophages and inhibiting all stages of T-cells activation	Induction, maintenance immunosuppression and protection from acute rejections	Cushing diseases, bone disease, glucose intolerance, infections
Muromonab-CD3 (OKT-3)	Monoclonal Antibody of IgG_{2A} clones to the CD3 portion of the T-cell recepto	Blocking T-cell function	Induction of immunosuppression and protection from acute rejection (primary treatment or steroid-resistant)	Cytokine release syndrome (fever, dyspnea, wheezes, headache, hypotension) and pulmonary edema.

Table 1. Immunosuppression regimens used for clinical applications on human patients

the risks of inducing a long-term immunosuppression represent a challenging issue for researches and clinicians. Total body radiation after organs' transplantation was among the first protocols of immunosuppression, but it resulted as extremely severe and led inexorably to the death of all the patients. Therefore, steroid alone were used without success. With the development of 6-mercaptopurine (Purinethol), followed by azathioprine (Imuran) in the 1960s, pharmacological immunosuppression became the standard protocol after both organs and cells transplantation until 1980s, when cyclosporine (Sandimmune and Neoral) was introduced as the first calcineurin inhibitor. Calcineurin is a protein phosphatase also known as protein phosphatase 3, PPP3CA, which activates the T cells of the immune system and can be blocked by drugs. Cyclosporine was initially used in combination with azathioprine and steroids and was credited with a dramatic improvement of graft survival. Cyclosporin is thought to bind to the cytosolic protein cyclophilin (an immunophilin) of immunocompetent lymphocytes, especially T-lymphocytes. This complex of ciclosporin and cyclophilin inhibits the phosphatase calcineurin, which under baseline conditions induces the transcription of interleukin-2. The drugs also inhibits lymphokine production and interleukin release, leading to a reduced function of effector T-cells. In 1994 another calcineurin inhibitor, the macrolide antibiotic Tacrolimus (or FK-506), active against helper T cells, became available and gradually supplanted cyclosporine in many clinical Institutes. It has been largely used for maintenance of the immunosuppression and for rescue therapy in patients with refractory rejection under cyclosporine-based therapy. However, the risk of both acute and chronic nephrotoxicity attributed to calcineurin inhibitors has strongly suggested the development of protocols free of these agents as most desirable.

At the present, numerous immunosuppressive drugs and protocols have been designed for transplantation (Table 1), but a protocol which is highly effective with minimal side effects has still to be identified. In this view, although the brain is commonly considered partially "immunoprivileged", a specific immunosuppression regimen has to provide the best conditions allowing graft survival, preventing the patient from the additional burden of an immune reaction against the graft (Barker and Widner 2004).

Actually, the precise sequelae of events leading from antigen recognition to lymphocyte activation and proliferation has still to be elucidated. However, recent findings, concerning the molecular actions of cyclosporine A (CsA) and the new immunosuppressive drugs, Tacrolimus and Rapamycin, have provided important novel breakthroughs in the biochemical processes involved. Interestingly, none of the T-cell directed immunosuppressants is, by itself, anti-lymphocyitic. Conversely, these molecules act as "molecular adaptors" which mediate the interaction between specific intracellular drug-binding proteins and target molecules. Several additional drugs are currently used as immunomodulatory agents, eventually in combination with Calcineurin inhibitors. Most of these, like steroids, azathioprine, MMF, sirolimus, are routinely used in peripheral organ allograft programs with a unique and different mode of action to that of tacrolimus and cyclosporin A (Table1). The use of adjuvants agents allows clinicians to achieve adequate immunosuppression while decreasing the dose and the toxicity of individual agents.

In neural transplantation, immunomodulators have been used experimentally, in particular with xenografts. Antibodies against T-cell receptor anti-TCR and T cells have been used to enhance the survival of intracerebral neural xenografts in rats (Okura et al. 1997;Wood et al. 1996). Also the use of blockers of T-cells costimulatory molecules have been explored as alternative route to tolerance, therefore highlighting the value of targeting this arm of the immune response for xenograft survival (Larsson et al. 2003;Larsson et al. 2002).

7. Low immunogenic potential of NSC

We already obtained some evidence of hNSCs efficacy and immunogenic tolerance upon transplantation into animal models of neurological disorders (Rota Nodari, et al. 2010) such as transient global ischemia, which is a model of vascular dementia and resembles several pathological features of AD. At 3 days from global ischemic injury, hNSC were unilaterally implantated into the corpus callosum or the hippocampal fissure of adult rat brains. After 1 month, hNSCs were detected to migrate through the corpus callosum (Fig.3), into the cortex or throughout the dentate gyrus of the hippocampus and by the fourth month, to reach the ipsilateral subventricular zone, the CA1-3 hippocampal layers and the controlateral hemisphere, showing to be non-tumorigenic and to undergo a proper regional differentiation into GABAergic and GLUTAmatergic neurons (Rota Nodari, et al. 2010). Notably, these results could be accomplished using transient immunosuppression, i.e administering cyclosporine for 15 days following the ischemic event. A wide array of studies have shown that NSCs are not susceptible to immunological rejection (Bjorklund et al. 2003;Mendez et al. 2008;Olstorn et al. 2007;Wennersten et al. 2006) even when transplanted in animal models like EAE, characterized by a constitutively activated immunological response(Pluchino, et al. 2003;Pluchino, et al. 2005). Similar results were also obtained in a different context: after transplantation into the adult rat brain lesioned by focal demyelination (Ferrari et al., submitted), hNSCs demonstrated to integrate into the NSC host niche and to migrate toward the lesioned corpus callosum, where they properly differentiated into myelinating oligodendrocytes. No sign of tumorigenicity was ever

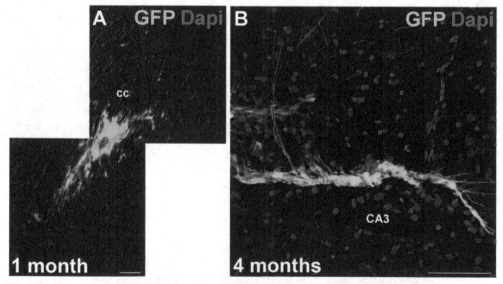

Fig. 3. hNSC transduced with a lentiviral vector carrying the reporter gene gfp were transplanted into the brain of adult rats after 3 days from lesioning by transient global ischemia. Confocal microscopy analysis showing hNSC-GFP integration into the corpus callosum (A) (1 month from transplantation) and in the hippocampal CA3 layer (B) (4 months from transplantation) under transient immunosuppression. Total nuclei are shown by dapi staining (blue). Scale Bar: 50μm. cc: corpus callosum; CA3: hippocampal layer

detected upon transplantation of hNSCs (unpublished observation) nor of hNSC immortalized with proliferating genes as c-myc, c-myc T58A and v-myc (De Filippis et al. 2008; De Filippis et al. 2007). These results have confirmed that hNSC are scarcely immunogenic. Consistently, parallel analysis of hNSC in vitro by cytofluorimetric assays showed that hNSC display only a very faint expression of HLA DR compared to a normal expression of HLA A, B and C (see Figure 1). Moreover, recent studies have shown that hNSCs may also exert their therapeutic potential through an immunomodulatory action (Bacigaluppi, et al. 2009; Pluchino, et al. 2009; Pluchino, et al. 2005).

8. NSC-mediated immunomodulation of the inflammatory component in neurodegenerative disorders

Besides neurodegeneration *per se*, one of the hallmarks characterizing most neurodegenerative disorders like stroke, AD, PD, ALS, MLD, is the development of an inflammatory environment, which can contribute to tissue damage (Glass et al. 2010). Although for a long time the NSC-mediated therapy was basically aimed at replacing damaged neural cells (Lindvall et al. 2004; Pluchino, et al. 2003), the local immune response has been shown to play a key role in recruitment of neural precursors to the lesion site. When neuroinflammation is prevailing over neurodegeneration, NSC have been shown to promote long-lasting neuroprotection and to exert unexpected immune-like functions (Pluchino, et al. 2005). Pluchino et al. (Pluchino, et al. 2005) showed that after systemic injection into a mouse model of multiple sclerosis, transplanted NSC are recruited into perivascular niche areas, where they retain undifferentiated features, proliferate and promote CNS repair through a cross-talk with inflammatory CNS-infiltrating T cells. A dual role in the regulation of both neurogenesis and oligodendrogenesis of adult neural progenitor cells is played by microglia (Streit 2002), so that the two physiological processes can be blocked by inflammation-associated microglia or induced by IL-4/IFN-γ associated to T-helper cells (Butovsky et al. 2006). Several studies have demonstrated that T cells able to recognize CNS antigens can foster spontaneous recovery from CNS injuries through an active cross-talk with local microglia (Hauben et al. 2000;Hofstetter et al. 2003;Moalem et al. 1999;Yoles et al. 2001). Consistently, T cell-based vaccination of mice with a myelin-derived peptide appeared to synergistically promote functional recovery after spinal cord injury when combined with transplantation of neural precursors into the cerebro-spinal fluid (Ziv, et al. 2006a). It's important to consider that immune cells are involved in the control of neurogenesis even under physiological conditions (Ziv, et al. 2006b). However, under pathological environment, the outcome of the interplay between inflammation, synaptic transmission and neurodegeneration is strongly conditioned by the short- or long-term persistence of inflammation (Centonze et al. 2010;Pluchino et al. 2008). Upon acute inflammatory injuries, such as stroke, neurogenesis is notably increased (Zhang et al. 2004). Conversely, a persistent brain inflammation in chronic inflammatory disorders, such as MS (Pluchino, et al. 2008) has been shown to alter both the proliferative and migratory capacities of NSCs in the SVZ, thus leading to a perpetuating non cell-autonomous dysfunction of the endogenous CNS stem cell compartment.

Both in the globally ischemic and focally demyelinated rat brains, we observed that transplantation of hNSCs can effectively decrease reactive astrogliosis and dampen microglial activation in the injuried areas (Rota Nodari, et al. 2010); unpublished results).

This phenomenon may, in fact, participate in the low immunogenic response that these cells seem to elicit in the CNS, together with the lack of expression of Molecular

Histocompatibility Complex class II components (MHCII) (Imitola et al. 2004a;Imitola, et al. 2004b)(see also Fig 1). Notwithstanding, it is also true that some level of immune surveillance is maintained in the adult brain upon NSC engraftment, which explains the widespread need to use immune suppression (Wennersten, et al. 2006) in experimental and clinical intracerebral transplantation (Bjorklund, et al. 2003;Olstorn, et al. 2007).The successful use of transient immunosuppression proposes a suitable milder approach to immunosuppression for the prospective use of hNSCs for clinical purposes. The fact that the discontinuous treatment with cyclosporine does not affect integration of transplanted cells in most of the brain regions, which to all effects emerge as immunoprivileged when considering hNSCs, is in good accordance with most recent findings (Wennersten, et al. 2006). These evidences are driving the progressive translation of the knowledge "from the bench to the bedside", thus leading to the use of hNSCs as a suitable tool to model transplantation in pre-clinical settings and to the promotion of GMP-grade hNSC for stem cell-mediated therapy of neurodegenerative disorders.

9. Transplanted NSC switch on or off the immune reactivity into host?

Usually, after the cell or tissue transplant into CNS, the intensity and rapidity of the rejection depend on the phylogenetic distance between donor and host (Dymecki et al. 1990;Mason et al. 1986;Pakzaban and Isacson 1994) and the status of the host immune system (Marion et al. 1990), but also from the nature and differentiation state of transplanted cells. Capetian and colleagues (Capetian et al. 2011) demonstrate that murine NSCs derived from newborn C57BL/6, cultured as neurospheres and placed into kidney capsule as a non-immunopriviliged site of BALB/c survived for 28 days without rejection although these 2 strains were been immunologically incompatible. However the graft were readly rejected when the recipient animal was either pre or post sensitized using donor splenocytes.

Also in these example, as well as in our human cells (Figure 1) the murine neural stem cells showed no expression of MHC I or II, in contrast with surrounding tissue or other terminally differentiated cells. This demonstrated that NSCs themselves are not attacked by immune defense mechanisms since they do not sensitize host (so they have a low immunogenicity), but can however be rejected if the host is or becomes sensitized.

In the past there have been concerns that the loss or lack of clinical improvement after neural grafting could be due to immunological rejection processes that compromise neural graft survival and function. However, autopsy findings of patients at long-term follow-up post-transplantation showed little evidence of immunological reactions (Freeman et al. 2000;Kordower et al. 2008;Kordower et al. 1996;Li et al. 2008;Mendez et al. 2005).

According to results of different clinical trials on Huntington Disease where all the patients received adequate immunosuppression for over 1 year, most of the patients developed anti HLA I antibodies but only few showed overt signs of immunological rejection.

Moreover there are accruing evidences (Pluchino, et al. 2009) that NSCs injected into CNS or intravenously in multiple sclerosis animal models are scarcely (if any) prone to differentiate, while they are able to exert a plethora of "healing actions", such as production of pleiotropic factors and cytokines, scavenging of toxic molecules and immunomodulation of the inflammatory environment. In addition Akesson and colleagues (Akesson, et al. 2009) have shown that human Neural stem cells derived from aborted fetuses of 5-12 weeks of gestation were able to inhibit lymphocyte proliferation induced by alloantigen and at NSC:Lymphomonocyte ratio of 1:1 a complete suppression was seen. These effect was clearly specific and mediated by cell-cell interactions as demonstrated by tha fact that the above mentioned proliferation was not affected by presence or absence of supernatants from NSCs cultures.

Moreover, recent evidence has suggested that the majority of the stem cell-mediated therapeutic effects in inflammatory CNS disorders are possibly taking place peripherally, at the level of immune relevant anatomical site, such as secondary lymphoid organs.

On the other hand the surgery could influence "per se" the fate of transplanted cells, albeit stereotactic techniques allow to inject NSCs by a minimally invasive procedure.

There are three main factors to be taken in account that can influence the extent of the host reaction and graft survival in an intraparenchimal cell graft: i) the extent of tissue trauma during injection, ii) cell suspension preparation and iii) the site of implantation.

The intraparenchymal injection lead to breakage of blood brain barrier at least for a couple of weeks facilitating the limphomonocyte patrolling and reaction against the graft. A low viability of cell suspensions could also trigger an immune reaction. Furthermore, the site of implantation can have a considerable effect on the host immune reaction. For example, peri- or intraventricular graft placement can lead to increased rates of immune response in terms of MHC class I expression inside the grafts and lymphocyte invasion (Oertel et al. 2004).

10. Conclusions

Although NSCs cell therapy seem to be a promising development for a number on neurological diseases, transplantation of NSC into the central nervous system is from an immunological viewpoint a true challenge both for the host as well as for the donor cells. Moreover more experiments are necessary to fully elucidate the mechanisms underlining the interactions between stem cells graft and host immune system. In conclusion, the mildest approach for clinical trials on humans is likely a transient immunosuppression regimen.

11. Acknowledgements

We thank Cristina Zalfa for image editing, Giuseppe Lamorte for FACS analysis and Prof. Angelo Vescovi for precious suggestions. This work was supported by Fondazione Borgonovo, Fondazione Neurothon ONLUS, Fondazione Cellule Staminali of Terni, Fondazione Milan.

12. References

Akesson E, Wolmer-Solberg N, Cederarv M, Falci S and Odeberg J. 2009. Human neural stem cells and astrocytes, but not neurons, suppress an allogeneic lymphocyte response. Stem Cell Res 2(1):56-67.

Alvarez-Buylla A and Garcia-Verdugo JM. 2002. Neurogenesis in adult subventricular zone. J Neurosci 22(3):629-34.

Alvarez-Buylla A, Garcia-Verdugo JM and Tramontin AD. 2001. A unified hypothesis on the lineage of neural stem cells. Nat Rev Neurosci 2(4):287-93.

Anderson DJ, Gage FH and Weissman IL. 2001. Can stem cells cross lineage boundaries? Nat Med 7(4):393-5.

Armstrong RC, Harvath L and Dubois-Dalcq ME. 1990. Type 1 astrocytes and oligodendrocyte-type 2 astrocyte glial progenitors migrate toward distinct molecules. J Neurosci Res 27(3):400-7.

Bacigaluppi M, Pluchino S, Peruzzotti Jametti L, Kilic E, Kilic U, Salani G, Brambilla E, West MJ, Comi G, Martino Gand others. 2009. Delayed post-ischaemic neuroprotection following systemic neural stem cell transplantation involves multiple mechanisms. Brain 132(Pt 8):2239-51.

Barker RA and Widner H. 2004. Immune problems in central nervous system cell therapy. NeuroRx 1(4):472-81.

Beers DR, Henkel JS, Xiao Q, Zhao W, Wang J, Yen AA, Siklos L, McKercher SR and Appel SH. 2006. Wild-type microglia extend survival in PU.1 knockout mice with familial amyotrophic lateral sclerosis. Proc Natl Acad Sci U S A 103(43):16021-6.

Behrstock S, Ebert A, McHugh J, Vosberg S, Moore J, Schneider B, Capowski E, Hei D, Kordower J, Aebischer Pand others. 2006. Human neural progenitors deliver glial cell line-derived neurotrophic factor to parkinsonian rodents and aged primates. Gene Ther 13(5):379-88.

Belmadani A, Tran PB, Ren D and Miller RJ. 2006. Chemokines regulate the migration of neural progenitors to sites of neuroinflammation. J Neurosci 26(12):3182-91.

Ben-Hur T. 2008. Immunomodulation by neural stem cells. J Neurol Sci 265(1-2):102-4.

Ben-Hur T, Ben-Menachem O, Furer V, Einstein O, Mizrachi-Kol R and Grigoriadis N. 2003. Effects of proinflammatory cytokines on the growth, fate, and motility of multipotential neural precursor cells. Mol Cell Neurosci 24(3):623-31.

Bjorklund A, Dunnett SB, Brundin P, Stoessl AJ, Freed CR, Breeze RE, Levivier M, Peschanski M, Studer L and Barker R. 2003. Neural transplantation for the treatment of Parkinson's disease. Lancet Neurol 2(7):437-45.

Butovsky O, Ziv Y, Schwartz A, Landa G, Talpalar AE, Pluchino S, Martino G and Schwartz M. 2006. Microglia activated by IL-4 or IFN-gamma differentially induce neurogenesis and oligodendrogenesis from adult stem/progenitor cells. Mol Cell Neurosci 31(1):149-60.

Cao QL, Zhang YP, Howard RM, Walters WM, Tsoulfas P and Whittemore SR. 2001. Pluripotent stem cells engrafted into the normal or lesioned adult rat spinal cord are restricted to a glial lineage. Exp Neurol 167(1):48-58.

Capetian P, Dobrossy M, Winkler C, Prinz M and Nikkhah G. 2011. To be or not to be accepted: the role of immunogenicity of neural stem cells following transplantation into the brain in animal and human studies. Semin Immunopathol.

Centonze D, Muzio L, Rossi S, Furlan R, Bernardi G and Martino G. 2010. The link between inflammation, synaptic transmission and neurodegeneration in multiple sclerosis. Cell Death Differ 17(7):1083-91.

Chu K, Kim M, Park KI, Jeong SW, Park HK, Jung KH, Lee ST, Kang L, Lee K, Park DKand others. 2004. Human neural stem cells improve sensorimotor deficits in the adult rat brain with experimental focal ischemia. Brain Res 1016(2):145-53.

Craig CG, Tropepe V, Morshead CM, Reynolds BA, Weiss S and van der Kooy D. 1996. In vivo growth factor expansion of endogenous subependymal neural precursor cell populations in the adult mouse brain. J Neurosci 16(8):2649-58.

De Filippis L, Ferrari D, Rota Nodari L, Amati B, Snyder E and Vescovi AL. 2008. Immortalization of human neural stem cells with the c-myc mutant T58A. PLoS One 3(10):e3310.

De Filippis L, Lamorte G, Snyder EY, Malgaroli A and Vescovi AL. 2007. A novel, immortal, and multipotent human neural stem cell line generating functional neurons and oligodendrocytes. Stem Cells 25(9):2312-21.

Doetsch F. 2003. A niche for adult neural stem cells. Curr Opin Genet Dev 13(5):543-50.

Dymecki J, Poltorak M and Freed WJ. 1990. The degree of genetic disparity between donor and host correlates with survival of intraventricular substantia nigra grafts. Reg Immunol 3(1):17-22.

Ebert AD, Beres AJ, Barber AE and Svendsen CN. 2008. Human neural progenitor cells over-expressing IGF-1 protect dopamine neurons and restore function in a rat model of Parkinson's disease. Exp Neurol 209(1):213-23.

Emsley JG, Mitchell BD, Magavi SS, Arlotta P and Macklis JD. 2004. The repair of complex neuronal circuitry by transplanted and endogenous precursors. NeuroRx 1(4):452-71.

Freeman TB, Cicchetti F, Hauser RA, Deacon TW, Li XJ, Hersch SM, Nauert GM, Sanberg PR, Kordower JH, Saporta Sand others. 2000. Transplanted fetal striatum in Huntington's disease: phenotypic development and lack of pathology. Proc Natl Acad Sci U S A 97(25):13877-82.

Gage FH. 2000. Mammalian neural stem cells. Science 287(5457):1433-8.

Gage FH, Kempermann G, Palmer TD, Peterson DA and Ray J. 1998. Multipotent progenitor cells in the adult dentate gyrus. J Neurobiol 36(2):249-66.

Garrido RS, Aguado JM, Diaz-Pedroche C, Len O, Montejo M, Moreno A, Gurgui M, Torre-Cisneros J, Pareja F, Segovia Jand others. 2006. A review of critical periods for opportunistic infection in the new transplantation era. Transplantation 82(11):1457-62.

Glass CK, Saijo K, Winner B, Marchetto MC and Gage FH. 2010. Mechanisms underlying inflammation in neurodegeneration. Cell 140(6):918-34.

Glezer I, Simard AR and Rivest S. 2007. Neuroprotective role of the innate immune system by microglia. Neuroscience 147(4):867-83.

Gritti A, Parati EA, Cova L, Frolichsthal P, Galli R, Wanke E, Faravelli L, Morassutti DJ, Roisen F, Nickel DDand others. 1996. Multipotential stem cells from the adult mouse brain proliferate and self-renew in response to basic fibroblast growth factor. J Neurosci 16(3):1091-100.

Guo J, Zeng Y, Liang Y, Wang L, Su H and Wu W. 2007. Cyclosporine affects the proliferation and differentiation of neural stem cells in culture. Neuroreport 18(9):863-8.

Hauben E, Butovsky O, Nevo U, Yoles E, Moalem G, Agranov E, Mor F, Leibowitz-Amit R, Pevsner E, Akselrod Sand others. 2000. Passive or active immunization with myelin basic protein promotes recovery from spinal cord contusion. J Neurosci 20(17):6421-30.

Hofstetter HH, Sewell DL, Liu F, Sandor M, Forsthuber T, Lehmann PV and Fabry Z. 2003. Autoreactive T cells promote post-traumatic healing in the central nervous system. J Neuroimmunol 134(1-2):25-34.

Imitola J, Comabella M, Chandraker AK, Dangond F, Sayegh MH, Snyder EY and Khoury SJ. 2004a. Neural stem/progenitor cells express costimulatory molecules that are differentially regulated by inflammatory and apoptotic stimuli. Am J Pathol 164(5):1615-25.

Imitola J, Raddassi K, Park KI, Mueller FJ, Nieto M, Teng YD, Frenkel D, Li J, Sidman RL, Walsh CAand others. 2004b. Directed migration of neural stem cells to sites of CNS injury by the stromal cell-derived factor 1alpha/CXC chemokine receptor 4 pathway. Proc Natl Acad Sci U S A 101(52):18117-22.

Jiang Q, Zhang ZG, Ding GL, Zhang L, Ewing JR, Wang L, Zhang R, Li L, Lu M, Meng H and others. 2005. Investigation of neural progenitor cell induced angiogenesis after embolic stroke in rat using MRI. Neuroimage 28(3):698-707.

Kim SU and de Vellis J. 2009. Stem cell-based cell therapy in neurological diseases: a review. J Neurosci Res 87(10):2183-200.

Kordower JH, Chu Y, Hauser RA, Freeman TB and Olanow CW. 2008. Lewy body-like pathology in long-term embryonic nigral transplants in Parkinson's disease. Nat Med 14(5):504-6.

Kordower JH, Rosenstein JM, Collier TJ, Burke MA, Chen EY, Li JM, Martel L, Levey AE, Mufson EJ, Freeman TBand others. 1996. Functional fetal nigral grafts in a patient with Parkinson's disease: chemoanatomic, ultrastructural, and metabolic studies. J Comp Neurol 370(2):203-30.

Kuhn HG, Winkler J, Kempermann G, Thal LJ and Gage FH. 1997. Epidermal growth factor and fibroblast growth factor-2 have different effects on neural progenitors in the adult rat brain. J Neurosci 17(15):5820-9.

Lalive PH, Paglinawan R, Biollaz G, Kappos EA, Leone DP, Malipiero U, Relvas JB, Moransard M, Suter T and Fontana A. 2005. TGF-beta-treated microglia induce oligodendrocyte precursor cell chemotaxis through the HGF-c-Met pathway. Eur J Immunol 35(3):727-37.

Larsson LC, Corbascio M, Pearson TC, Larsen CP, Ekberg H and Widner H. 2003. Induction of operational tolerance to discordant dopaminergic porcine xenografts. Transplantation 75(9):1448-54.

Larsson LC, Corbascio M, Widner H, Pearson TC, Larsen CP and Ekberg H. 2002. Simultaneous inhibition of B7 and LFA-1 signaling prevents rejection of discordant neural xenografts in mice lacking CD40L. Xenotransplantation 9(1):68-76.

Li JY, Englund E, Holton JL, Soulet D, Hagell P, Lees AJ, Lashley T, Quinn NP, Rehncrona S, Bjorklund Aand others. 2008. Lewy bodies in grafted neurons in subjects with Parkinson's disease suggest host-to-graft disease propagation. Nat Med 14(5):501-3.

Lindvall O and Kokaia Z. 2010. Stem cells in human neurodegenerative disorders--time for clinical translation? J Clin Invest 120(1):29-40.

Lindvall O, Kokaia Z and Martinez-Serrano A. 2004. Stem cell therapy for human neurodegenerative disorders-how to make it work. Nat Med 10 Suppl:S42-50.

Madri JA. 2009. Modeling the neurovascular niche: implications for recovery from CNS injury. J Physiol Pharmacol 60 Suppl 4:95-104.

Marion DW, Pollack IF and Lund RD. 1990. Patterns of immune rejection of mouse neocortex transplanted into neonatal rat brain, and effects of host immunosuppression. Brain Res 519(1-2):133-43.

Mason DW, Charlton HM, Jones AJ, Lavy CB, Puklavec M and Simmonds SJ. 1986. The fate of allogeneic and xenogeneic neuronal tissue transplanted into the third ventricle of rodents. Neuroscience 19(3):685-94.

Mendez I, Sanchez-Pernaute R, Cooper O, Vinuela A, Ferrari D, Bjorklund L, Dagher A and Isacson O. 2005. Cell type analysis of functional fetal dopamine cell suspension transplants in the striatum and substantia nigra of patients with Parkinson's disease. Brain 128(Pt 7):1498-510.

Mendez I, Vinuela A, Astradsson A, Mukhida K, Hallett P, Robertson H, Tierney T, Holness R, Dagher A, Trojanowski JQand others. 2008. Dopamine neurons implanted into people with Parkinson's disease survive without pathology for 14 years. Nat Med 14(5):507-9.

Moalem G, Leibowitz-Amit R, Yoles E, Mor F, Cohen IR and Schwartz M. 1999. Autoimmune T cells protect neurons from secondary degeneration after central nervous system axotomy. Nat Med 5(1):49-55.

Neumann J, Gunzer M, Gutzeit HO, Ullrich O, Reymann KG and Dinkel K. 2006. Microglia provide neuroprotection after ischemia. FASEB J 20(6):714-6.

Odeberg J, Piao JH, Samuelsson EB, Falci S and Akesson E. 2005. Low immunogenicity of in vitro-expanded human neural cells despite high MHC expression. J Neuroimmunol 161(1-2):1-11.

Oertel J, Samii M and Walter GF. 2004. Fetal allogeneic dopaminergic cell suspension grafts in the ventricular system of the rat: characterization of transplant morphology and graft-host interactions. Acta Neuropathol 107(5):421-7.

Okura Y, Tanaka R, Ono K, Yoshida S, Tanuma N and Matsumoto Y. 1997. Treatment of rat hemiparkinson model with xenogeneic neural transplantation: tolerance induction by anti-T-cell antibodies. J Neurosci Res 48(5):385-96.

Olstorn H, Moe MC, Roste GK, Bueters T and Langmoen IA. 2007. Transplantation of stem cells from the adult human brain to the adult rat brain. Neurosurgery 60(6):1089-98; discussion 1098-9.

Pakzaban P and Isacson O. 1994. Neural xenotransplantation: reconstruction of neuronal circuitry across species barriers. Neuroscience 62(4):989-1001.

Pastrana E, Cheng LC and Doetsch F. 2009. Simultaneous prospective purification of adult subventricular zone neural stem cells and their progeny. Proc Natl Acad Sci U S A 106(15):6387-92.

Pluchino S, Gritti A, Blezer E, Amadio S, Brambilla E, Borsellino G, Cossetti C, Del Carro U, Comi G, t Hart Band others. 2009. Human neural stem cells ameliorate autoimmune encephalomyelitis in non-human primates. Ann Neurol 66(3):343-54.

Pluchino S, Muzio L, Imitola J, Deleidi M, Alfaro-Cervello C, Salani G, Porcheri C, Brambilla E, Cavasinni F, Bergamaschi Aand others. 2008. Persistent inflammation alters the function of the endogenous brain stem cell compartment. Brain 131(Pt 10):2564-78.

Pluchino S, Quattrini A, Brambilla E, Gritti A, Salani G, Dina G, Galli R, Del Carro U, Amadio S, Bergami Aand others. 2003. Injection of adult neurospheres induces recovery in a chronic model of multiple sclerosis. Nature 422(6933):688-94.

Pluchino S, Zanotti L, Rossi B, Brambilla E, Ottoboni L, Salani G, Martinello M, Cattalini A, Bergami A, Furlan Rand others. 2005. Neurosphere-derived multipotent precursors promote neuroprotection by an immunomodulatory mechanism. Nature 436(7048):266-71.

Popa-Wagner A, Buga AM and Kokaia Z. 2009. Perturbed cellular response to brain injury during aging. Ageing Res Rev.

Reynolds BA and Weiss S. 1992. Generation of neurons and astrocytes from isolated cells of the adult mammalian central nervous system. Science 255(5052):1707-10.

Rezzani R. 2006. Exploring cyclosporine A-side effects and the protective role-played by antioxidants: the morphological and immunohistochemical studies. Histol Histopathol 21(3):301-16.

Romanko MJ, Rola R, Fike JR, Szele FG, Dizon ML, Felling RJ, Brazel CY and Levison SW. 2004. Roles of the mammalian subventricular zone in cell replacement after brain injury. Prog Neurobiol 74(2):77-99.

Rota Nodari L, Ferrari D, Giani F, Bossi M, Rodriguez-Menendez V, Tredici G, Delia D, Vescovi AL and De Filippis L. 2010. Long-Term Survival of Human Neural Stem Cells in the Ischemic Rat Brain upon Transient Immunosuppression. PLoS One 5(11):e14035.

Schwartz M and Moalem G. 2001. Beneficial immune activity after CNS injury: prospects for vaccination. J Neuroimmunol 113(2):185-92.

Shihabuddin LS, Horner PJ, Ray J and Gage FH. 2000. Adult spinal cord stem cells generate neurons after transplantation in the adult dentate gyrus. J Neurosci 20(23):8727-35.

Streit WJ. 2002. Microglia and the response to brain injury. Ernst Schering Res Found Workshop(39):11-24.

Suhonen JO, Peterson DA, Ray J and Gage FH. 1996. Differentiation of adult hippocampus-derived progenitors into olfactory neurons in vivo. Nature 383(6601):624-7.

Temple S. 2001. The development of neural stem cells. Nature 414(6859):112-7.

Temple S and Alvarez-Buylla A. 1999. Stem cells in the adult mammalian central nervous system. Curr Opin Neurobiol 9(1):135-41.

Ubiali F, Nava S, Nessi V, Frigerio S, Parati E, Bernasconi P, Mantegazza R and Baggi F. 2007. Allorecognition of human neural stem cells by peripheral blood lymphocytes despite low expression of MHC molecules: role of TGF-beta in modulating proliferation. Int Immunol 19(9):1063-74.

Weiss S, Reynolds BA, Vescovi AL, Morshead C, Craig CG and van der Kooy D. 1996. Is there a neural stem cell in the mammalian forebrain? Trends Neurosci 19(9):387-93.

Wennersten A, Holmin S, Al Nimer F, Meijer X, Wahlberg LU and Mathiesen T. 2006. Sustained survival of xenografted human neural stem/progenitor cells in experimental brain trauma despite discontinuation of immunosuppression. Exp Neurol 199(2):339-47.

Wood MJ, Sloan DJ, Wood KJ and Charlton HM. 1996. Indefinite survival of neural xenografts induced with anti-CD4 monoclonal antibodies. Neuroscience 70(3):775-89.

Yoles E, Hauben E, Palgi O, Agranov E, Gothilf A, Cohen A, Kuchroo V, Cohen IR, Weiner H and Schwartz M. 2001. Protective autoimmunity is a physiological response to CNS trauma. J Neurosci 21(11):3740-8.

Zhang R, Zhang Z, Wang L, Wang Y, Gousev A, Zhang L, Ho KL, Morshead C and Chopp M. 2004. Activated neural stem cells contribute to stroke-induced neurogenesis and neuroblast migration toward the infarct boundary in adult rats. J Cereb Blood Flow Metab 24(4):441-8.

Ziv Y, Avidan H, Pluchino S, Martino G and Schwartz M. 2006a. Synergy between immune cells and adult neural stem/progenitor cells promotes functional recovery from spinal cord injury. Proc Natl Acad Sci U S A 103(35):13174-9.

Ziv Y, Ron N, Butovsky O, Landa G, Sudai E, Greenberg N, Cohen H, Kipnis J and Schwartz M. 2006b. Immune cells contribute to the maintenance of neurogenesis and spatial learning abilities in adulthood. Nat Neurosci 9(2):268-75.

5

Radiotherapy and Immunity – A Mini Review

Rosangela Correa Villar

Department of Radiation Oncology, University of Sao Paulo, Medicine School
Brasil

1. Introduction

Slavin *et al.* in [1976], were the first to found that rejection of skin and heart allograft was greatly delayed in rodents treated with Total Lymphoid Irradiation (TLI). Since 1980, the immunosupression of TLI has been applied in transplants and autoimmune diseases. However, the development of immunosuppressive drugs decreased the use of radiotherapy for immunosuppressive finality except for the use of total body irradiation (TBI) or TLI as myeloablative treatment before bone marrow transplantation

The mechanism by which TLI-treated patients have a graft prolongation is not entirely understood. During many years of its use many changes has been observed specially in lymphocytes counts. The majority of the studies, however, were done without modern techniques to characterize the fate of different subtypes of lymphocytes and is difficult to compare the results. The majority of the studies has been done *in vitro* and in regimes using TBI and bone marrow transplants. There is some evidence that suppressor T-cells might be involved in the long term maintenance of allografts in these patients [Gray et al, 1989]. TLI provokes a more pronounced impairment of T-dependent immunological functions, as measured with phytohemaglutinin- (PHA), concanavalin A- (Con A), and pokeveed-induced (PWM) blastogenesis than does conventional immunosuppression. The more profound changes in the balance between T helper and T suppressor cells after TLI are also associated with a more pronounced suppressor cell activity, as measured with different functional suppressor cell assays. [Fergunson et al, 1981; Waer et al, 1987]. The TLI seems to produce an "amnesic state" and the autoantigens cannot be recognized by the host anymore. In the past, radiation therapy had traditionally been viewed as immunosuppressive (Cole, 1986; James et al., 1989; Wasserman et al., 1989). Lymphocyte radiosensitivity is well established and remains the dominant explanation for this effect. However, substantial evidence suggests more varied effects of radiation on the immune system, prompting the re-characterization of radiation as 'immunomodulatory' rather than immunosuppressive (McBride et al., 2004).

Ionising radiation induces diverse effects on cell survival, apoptosis, proliferation and differentiation depending on the dosage and target cell (Jonathan et al. 1999). High dose of radiation often results in massive DNA damage that involves double-strand breaks and subsequent cell death. Low dose of irradiation induces reactive oxygen species (ROS) and the activation of specific intracellular signaling pathways and transcription factors leading to proliferation and differentiation of target cells (Kasid et al. 1996, Lander et al. 1997, Finkel 1998). Therefore, irradiation can modulate immune response via its variable effects on immune cell survival and differentiation (Shankar et al. 1999, Rho et al. 2004, Liu 2007, Shan et al.2007).

The immune system responds to ionizing radiation with distinct characteristics depending on multiple factors such as dose and dose rate, tissue and cell types. Overall, immune cells are susceptible to radiation-induced damage and readily undergo apoptosis in response to small doses of radiation. Cellular apoptosis is critically regulated by various intracellular and extracellular signaling mechanisms. CD95 (Apo-1/Fas) is a homotrimeric tumour necrosis factor receptor (TNFR) family member characterised by the presence of a death domain in its cytoplasmic tail. CD95-mediated apoptosis is an important process with enormous physiological and pathophysiological impact and cell-type-specific features. CD95 molecules have been implicated in the maintenance of self-tolerance and T-cell homeostasis by transmitting apoptotic signals to repeatedly activated antigen-specific T cells, as well as to antigen-presenting dendritic cells (DCs) and activated B cells. (Schu" tze et al. 2008). For example, It has been described that Treg maintain immunological tolerance by suppression of autoreactive T cells but it was also shown that low dose total body irradiation (LTBI) selectively decreased the proportion and absolute number of Treg and enhanced antitumor immunity in murine model. It occurs because Treg displaying much higher apoptotic baseline and apoptosis-related proteins are more radiosensitive than its effector counterpart CD4pCD257T cells (Mendge et al, 2011) An important finding to help explain the immune 'stimulating' effect of low dose irradiation is the differential impact on Treg vs. CD4þ CD257 cell population. These relevant findings appoint to the hypotheses that the net balance for the immune system may be a relative decrease in Treg-mediated suppression and a net increase in effector T cell activity. Similar effect was confirmed in in-vivo that LTBI is a very attractive adjuvant strategy to enhance overall cancer immunotherapy or vaccine responses (Liu et al.2010). Other possible mechanisms of immune enhancement are elimination of suppressor cells as Treg and myeloid suppressor cells and augmentation of the immune response including natural killer (NK) cells, B cells and T cells activation, costimulatory molecules upregulation, IFNg and IL-2 production and release, and enhanced proliferative activity of lymphocytes to mitogenic stimuli (Belka et al, 1999; Hashimoto et al, 1999; Safwat 2000a; 2000b; Liu et al, 2001; Kipnis et al, 2004; Jin et al, 2007; Shan et al, 2007)

Although the effects of radiation on the survival of lymphocytes have been extensively studied *in vitro*, a correlation of the frequency of radiation-induced apoptosis in human peripheral blood lymphocytes during TLI have not previously been performed. In 2008 we published the clinical results of a protocol using TLI plus immunosuppressive agents to prevent recurrence after renal transplant in patients with focal and segmental glomerulosclerosis (FSGS) (Villar et al, 2008). This disease presents with early recurrence after renal transplants and an involvement of the immune system has been implicated in its pathogenesis. During the study the purpose was also to investigate the changes in peripheral blood monocyte and lymphocyte subpopulations and the role of the *in vivo* induction of apoptosis in patients undergoing TLI pre renal transplant (TX) (unpublished data). It was a very rare opportunity to study *in vivo* the immunosuppressant effect caused by TLI during each week of the treatement in patients that had not received any immunosuppressive drug or chemotherapy before. We studied 9 patients and they were treated with aggressive immunosuppressive treatment associating TLI with the drugs mycophenolate mofetil (MMF), prednisone (PRED) and cyclosporine (CsA) commonly used in conventional immunosuppressive treatments. TLI were performed as described in Villar et al, 2008. Immunophenotyped peripheral blood T and B lymphocyte subsets and monocytes were performed before treatment (control) and followed during each week of

TLI (after each 9 Gy), on TX´s day and after TX (30, 60 and 90 days) using flow cytometry. The percentages of T-helper, T-suppressor, B-lymphocytes and monocytes/macrophages cells, were determined on the cells in the lymphogate. Mitogen stimulation tests in lymphocytes culture using phytohemaglutinin (PHA) and pokeweed mitogen (PWM) were performed before and after completion of TLI, at the TX day and at 1 month interval up to three months post-transplantation.

1.1 Isolation of lymphocytes and detection of apoptosis

The *in vivo* radiation-induced apoptosis in lymphocytes was investigated in blood samples of 9 patients before TLI, pre and pos-hemodyalisis (controls 1 and 2) and 6h and 24h after the first and the second fraction of TLI and 6h after each 9 Gy until the end of TLI. The observation of apoptosis on freshly blood samples (2 patients) were insignificant then in the others (7 patients), we decided to observe the commitment to apoptosis of the lymphocytes irradiated *in vivo* after 72h in cell culture with and without mitogen (PHA) using an *ex vivo* test. After the cells were kept in culture they were assessed for binding of Annexin by resuspending 2×10^5 cel/100µl and subsequently by incubating with 10µl Annexin V-FITC for 30min. In order to distinguish between apoptotic (Annexin V+/PI-) and secondary necrotic (Annexin V +/PI+) cells, 10µl of propidiun iodeto (PI) (2µg/ml) was also added before analyzing on a Coulter Epics XL-MCL flow cytometer. Two-colour flow-cytometric analyses were performed on a FACSort. A gate was put on Annexin V + (green) cells and a backgating performed on the scatter plot in order to discriminate optimally platelets and debris from smaller apoptotic cells with exclusion of monocytes (increased side scatter). In cells with a damaged membrane PI cannot be excluded anymore and a red fluorescent signal was observed indicating secondary necrotic cells. The results were expressed as percentage of apoptotic cells in 10.000 cells counted in the pre-determined window. All the results were expressed as the percentage of the pre-treatment value. Statistical analysis was performed comparing the values before and after treatment (Friedman´s ANOVA – p ≤ 0.05). We observed significant reduction of all parameters analysed after treatment. Leukocytes decreased 55%, lymphocytes had a reduction of 60%, 70 % and 97 % for CD3/CD4, CD8 and CD19, respectively, at the transplant's day (p<0,05) The statistical analysis showed a significant decrease since the first week of TLI (p<0,05). The steep decrease for T cells was not significantly different between CD4 and CD8, but the decrease of B-cells was significantly more important than T-cells **(fig.1)**. The decrease observed in CD14 cells was not significant (p=0,569). Lymphocytes proliferative activity decrease 60% (with PHA) and 67% (with PWM) after TLI. The PWM response was less expressive (p = 0,09), statistical analysis showed reduction significantly maintained after TX only with PHA (p=0,009) **(fig 2,3)**.

There was significant increase of apoptosis *in vivo* in peripheral blood lymphocytes (PBL) in the beginning of TLI, (6h after first fraction of TLI) and necrosis at the end of TLI (10 and 15 fractions of TLI) **(fig. 4,5)**. The phenomenon (apoptosis) was significantly increased by PHA stimulus **(fig.6)**.

In our experience TLI provide important immunosuppresion with a significant fall in T and B lymphocytes and functional response to PHA. The B lymphocytes were the more radiosensitive and the monocyte the most radioresistant cells. No significant differences between T-helper and T-supressor/cytotoxic cells were observed.TLI induced significant increase of apoptosis *in vivo* in PBL after low doses and necrosis after high doses of TLI.

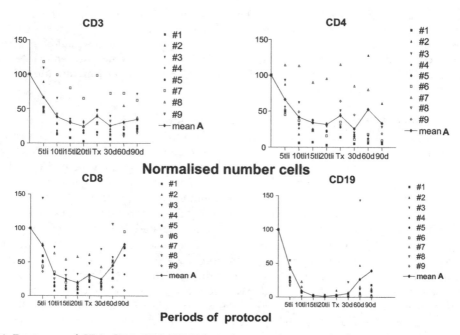

Fig. 1. Response of CD3, CD4, CD8, CD19 lymphocytes during radiotherapy and after transplant. The results were normalized to the values obtained before the treatment and plotted against the equivalent period of evaluation. A mean time-response curve resulting from statistical analyse to the data of all patients (mean A). Individual patients results are indicated on the figures

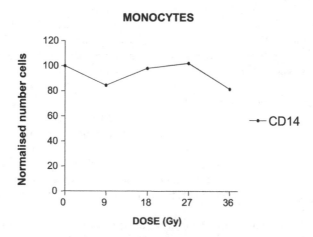

Fig. 2. Response of monocytes (CD14) with dose (Gy) in the nine (9) patients. The results were normalised to the values obtained before the start of the TLI and plotted against the equivalent period of the irradiation (first to fourth week).

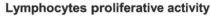

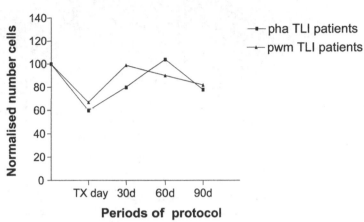

Fig. 3. Lymphoproliferative activity of 9 patients during the periods of protocol: control, after TLI (day of TX), 30, 60 and 90 days after TX. PHA = lymphocytes culture with phitohemaglutinin mitogen stimulation. PWM = lymphocytes culture with pokeweed mitogen stimulation

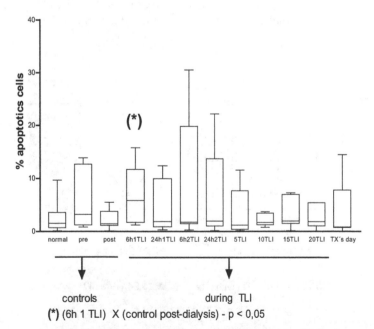

Fig. 4. Percentagem of apoptotic cells (Annexin+) observed in culture of lymphocytes without PHA. Results of controls (normal subjects, patients pre and post-dialysis and before TLI) , patients during TLI and on TX's day

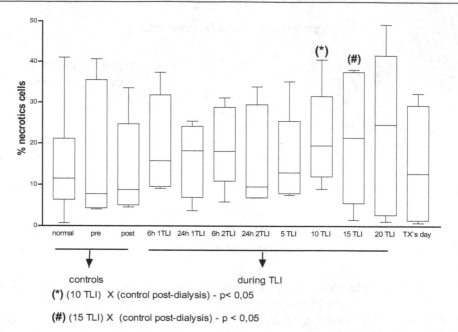

Fig. 5. Percentagem of necrotic cells (Pi +) observed in culture of lymphocytes without PHA. Results of controls (normal subjects, patients pre and post-dialysis and before TLI) , patients during TLI and on TX´s day. Necrotics cells increased at the end of TLI

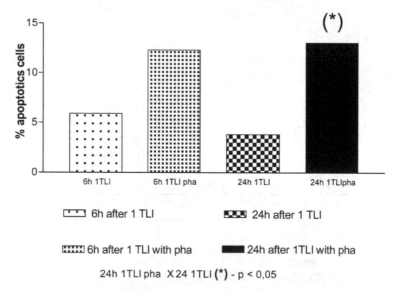

Fig. 6. Comparative analyse of percentagem of apoptotics cells observed in the periods of 6h and 24h after first fraction of TLI in culture of lymphocites with and without PHA.The percentagem of apoptosis was higher in the presence of PHA

2. Mini review

Lymphocyte radiosensitivity is well established and remains the dominant explanation for the immunosuppressive effect of radiotherapy. However, substantial evidence suggests more varied effects of radiation on the immune system, prompting the re-characterization of radiation as 'immunomodulatory' rather than immunosuppressive (McBride et al., 2004). The effect of radiotherapy in microenviroment, cytokines, gene expressions and the importance of the dose in the immunossuprressive effect has emerging as new and important concepts. The use of the immunomodulatory effect of radiation in oncology has been pointed as a new perspective and its participation has again increasing in transplants tolerance and in treatment of autoimmune diseases. In the next pages we describe the new and important concepts recently acquired in radiotherapy and immunity

2.1 The role of radiation
2.1.1 Immunomodulatory effects of radiation
Increased expression of proinflammatory cytokines, including TNF-a and IL-1b following radiation has been reported by some authors (Hallahan et al.,1989; Ishihara et al., 1995; Nemoto et al., 1995). These observations suggest a potential role for radiation in signaling 'danger' and, perhaps, in the activation of antigen presenting cells (McBride et al., 2004). However, studies aimed at determining the effects of radiation on antigen-presenting cell phenotype, cytokine expression and function have been contradictory. While alterations in dendritic cells (DC) phenotype have been demonstrated infrequently (Cao et al.,2004), a number of investigators have noted changes in the cytokine secretory profile and function of DCs following irradiation. For example, Shigematsu et al. (2007), reported enhanced expression of IL-2, IL-12 and IFN-g by irradiated DCs and it was correlated with greater T-cell proliferation compared to non-irradiated DCs. In contrast, Merrick et al. (2005) reported decreased IL-12 production and impaired naive T-cell priming by irradiated compared to non-irradiated DCs. These contradictory findings may be attributable to the different irradiation strategies and models utilized in these studies. The effect of radiation on DC antigen presentation also remains controversial with a number of studies suggesting significant modulation of, or no effect on, T-cell stimulatory capacity. Interestingly, Liao et al. (2004) reported impaired T-cell priming against endogenously processed antigen and enhanced priming against exogenous peptide pointing to a more complex interplay between radiation and DC function. A number of factors may explain why the consistent characterization of immune responses to radiation remains elusive including differences in radiosensitivity or reactivity of different cell and tissue types, and dose-dependent effects. For example, the dose effect has been explored in a number of studies, some of which suggesting that lower doses of radiation have a greater potential to enhance immune responses (Hashimoto et al., 1999; Cao et al., 2002; Shigematsu et al., 2007)

3. Irradiation and transplants

Recently, the approach of combined organ and hematopoietic cell transplantation has been successfully applied to tolerance induction in humans (Fudaba el al., 2006; Scandling et al., 2008; Kawai et al., 2008). Conditioning regimens used to achieve mixed chimerism and tolerance include lethal and sublethal total body irradiation (TBI) with or without thymic irradiation and anti-T cell antibodies (Ildstad & Sachs 1984; Kawai et al., 2002; Stykes 2001),

TLI with and without anti-T cell antibodies (Slavin et al., 1976; Slavin et al., 1978; Slavin et al, 1977; Scandling et al., 2008 ;Hayamizu et al, 1999; Lan et al, 2000; Higuchi et al, 2002), costimulatory blockade with or without rapamycin therapy or cytoreduction (Wekerle et al, 2000; Durhan et al, 2000; Lambert et al., 2002;Graca et al., 2006), injection of naturally occurring CD4+CD25+ Treg (nTreg) cells combined with radiation cytoreduction (Golshayn et al., 2007; Wood & Sakaguchi, 2003), and chemical cytoreduction combined with thymic irradiation, and anti-T cell antibodies (Fudaba et al, 2006; Kawai et al 2008,).

Although central and peripheral clonal deletion in chimeras can explain the lack of reactivity of host immune cells to donor alloantigens (Stikes 2001; Wekerle et al, 1998), host regulatory T cells that remain after cytoreduction or that are injected after cytoreduction can also play an important role in the engraftment of the donor organ and hematopoietic cells (Higushi 2002, Golshayn et al, 2007; Wood & Sakaguchi 2003).

In the mixed chimera and tolerance induction model with TLI, anti-thymocyte serum (ATS),and bone marrow transplantation, tolerance is dependent on the residual host natural killer (NK) T cells . However,CD4 regulatory T cells, (Tregs) and nTregs induced from CD4+CD25- T cell precursors (iTregs) have been shown to play an important role in promoting tolerance to allografts in both chimeric and non-chimeric mouse models (Lambert et al., 2002,Chai et al, 2005,Graca et al., 2002, Sakaguchi, 2005, Kang et al, 2007). Nador et al, 2010 has been studying the role of residual host Tregs in the mixed chimera model using TLI and ATS conditioning. They demonstrated the requirement for host Tregs selectively depleting these cells pretransplant with a single injection of anti-CD25 mAb. The experiment results showed that deficiency in either NK T cell or Tregs prevents chimerism and tolerance in the TLI and ATS model. This lymphodepletive-conditioning regimen facilitated tolerance by altering the balance of host T cell subsets to markedly favor the NKT cells and Tregs over alloreactive host naïve (CD62LhiCD44lo) T cells. Therefore, the changes in the balance of regulatory and naïve T cell subsets and their contributions to graft acceptance or rejection using a TLI and ATS conditioning regimen is the responsible to induce mixed chimerism and tolerance after combined heart and bone marrow transplantation (Hayamizu et al., 1999; Lan et al., 2000; Higuchi et al., 2002).

It was demonstrated that one day after the completion of TLI and ATS conditioning (time point of donor bone marrow infusion) there was a marked increase in the ratio of CD4+ CD25+Foxp3+ Treg cells and NKT cells to naïve conventional T cells. The change in the balance of T cell subsets is best explained by their differential resistance to radiation induced cell death due to differential expression of the anti-apoptotic protein, Bcl-2, as reported previously (Yao et al., 2009). Nador et al, 2010 showed thatp53-/- mice had no change in the balance after TLI. T cell proliferation and thymic generation of T cells play a minimal role whereas the p53/Bcl-2 apoptotic pathway plays the dominant role in the changes (Yao et al, 2009). The considerable resistance of Treg cells to apoptosis induced by ATS as compared to conventional T cells has been reported to be due to high levels of expression of the anti-apoptotic protein, BCLXL (Ninamimura et al, 2006). It is of interest that the altered balance of T cell subsets favoring Treg and NKT cells returned to normal about 6 weeks after conditioning, and by that time the stable mixed chimeras are tolerant to the heart allografts due to clonal deletion (Higuchi et al, 2002).

The relationship between NKT cells and Tregs in responses to alloantigens has been reported recently (Pillai et al, 2009). Naïve but not memory phenotype CD4+ T cells from untreated mice show alloreactivity in the MLR, and alloreactivity by conventional T cells in the MLR is suppressed by Treg cells at a 1:1 ratio (Dutt et al., 2007; Schiopu, A. & Wood, 2008). The changed ratio of these cells on day 1 was likely to have prevented the hosts from rejecting bone marrow and heart allografts acutely. In another experiment, the ability of naïve and memory phenotype T cells from untreated BALB/c mice to reject C57BL/6 heart allografts was compared by transferring equal numbers of sorted cells to immunodeficient RAG-2-/- BALB/ c hosts bearing the grafts. Whereas the naïve cell injection resulted in rejection of all grafts, the memory phenotype cell injection obtained from donors that had not been exposed to alloantigens resulted in no rejection over a 100-day observation period. In conclusion, the TLI and ATS tolerance induction model requires both regulatory NKT cells and Tregs for graft acceptance. Tolerance is promoted by profound but transient changes in the balance of regulatory and naive T cells of host origin favoring the regulatory cells. (Nador et al, 2010)

4. Irradiation and self-reactive immune response

CD4 regulatory T cells (Tregs) are the main effectors of immunological tolerance in adult life. Several studies have indicated that quantitative and qualitative abnormalities of regulatory Tregs contribute to the pathogenesis of autoimmune diseases as collagen-induced disease arthritis (CIA) (Morgan et al, 2003; Morgan et al, 2005) and in a spontaneous model of Rheumatoid Arthritis (RA).(Sakaguchi et al, 2003) There is evidence that the local proinflammatory environment is fundamental in imparting a Treg defect, because the treatment with anti-tumour necrosis factor (TNF)α may restore their function by generating transforming growth factor (TGF)β producing Tregs.(Nadkarmi et al, 2007). Therefore, generating functionally effective Tregs may provide an effective approach for the treatment of collagen-induced disease.

The adoptive transfer of Tregs can be efficacious in the treatment of autoimmune diseases in preclinical models,(Tang Q, 2004) but the major limitation of such a strategy is that, in order to obtain a dose sufficient for clinical use, Tregs need to be expanded in vitro with implications on their functionality (Hoffman et al, 2009). An alternative strategy is to increase the number of Tregs by exploiting the selective advantage of Tregs over conventional T cells during homeostatic reconstitution following cell ablative treatments (Cox et al., 2005; Nadal et al., 2007). It was previously reported that even non-myeloablative doses of irradiation are sufficient to determine a selective retention/expansion of Tregs capable of producing an immunosuppressive activity against donor haematopoietic antigens, thus facilitating their engraftment (Weng et al, 2007). Therefore, one very possible hypothesis is that partial myeloablation could also generate the conditions to control autoimmune diseases.

Myeloablative regimens have successfully been used for the treatment of severe forms of autoimmune arthritis (Dazzi et al.; 2007) whereby the consequent haematopoietic reconstitution is associated with a comprehensive renewal of the T cell repertoire (Murano et al, 2005). The major drawback of these approaches is toxicity. Mild myeloablation appears to be sufficient to modulate pathogenic immune responses and produce beneficial effects on CIA (Nakatsukasa et al, 2008) but the mechanisms remain to be clarified.

Weng et al., 2010 demonstrated that low-dose irradiation ameliorates CIA at the time of disease induction and if used when clinical signs of the disease are detectable. They established a causative relationship between the therapeutic efficacy of irradiation and Treg mediated tolerance. Irradiation induced immune tolerance to the immunizing collagen through modalities that require the presence of Tregs. The therapeutic activity is associated with the development of Treg immunosuppressive activity and the in vivo depletion of Tregs prevents the beneficial effects of irradiation.

Tregs selectively survive myeloablative regimens and undergo a marked expansion while retaining their functional activity (Bayer et al., 2009). The same mechanisms might account for the therapeutic efficacy of autologous BM transplantation in autoimmune arthritis (Roord et al., 2008). In a proteoglycan-induced arthritis, the conditioning of recipient mice with a lethal irradiation dose (7.5 cGy) and subsequent syngeneic BM transplantation significantly reduced the severity of arthritis. This study observed an increment in the proportion of CD4CD25 T cells and the clinical improvement was prevented if recipient mice received anti-CD25 depleting antibodies 1 week after the transplant. In contrast to other results, the investigators did not observe any effect if anti-CD25 antibodies were given on the day of the transplant. The disparity should be ascribed to the different intensity of the conditioning regimen (7.5 cGy vs 4 cGy) that delayed Treg homeostatic reconstitution as demonstrated by the delayed peak of Treg expansion following the myeloablative dose (Bayer et al, 2009).

The transient nature of the therapeutic effect induced by low-dose irradiation in the CIA model can result from the contribution of various factors. Firstly, the Tregs that are proportionally expanded following the non-myeloablative regimen are of recipient origin and, because of the rapid expansion kinetics, of the memory type. Their effect could be less durable and/or less potent than the naive Tregs that are generated at a later stage during the haematopoietic reconstitution following full myeloablation (Roord et al., 2008). However, to our knowledge there is no evidence of such at difference in the activity of different Treg subtypes and it is more likely that the magnitude of myeloablation differently influences the duration and thus the efficacy of the Tregs proportional increment (Weng et al., 2007; Laylor et al, 2005). The quantization of CD4CD25FoxP3+ following low-dose irradiation indicated that the percentage of Tregs increased at 12 days and, although less so, also remained elevated a week later. However, when we enumerated the absolute values, the numbers of CD4CD25FoxP3+ were much reduced as compared to CIA controls. Since the absolute number of CD4FoxP3−T cells, which contain the fraction responsible for mediating the disease, was equally reduced, it is the resulting change in the ratio between effectors and Tregs that should account for the therapeutic effect. The characterization of the effector cells in treated mice suggests that the dose of irradiation used did not affect the proportion of IL17 producing T cells. Since IL17 has been suggested to play an important role in RA and CIA (Fugimoto et al, 2008), it appears that neither irradiation nor the proportional Treg expansion is sufficient to interfere with IL17 production. Although this could justify the incomplete therapeutic effect, the levels of T helper 17 cells (Th17) in peripheral lymphoid tissues do not correlate with their levels in the injured tissues. It has been reported that anti-TNFα treatment, despite its ability to prevent Th17 in the joints increases their numbers in draining LNs.(Notley et al., 2008) We also observed that the numbers of IFNγ-producing cells are reduced in the irradiated animals. While reducing the inflammatory activity, the inhibition of IFNγ production also limits the potential to convert effector to FoxP3+ cells.(Xiao et al., 2008) The interpretation of the data is complicated by the fact that the pathogenic or protective effects of these cytokines are dependent on the timing of their production.(Lohr et al., 2006) The evidence provided the rationale to exploit the selective Treg activation induced by partial immunoablation for the treatment of autoimmune diseases. Further studies are however warranted to improve the duration of the therapeutic efficacy (Weng et al., 2010).

5. Radiotherapy and immunomodulation in cancer

Radiation is commonly used as a method of decreasing lymphocyte numbers via cytotoxicity for the purpose of bone marrow transplantation (BMT). CD25þCD4þ regulatory T cells (Treg) comprise 5–10% of the circulating CD4þ T cell population and suppress immune responses. A large body of experimental data suggests an essential role played by these cells in self-tolerance, transplantation, allergy and tumor/microbial immunity (Wing et al. 2006). Currently, many investigators are pursuing strategies to modulate the function or the number of Treg, which may offer a means to regulate host immunity for therapeutic effect in autoimmune diseases and cancers (Zou 2006). However, previous investigators have also suggested that low-dose whole-body irradiation (LTBI) results in immune enhancement in the treatment of chronic lymphocytic leukemia (CLL) and lymphoma (Safwat 2000a, 2000b). Accumulating evidence shows that irradiation influences the phenotype and function of immune cells (Cao et al. 2004, 2009, Reuben et al. 2004, Merrick et al. 2005). For example, Cao et al, showed that irradiation inhibited proliferation and suppressive ability of Treg with dose-dependent decrease of FOXP3 expression (Cao et al. 2009). A differential radiosensitivity and apoptosis-related proteins expression exist at varying doses of radiation between human Treg and effector T cells. LTBI is successful in inducing long-term remissions and has been shown to be as effective as the chemotherapy to which it has been compared in lymphoma (Safwat 2000a). However, the mechanism of this effect is unknown. The efficacy of LTBI could be partly attributed to a radiation-induced immune enhancement rather than to direct killing of tumor cells by radiation. This type of immune enhancement could be induced by two mechanisms: a differential elimination of the suppressive T subset of lymphocytes or an augmentation of the immune response through direct and/or indirect stimulation of T lymphocytes. RT can also theoretically enhance anti-tumor immunity via increasing the expression of tumor-associated antigens, inducing immune-mediated targeting of the tumor stroma, and diminishing regulatory T cell activity. Recent evidence suggests that RT may also activate effectors of innate immunity through Toll-like receptor (TLR)-dependent mechanisms, thereby augmenting the adaptive immune response to cancer (Roses et al. 2008). Thus RT can be better-characterized as having immunomodulatory properties that can allow its use as adjunct to immunotherapy (McBride et al. 2004).

6. Enhancement of antitumor effectors mechanisms

The efficacy of radiation therapy in the treatment of many tumor types is well established. While radiation induced tumor regression is largely the result of directed damage to radiosensitive tumor cells, evidence points to a number of additional immune-mediated mechanisms. Suppressor populations of T cells may be more radiosensitive than their effector counterparts and, conversely, tumor-specific effector T cells may be relatively radio-resistant (North, 1986; Dunn and North, 1991). This notion, as it relates to contemporary definitions of regulatory T cells (Tregs), has not been extensively explored. However, one recent study implicated Treg depletion in the enhanced efficacy of adoptive T-cell immunotherapy for transplanted melanomas following whole-body irradiation in a murine model (Antony et al., 2005). Enhanced functionality of adoptively transferred T cells following radiation induced lympho-depletion has also been linked to increased availability of homeostatic cytokines (Wrzesinski et al., 2007). A number of studies have measured the effects of low-dose total-body irradiation on the relative size of T-cell subpopulations and expression of cytokines associated with T-cell activation. In one report, low dose irradiation following transplantation of a hepatoma cell line in a rat model resulted in an increased proportion of CD8-positive splenocytes, increased numbers of tumor infiltrating lymphocytes, increased TNF-a and IFN-g expression and decreased TGF-b expression This response correlated with a reduction in metastases (Hashimoto et al., 1999). Another study demonstrated an increased CD4:CD8 T cell ratio, and decreased expression of TGF-b and VEGF following low-dose total body-irradiation, which correlated with delayed tumor growth in mice transplanted with the Lewis lung carcinoma cell line (Miller et al., 2003). The so-called 'abscopal effect', whereby radiation results in reduced tumor growth outside the direct radiation field, suggests radiation-induced immune-mediated mechanisms. The fact that this effect may be enhanced with Fms-like tyrosine kinase receptor 3 ligand (Flt-3L), a stem cell mobilizing factor that augments the number of circulating DC precursors, in immunocompetent mice and abrogated in T-cell-deficient mice lends additional support to this contention (Demaria et al., 2004).

7. Stromal effects

Radiation may induce immune-mediated targeting of tumor stroma. Antigen released following tumor irradiation may be presented by stromal cells for subsequent destruction by CTLs. This mechanism was recently demonstrated by Zhang et al. (2007) in experiments utilizing immunodeficient mice given tumor transplants. Only the combination of irradiation and adoptive transfer of CTLs resulted in tumor regression. This regression correlated with increased expression of tumor-specific peptide-MHC complexes as delineated using a tumor antigen/MHC complex-specific TCR tetramer. Direct effects of radiation on the stroma may play a role in enhancing immune-mediated tumor regression as well. Induced modulation of the expression of adhesion molecules, such as accumulation of P-selectin in the lumen of tumor vasculature, may enhance infiltration of immune effectors into the tumor stroma (Hallahan et al., 1998; Hallahan and Virudachalam, 1999). Enhancement of tumor antigen recognition Induction of antitumor immunity by radiation may result from enhanced tumor antigen recognition. Irradiation induces tumor cell apoptosis, or necrosis secondary to vascular injury (Acker et al., 1998). Subsequent phagocytosis of apoptotic bodies by DCs and initiation of antitumor T-cell responses through cross presentation may ensue if DC maturation signals are concomitantly present. A number of studies have suggested that necrosis, but not apoptosis, is associated with DC maturation signals (Basu et al., 2000; Sauter et al., 2000) However, more recently evidence that some apoptotic pathways do induce DC maturation and antitumor immunity has emerged (Scheffer et al., 2003). Sublethal irradiation of tumors may also result in enhanced expression of surface molecules recognized or targeted by immune effectors, as is suggested by studies demonstrating increased expression of the MHC class I antigen, H-2D, by melanoma cells (Hauser et al., 1993) and tumor associated antigens including carcinoembryonic antigen by gastric adenocarcinoma cells (Hareyama et al., 1991). Increased expression of the death receptor Fas following radiation has also been demonstrated in a transgenic carcinoembryonic antigen-expressing tumor model and associated with greater susceptibility to CTL mediated tumor cell lysis (Chakraborty et al., 2003). Combining immunotherapy and radiation building upon the hypothesis that radiation can enhance anti-tumor immunity, investigators have begun to combine radiation therapy with immunotherapies as was recently reviewed (Demaria et al., 2005a). Generally, such efforts employ radiation to induce tumor cell apoptosis or necrosis with resultant antigen release for subsequent presentation by DCs. Several investigators have studied combinations of intra-tumoral or peri-tumoral DC administration (Nikitina and), or administration of Flt-3L (Chakravarty ct al., 1999, 2006; Demaria et al., 2004) combined with irradiation, yielding promising results. Administration of a recombinant viral vaccine-expressing tumor-associated antigen(s) and costimulatory molecules in combination with tumor irradiation may capitalize on the capacity of radiation to enhance immune recognition of antigen-expressing tumor cells. Such an effect was recently demonstrated and linked to radiation induced up regulation of Fas on tumor cells (Chakraborty et al., 2004). A number of investigators have explored combinations of cytokine therapy and irradiation; studied cytokines include IL-3 (Chiang et al., 2000), IL-12 (Seetharam et al., 1999; Lohr et al., 2000) and TNFa (Weichselbaum et al., 1994). Local radiation therapy in combination with CTLA-4 blockade is an additional novel approach for overcoming mechanisms of tumor tolerance. This combination was recently demonstrated to induce anti-tumor CD8 T cells in a poorly immunogenic murine adenocarcinoma model, whereas CTLA-4 blockade alone did not (Demaria et al., 2005b). Collectively, these studies encourage optimism regarding the potential of combined immunotherapy and radiotherapy.

The 'innate' components of the mammalian immune system has been reviewed and new concepts introduced; the discovery of Toll-like receptors (TLRs) is a notable example. These receptors recognize highly conserved molecular patterns common to pathogens, termed pathogen-associated molecular patterns (Janeway and Medzhitov, 2002). Examples of pathogen-associated molecular patterns and corresponding TLRs include:doublestranded RNA, which is recognized by TLR3 (Alexopoulou et al., 2001), Lipopolysaccharide (LPS), which is recognized by TLR4 (Poltorak et al., 1998) and many others (Roses et al., 2008).

An extensive investigation into the molecular basis of TLR function has been undertaken in recent years (Akira and Takeda, 2004). Though considerable overlap exists between implicated pathways, signaling through the various TLRs may initiate discreet downstream molecular events. Most TLRs act through the myeloid differentiation primary response protein 88 (MyD88) and tumor necrosis factor receptor-associated factor 6 to activate nuclear factor kB (NF-kB) and mitogen-activated protein kinases and induce gene transcription. At the cellular level, TLR binding results not only in the activation of effectors of innate immunity, but also in the induction of adaptive responses. Ligation of TLRs expressed by antigen presenting cells may result in the expression of co-stimulatory molecules (for example, CD80 and CD86) and cytokines (for example, IL-6 and IL-12) (Macagno et al., 2007). Moreover, TLR-primed dendritic cells induce antigen-specific high avidity CD8 (Xu et al., 2003, 2006) and type-I polarized CD4 T-cell responses (Wesa et al., 2007). These findings have provided a foundation for immunotherapeutic strategies targeting tumor-associated antigens for the treatment of malignancies

Through the induction of antigen-presenting cell maturation and secretion of proinflammatory chemokines and cytokines, TLRs provide a link between innate and adaptive immunity, which may be exploited to induce robust immune responses against specific antigens, the therapeutic potential of TLR-targeted therapies. Conversely, TLR-targeted therapy may enhance subsequent responses to chemotherapy. Such combinations have been explored in a number of preclinical studies, sometimes with promising results (Lake and Robinson, 2005; Bourquin et al., 2006; Shi et al., 2007). While radiation therapy has not been explored as extensively, it too is emerging as a potentially powerful tool when combined with immunotherapies.

8. Radiation-induced TLR signaling

Investigations into the function TLRs have provided mechanistic insight into the actions of several established cancer therapies. Recent evidence suggests that TLR-dependent mechanisms contribute to the therapeutic effects of radiation as well. It has been widely hypothesized that tumor irradiation activates effectors of innate immunity through the induction of tumor cell apoptosis and the release of endogenous TLR agonists. The observation that such ubiquitous factors heat-shock proteins and uric acid can act through TLRs and induce DC maturation (Gallucci et al., 1999) supports this mechanism as does the demonstration that immature DCs, when administered into irradiated tumors, induce antitumor immunity (Kim et al., 2004).Most recently, the high-mobility-group box 1 alarmin protein, released by dying tumor cells, was shown to act on TLR4 expressed by DCs. Moreover, binding of TLR4 was demonstrated to increase the efficiency of tumor antigen processing and presentation (Apetoh et al., 2007). TLR dependent mechanisms may play a role in systemic therapies as well. Whole body irradiation was recently shown to increase bacterial translocation and circulating levels of the TLR 4 agonist lipopolysaccharide. This phenomenon was associated with enhanced anti-tumor immunity in an adoptive transfer model (Paulos et al., 2007). When considered together, such evidence provides a strong rationale for the use of radiation therapy as an immune intervention; a paradigm shift from the traditional view of radiation therapy as a cytotoxic therapy. The capacity of radiation to elicit the expression of TLR ligands systemically after gastrointestinal tract irradiation, or locally after tumor irradiation, may prove valuable in conjunction with other immunotherapies.

Potentiating anti-tumor immunity with radiation therapy and TLR agonists

Few investigators have directly studied the combination of radiation and TLR-targeted therapies; this despite recognition that the therapeutic effects of radiation maybe dependent upon TLR signaling. Mason et al. (2005) recently demonstrated a markedly enhanced tumor response to radiation therapy following peri- and intratumoral injections of the TLR agonist, CpG, in a murine fibrosarcoma model (Milas et al., 2004). In light of the recently elucidated role of TLRs in radiation induced responses, this effect may reflect synergy at the level of TLR signaling. Further investigations are required to determine the applicability of such approaches but potential implications of these findings are broad. TLR-targeted therapy may sensitize a wide range of tumor types to radiation therapy and result in a reduction of the radiation dose necessary to achieve a therapeutic effect. Such approaches may become increasingly important as new TLR-targeted therapies emerge.

9. Conclusions

Definitely, radiotherapy has been seen now as a immunomodulatory treatment. Many concepts has been changing during the past few years. A role for novel neoadjuvant immunotherapies is emerging and will result in opportunities to study their interplay with conventional treatments, such as chemotherapy and radiation and immunosuppressive drugs. Radiation therapy may be an important adjunct to immunotherapies with the potential to enhance the antigenicity of tumors and promote stromal targeting. Perhaps more importantly, radiation therapy may activate effectors of innate immunity through TLR-dependent mechanisms. The relative contributions of these distinct radiation-induced mechanisms remain unclear. As we learn more about the immune-mediated mechanisms we will be better able to utilize these modalities and emerging immunotherapies in combination (Roses et al, 2008).

10. References

Acker, J.C.; Marks, L.B.; Spencer, D.P.; et al. (1998). Serial in vivo observations of cerebral vasculature after treatment with a large single fraction of radiation. Radiat Res 149:350–359.

Akira, S. & Takeda, K. (2004). Toll-like receptor signalling. Nat Rev Immunol 4:499–511.

Alexopoulou, L.; Holt, A.C.; Medzhitov, R; et al. (2001). Recognition of double-stranded RNA and activation of NF-kappaB by Toll-like receptor 3. Nature 413:732–738.

Antony, P.A; Piccirillo, C.A; Akpinarli, A, et al. (2005). CD8+ T cell immunity against a tumor/self-antigen is augmented by CD4+ T helper cells and hindered by naturally occurring T regulatory cells. J Immunol 174: 2591–2601.

Apetoh, L.; Ghiringhelli, F; Tesniere, A.; et al. (2007). Toll-like receptor 4-dependent contribution of the immune system to anticancer chemotherapy and radiotherapy. Nat Med 13:1050–1059.

Basu, S.; Binder R.J.; Suto, R.;et al. (2000). Necrotic but not apoptotic cell death releases heat shock proteins, which deliver a partial maturation signal to dendritic cells and activate the NF-kappa B pathway. Int Immunol 12:1539–1546.

Bayer, A.L.; Jones, M.; Chirinos, J.; et al. (2009) Host CD4+CD25+ T cells can expand and comprise a major component of the Treg compartment after experimental HCT. Blood; 113:733–43.

Bourquin, C.; Schreiber, S.; Beck, S. ; et al. (2006). Immunotherapy with dendritic cells and CpG oligonucleotides can be combined with chemotherapy without loss of efficacy in a mouse model of colon cancer. Int J Cancer 118:2790–2795.

Belka, C.; Ottinger, H.; Kreuzfelder, E.; et al. (1999). Impact of localized radiotherapy on blood immune cells counts and function in humans. Radiotherapy & Oncology, 50:199–204.

Cao, M.D.; Chen, Z.D.; Xing, Y. (2004). Gamma irradiation of human dendritic cells influences proliferation and cytokine profile of T cells in autologous mixed lymphocyte reaction. Cell Biol Int 28:223–228.

Cao, Z.A.; Daniel, D.; Hanahan D. (2002). Sub-lethal radiation enhances anti-tumor immunotherapy in a transgenic mouse model of pancreatic cancer. BMC Cancer 2:11.

Cao, M.; Cabrera, R.; Xu, Y; et al. (2009). Gamma irradiation alters phenotypes and function of CD4þCD25þ regulatory T cells. Cell Biology International 33:565–571.

Chai, J.G.; Xue, S.A.; Coe D.; et al. (2005) Regulatory T cells, derived from naiveCD4+CD25- T cells by in vitro Foxp3 gene transfer, can induce transplantation tolerance. Transplantation; 79(10):1310–1316.

Chakraborty, M.; Abrams, S.I.; Camphausen, K.; et al. (2003). Irradiation of tumor cells up-regulates Fas and enhances CTL lytic activity and CTL adoptive immunotherapy. J Immunol 170:6338–6347.

Chakravarty, P.K.; Alfieri, A.; Thomas, E.K.; et al. (1999). Flt3-ligand administration after radiation therapy prolongs survival in a murine model of metastatic lung cancer. Cancer Res 59:6028–6032.

Chakravarty, P.K.; Guha, C.; Alfieri, A. et al. (2006). Flt3L therapy following localized tumor irradiation generates long-term protective immune response in metastatic lung cancer:its implication in designing a vaccination strategy. Oncology 70:245–254.

Chiang, C.S.; Hong, J.H.; Wu, Y.C.; et al. (2000). Combining radiation therapy with interleukin-3 gene immunotherapy. Cancer Gene Ther 7:1172–1178.

Cole, S. (1986). Long-term effects of local ionizing radiation treatment on Langerhans cells in mouse footpad epidermis. J Invest Dermatol, 87:608–612.

Cox, A.L., Thompson, S.A., Jones, J.L., et al. (2005) Lymphocyte homeostasis following therapeutic lymphocyte depletion in multiple sclerosis. Eur J Immunol ;35:3332–3342.

Dazzi, F.; van Laar J.M.; Cope, A.; et al. (2007) Cell therapy for autoimmune diseases. Arthritis Res Ther 2007;9:206.

Demaria, S.; Ng B.; Devitt, M.L.; et al. (2004). Ionizing radiation inhibition of distant untreated tumors (abscopal effect) is immune mediated. Int J Radiat Oncol Biol Phys 58:862–870.

Demaria, S.; Bhardwaj, N.; McBride, W.H.; et al. (2005a). Combining radiotherapy and immunotherapy:a revived partnership. Int J Radiat Oncol Biol Phys 63:655–666.

Demaria, S.; Kawashima, N.; Yang, A.M.; et al. (2005b). Immune-mediated inhibition of metastases after treatment with local radiation and CTLA-4 blockade in a mouse model of breast cancer. Clin Cancer Res 11:728–734.

Dunn, P.L. & North RJ. (1991). Selective radiation resistance of immunologically induced T cells as the basis for irradiationinduced T-cell-mediated regression of immunogenic tumor. J Leukoc Biol 49:388–396.

Durham, M.M.; Bingaman, A.W.; Adams, A.B.; et al.(2000) Cutting edge: administration of anti-CD40 ligand and donor bone marrow leads to hemopoietic chimerism and donor-specific tolerance without cytoreductive conditioning. J Immunol;165(1):1–4.

Dutt, S.; Tseng, D.; Ermann, J.; et al.(2007) Naive and memory T cells induce different types of graft-versus-host disease. J Immunol 2007;179(10):6547–6554.

Ferguson, R.M.; Sutherland D.E.R.; Kim, T., et al (1981) The in vitro assessment of the immunosuppressive effect of fractionated total lymphoid irradiation in renal allotransplantation. Transplant Proc, 3:1673-1675.

Finkel, T. (1998). Oxygen radicals and signaling. Current Opinion in Cell Biology, 10:248–253.

Fudaba, Y.; Spitzer ,T.R.; Shaffer, J., et al.(2006) Myeloma responses and tolerance following combined kidney and nonmyeloablative marrow transplantation: in vivo and in vitro analyses. Am J Transplant ;6(9):2121–2133.

Fujimoto M, Serada S, Mihara M, et al (2008) Interleukin-6 blockade suppresses autoimmune arthritis in mice by the inhibition of infl ammatory Th17 responses. Arthritis Rheum; 58:3710-9.

Gallucci, S. ; Lolkema, M. ; Matzinger, P. (1999). Natural adjuvants:endogenous activators of dendritic cells. Nat Med 5:1249–1255.

Golshayan, D.; Jiang, S.; Tsang, J.; et al.(2007) In vitro-expanded donor alloantigenspecific CD4+CD25+ regulatory T cells promote experimental transplantation tolerance. Blood;109(2):827–835.

Graca L, Cobbold SP, Waldmann H. (2002) Identification of regulatory T cells in tolerated allografts. J Exp Med ;195(12):1641–1646.

Graca, L., Daley, S., Fairchild, P.J.,et al. (2006) . Co-receptor and co-stimulation blockade for mixed chimerism and tolerance without myelosuppressive conditioning. BMC Immunol;7:9.

Gray, C.M; Smit Jam; Myburgh J.A (1989): Function and Numbers of natural killer (NK) cells in patients conditioned with total lymphoid irradiation (TLI). Tranplant Proc; 21(1):1980-1981.

Hallahan, D.E. & Virudachalam, S. (1999). Accumulation of P-selectin in the lumen of irradiated blood vessels. Radiat Res 152:6–13.

Hallahan, D.E.; Spriggs, D.R.; Beckett, M.A et al. (1989). Increased tumor necrosis factor alpha mRNA after cellular exposure to ionizing radiation. Proc Natl Acad Sci USA 86:10104–10107.

Hashimoto, S.; Shirato, H.; Hosokawa, M.; et al. (1999). The suppression of metastases and the change in host immune response after low-dose total-body irradiation in tumor-bearing rats. Radiation Research, 151:717-724.

Hauser SH, Calorini L, Wazer DE; et al. (1993). Radiation-enhanced expression of major histocompatibility complex class I antigen H-2Db in B16 melanoma cells. Cancer Res 53:1952-1955.

Hayamizu, K.; Lan, F.; Huie, P., Sibley,R.K.; et al. (1999) Comparison of chimeric acid and non-chimeric tolerance using posttransplant total lymphoid irradiation: cytokine expression and chronic rejection.Transplantation ;68(7):1036–1044.

Higuchi, M.; Zeng, D.; Shizuru, J.; et al. (2002). Immune tolerance to combined organ and bone marrow transplants after fractionated lymphoid irradiation involves regulatory NK T cells and clonal deletion. J Immunol 2002;169(10):5564–5570.

Hoffmann P, Boeld TJ, Eder R, et al. (2009) Loss of FOXP3 expression in natural human CD4+CD25+ regulatory T cells upon repetitive in vitro stimulation. Eur J Immunol ;39:1088–97.

Ildstad ST, Sachs DH (1984). Reconstitution with syngeneic plus allogeneic or xenogeneic bone marrow Leads to specific acceptance of allografts orxenografts. Nature;307(5947):168-170.

Ishihara, H., Tanaka, I.; Nemoto, K.; et al. (1995). Immediate-early, transient induction of the interleukin-1 beta gene in mouse spleen macrophages by ionizing radiation. J Radiat Res (Tokyo) 36:112-124.

Janeway Jr, C.A. & Medzhitov, R. (2002). Innate immune recognition. Annu Rev Immunol 20:197-216.

James,R.F.; Lake, S.P.; Chamberlain J., et al. (1989). Gamma irradiation of isolated rat islets pretransplantation produces indefinite allograft survival in cyclosporine-treatedrecipients. Transplantation, 47:929-933.

Jin, S.Z.; Pan, X.N.; Wu N.; et al. (2007). Whole-body low dose irradiation promotes the efficacy of conventional radiotherapy for cancer and possible mechanisms. Dose Response 5:349–358.

Jonathan, E.C.; Bernhard, E.J; McKenna, W.G. (1999). How does radiation kill cells? Current Opinion in Chemical Biology, 3:77–83.

Kang,S.M.; Tang, Q.; Bluestone, J.A. (2007)CD4+CD25+ regulatory T cells in transplantation: progress, challenges and prospects. Am J Transplant ;7(6):1457–1463.

Kasid, U.; Suy, S.; Dent, P., et al. (1996). Activation of Raf by ionizing radiation. Nature, 382:813–816.

Kawai, T.; Cosimi, A.B; Wee, S.L.; et al. (2002). Effect of mixed hematopoietic chimerism on cardiac allograft survival in cynomolgus monkeys.Transplantation ; 73(11):1757–1764.

Kawai T.; Cosimi A.B.; Spitzer, T.R.; et al (2008). HLA mismatchedrenal transplantation without maintenance immunosuppression. N Engl J Med 2008;358 (4):353–361.

Kim, K.W.; Kim, S.H.; Shin, J.G.; et al. (2004). Direct injection of immature dendritic cells into irradiated tumor induces efficient antitumor immunity. Int J Cancer 109:685–690.

Kipnis, J.; Avidan, H.; Markovich, Y.; et al. (2004). Low-dose gamma-irradiation promotes survival of injured neurons in the central nervous system via homeostasis-driven proliferation of T cells. European Journal of Neuroscience 19:1191–1198.

Lake, R.A. & Robinson, B. W. (2005). Immunotherapy and chemotherapy – a practical partnership. Nat Rev Cancer 5: 397–405.

Lambert, J.F., Colvin, G.A.; Zhong S., et al (2002). H2-mismatched transplantation with repetitive cell infusions and CD40 ligand antibody infusions without myeloablation. Br J Haematol ;119(1):155–163.

Lan F, Hayamizu K, Strober S (2000). Cyclosporine facilitates chimeric and inhibits nonchimeric tolerance after posttransplant total lymphoid irradiation. Transplantation;69(4):649–655.

Lander, H.M.; Tauras, J.M.; Ogiste, J.S., et al(1997). Activation of the receptor for advanced glycation end products triggers a p21(ras)-dependent mitogen-activated protein kinase pathway regulated by oxidant stress. Journal of Biological Chemistry, 272:17810–17814.

Laylor R, Dewchand H, Simpson E, et al. (2005). Engraftment of allogeneic hematopoietic stem cells requires both inhibition of host-versus-graft responses and 'space' for homeostatic expansion. Transplantation;79:1484–91.

Liao , Y.P.; Wang, C.C.; Butterfield, L.H.; et al. (2004). Ionizing radiation affects human MART-1 melanoma antigen processing and presentation by dendritic cells. J Immunol 173:2462–2469.

Liu, R.; Xiong, S.; Zhang, L.; et al.(2010). Enhancement of antitumor immunity by low-dose total body irradiationis associated with selectively decreasing the proportion and number of T regulatory cells. Cellular & Molecular Immunology, 7:157–162.

Liu, S.Z.; Jin, S.Z;, Liu, X.D.; et al. (2001). Role of CD28/B7 costimulation and IL-12/IL-10 interaction in the radiationinduced immune changes. BMC Immunology 2:8.

Lohr, F.; Hu, K.; Haroon Z.; et al. (2000). Combination treatment of murine tumors by adenovirus-mediated local B7/IL12 immunotherapy and radiotherapy. Mol Ther 2:195–203.

Lohr, J.; Knoechel, B.; Wang, J.J.; et al (2006). Role of IL-17 and regulatory T lymphocytes in a systemic autoimmune disease. J Exp Med ;203:2785–91.

Macagno, A.; Napolitani, G.; Lanzavecchia, A. ; et al., (2007). Duration, combination and timing:the signal integration model of dendritic cell activation. Trends Immunol 28:227–233.

Mason, K.A.; Ariga, H. ; Neal, R. ; et al. (2005). Targeting toll-like receptor 9 with CpG oligodeoxynucleotides enhances tumor response to fractionated radiotherapy. Clin Cancer Res 11:361–369.

Mcbride, W.II.; Chiang, C.S.; Olson, J.L, et al (2004). A sense of danger from radiation. Radiat Res 2004, 162:1-19.

Mengde, C., et al. (2011). Different radiosensitivity of CD4þCD25þ regulatory T cells and effector T cells to low dose gamma irradiation in vitro. Int. J. Radiat. Biol., 87(1) : 71–80.

Merrick, A.; Errington, F.; Milward, K.; et al. (2005). Immunosuppressive effects of radiation on human dendritic cells:reduced IL-12 production on activation and impairment of naive T-cellpriming. Br J Cancer 92:1450–1458.

Milas, L.; Mason, K.A.; Ariga, H. ; et al. (2004). CpG oligodeoxynucleotide enhances tumor response to radiation. Cancer Res 64:5074–5077.

Miller GM, Kim DW, Andres ML; et al. (2003). Changes in the activation and reconstitution of lymphocytes resulting from total-body irradiation correlate with slowed tumor growth. Oncology 65:229–241.

Minamimura, K., Gao, W., Maki, T. (2006) CD4+ regulatory T cells are spared from deletion by antilymphocyteserum, a polyclonal anti-T cell antibody.J Immunol;176(7):4125–4132.

Morgan ME, Sutmuller RP, Witteveen HJ, et al.(2003) CD25+ cell depletion hastens the onset of severe disease in collagen-induced arthritis. Arthritis Rheum ;48:1452–60.

Morgan ME, Flierman R, van Duivenvoorde LM, et al. (2005) Effective treatment of collageninduced arthritis by adoptive transfer of CD25+ regulatory T cells. Arthritis Rheum 52:2212–21.

Muraro, P.A., Douek, D.C., Packer, A.; et al (2005). Thymic output generates a new and diverse TCR repertoire after autologous stem cell transplantation in multiple sclerosis patients. J Exp Med 2005;201:805–16.

Nadal E, Garin M, Kaeda J, et al (2007) Increased frequencies of CD4(+)CD25(high) T(regs) correlate with disease relapse after allogeneic stem cell transplantation for chronic myeloid leukemia. Leukemia ;21:472–9.

Nadkarni S, Mauri C, Ehrenstein MR.(2007) Anti-TNF-alpha therapy induces a distinct regulatory T cell population in patients with rheumatoid arthritis via TGF-beta. J Exp Med;204:33–9.

Nador, R.G; Hongo, D; Yao, Z et al.; (2010) The Changed Balance of Regulatory and Naive T Cells Promotes Tolerance After TLI and Anti-T Cell Antibody Conditioning. Am J Transplant.; 10(2): 262–272.

Nakatsukasa H, Tsukimoto M, Ohshima Y, et al. (2008) Suppressing effect of low-dose gamma-ray irradiation on collagen-induced arthritis. J Radiat Res 2008;49:381–389.

Nemoto K, Ishihara, H., Tanaka, I.; et al. (1995). Expression of IL-1 beta mRNA in mice after whole body X-irradiation. J Radiat Res (Tokyo) 36:125–133.

Nikitina EY, Gabrilovich DI. (2001). Combination of gammairradiation and dendritic cell administration induces apotent antitumor response in tumor-bearing mice:approach to treatment of advanced stage cancer. Int J Cancer 94: 825–833.

North RJ. (1986). Radiation-induced, immunologicallymediated regression of an established tumor as an example of successful therapeutic immunomanipulation Preferential elimination of suppressor T cells allows sustained production of effector T cells. J Exp Med 164: 1652–1666.

Notley CA, Inglis JJ, Alzabin S, et al. (2008). Blockade of tumor necrosis factor in collageninduced arthritis reveals a novel immunoregulatory pathway for Th1 and Th17 cells. J Exp Med;205:2491–2497.

Paulos, C.M.; Wrzesinski, C.; Kaiser, A., et al. (2007). Microbial translocation augments the function of adoptively transferred self/tumor-specific CD8 T cells via TLR4 signaling. J Clin Invest 117: 2197–2204.

Pillai, A.B.; George, T.I., Dutt, S.; et al. (2009) Host natural killer T cells induce an IL-4 dependent expansion of donor CD4+CD25+Foxp3+ Tregs that protects against graft-versus-host disease. Blood.

Poltorak, A.; He, X.; Smirnova, I.; et al. (1998). Defective LPS signaling in C3H/HeJ and C57BL/10ScCr mice:mutations in Tlr4 gene. Science 282: 2085–2088.

Reuben JM; Korbling M; Gao H, et al.; (2004). The effect of low dose gamma irradiation on the differentiation and maturationof monocyte derived dendritic cells. Journal of Gravitational Physiology 11:P49–52.

Rho, H.S.; Park S.S.; Lee, C.E. (2004). Gamma irradiation up-regulatesexpression of B cell differentiation molecule CD23 by NFkappaB activation. Journal of Biochemistry and Molecular Biology 37:507–514.

Roord ST, de Jager W, Boon L, et al.(2008) Autologous bone marrow transplantation in autoimmune arthritis restores immune homeostasis through CD4+CD25+Foxp3+ regulatory T cells. Blood;111:5233–41.

Roses R E; Xu M; Koski GK; et al. (2008). Radiation therapy and Toll-like receptor signaling: Implications for the treatment of cancer. Oncogene 27:200–207.

Safwat A. (2000a). The immunobiology of low-dose total-body irradiation: More questions than answers. Radiation Research 153(5 Pt 1):599–604.

Safwat A.(2000b). The role of low-dose total body irradiation in treatment of non-hodgkin's lymphoma: A new look at an old method. Radiotherapy & Oncology 56:1–8.

Sakaguchi N, Takahashi T, Hata H, et al. (2003) Altered thymic T-cell selection due to a mutation of the ZAP-70 gene causes autoimmune arthritis in mice. Nature;426:454–60.

Sakaguchi S. (2005) Naturally arising Foxp3-expressing CD25+CD4+ regulatory T cells in immunological tolerance to self and non-self. Nat Immunol 2005;6(4):345–352.

Sauter B, Albert ML, Francisco L.; et al. (2000). Consequences of cell death:exposureto necrotic tumor cells, but not primary tissue cells orapoptotic cells, induces the maturation of immunostimulatory dendritic cells. J Exp Med 191:423–434.

Seetharam, S.; Staba, M.J.; Schumm, L.P. ; et al. (1999). Enhanced eradication of local and distant tumors by genetically produced interleukin-12 and radiation. Int J Oncol 15:769–773.

Scandling, J.D.; Busque S.; Dejbakhsh-Jones S.; et al (2008). Tolerance and chimerism after renal and hematopoietic-cell transplantation. N Engl J Med 2008;358(4):362–368.

Scheffer SR, Nave H, Korangy F, et al. (2003). Apoptotic, but not necrotic, tumor cell vaccines induce a potent immune response in vivo. Int J Cancer 103:205–211.

Schiopu, A. & Wood, K.J. (2008) Regulatory T cells: hypes and limitations. Curr Opin Organ Transplant 2008;13 (4):333–338.

Schu¨ tze S.; Tchikov, V.; Schneider-Brachert, W. (2008). Regulation of TNFR1 and CD95 signalling by receptor compartmentalization. Nature Reviews. Molecular Cell Biology 9:655–662.

Shan, Y.X.; Jin, S.Z.; Liu, X.D.; et al. (2007). Ionizing radiation stimulates secretion of pro-inflammatory cytokines: Dose response relationship, mechanisms and implications.Radiation and Environmental Biophysics 46:21–29.

Shankar, B.; Premachandran, S.; Bharambe, S.D.; et al. (1999). Modification of immune response by low dose ionizing radiation: Role of apoptosis. Immunology Letters 68:237–245.

Shi, Y.; White, D.; He, L. ; et al.; (2007). Toll-like receptor-7 tolerizes malignant B cells and enhances killing by cytotoxic agents. Cancer Res 67:1823–1831.

Shigematsu, A., Adachi, Y., Koike-Kiriyama, N., et al. (2007). Effects of low- dose irradiation on enhancement of immunity by dendritic cells. J Radiat Res (Tokyo) 48:51–55.

Slavin S, Strober S, Fuks Z (1977), et al. Induction of specific tissue transplantation tolerance using fractionated total lymphoid irradiation in adult mice: long-term survival of allogeneic bone marrow and skin grafts. J Exp Med;146(1):34–48.

Slavin, S.; Reitz, B.; Bieber, C.P.; et al (1978). Transplantation tolerance in adult rats using total lymphoid irradiation: permanent survival of skin, heart, and marrow allografts. J Exp Med;147(3):700–707.

Slavin, S.; Strober, S.; Fuks, Z.; Kapla, H.S. (1976). Long-term survival of skin allografts in mice treated with fractionated total lymphoid irradiation. Science ;193(4259):1252–1254.

Sykes M. (2001) Mixed chimerism and transplant tolerance. Immunity 2001;14(4):417–42.

Tang Q, Henriksen KJ, Bi M, et al. In vitro-expanded antigen-specifi c regulatory T cells suppress autoimmune diabetes. J Exp Med 2004;199:1455–65.

Villar, R.C.; Chocair, P.R.; Nadalin, W.; et al (2008). Total Lymphoid Irradiation for pretransplant immunossuppression and reccurrence of focal segmental glomerulosclerosis Transpl Int., Mar;21(3):286-9.

Waer, M.; Vanrenterghen, E.; Van der schueren, E., et al (1987). Identification and function of a major OKT3, OKT8, Leu-7, posiitve lymphocyte subpopulation in renal transplant recipients treated with total lymphoid irradiation. Transplant Proc 19(1):1570-1571.

Wasserman, J.; Blomgren, H; Rotstein, S; et al. (1989). Immunosuppression in irradiated breastcancer patients: in vitro effect of cyclooxygenase inhibitors. Bull N Y Acad Med, 65:36–44.

Wekerle T.; Sayegh, M.H.;Hill J.; et al.(1998) Extrathymic T cell deletion and allogeneic stem cell engraftment induced with costimulatory blockade is followed by central T cell tolerance. J Exp Med 187(12):2037–2044.

Wekerle, T.; Kurtz, J.; Ito, H.; et al. (2000) Allogeneic bone marrow transplantation with co-stimulatory blockade induces macrochimerism and tolerance without cytoreductive host treatment. Nat Med 2000;6(4):464–469.

Weng L, Dyson J, Dazzi F. (2007) Low-intensity transplant regimens facilitate recruitment of donor- specific regulatory T cells that promote hematopoietic engraftment. Proc Natl Acad Sci USA;104:8415–20.

Weng, L.; Willians, O.S.; Vieira, P.L. et al., (2010). The therapeutic activity of low-dose irradiation on experimental arthritis depends on the induction of endogenous regulatory T cell activity Ann Rheum Dis 2010;69:1519–1526.

Weichselbaum, R.R.; Hallahan, D. E.; Beckett, M.A. ; et al. (1994). Gene therapy targeted by radiation preferentially radiosensitizes tumor cells. Cancer Res 54:4266–4269.

Wesa, A.; Kalinski, P.; Kirkwood, J.M. , et al. (2007). Polarized type-1 dendritic cells (DC1) producing high levels of IL-12 family members rescue patient TH1-type antimelanoma CD4+ T cell responses in vitro. J Immunother 30:75– 82.

Wing K, Fehervari Z, Sakaguchi S. (2006). Emerging possibilities in the development and function of regulatory T cells. International Immunology 18:991–1000.

Wood,K.J.; Sakaguchi, S. (2003). Regulatory T cells in transplantation tolerance. Nat Rev Immunol 2003;3(3):199–210.

Wrzesinski C, Paulos CM, Gattinoni L et al. (2007). Hematopoietic stem cells promote the expansion and function of adoptively transferred antitumor CD8 T cells. J Clin Invest 117:492–501.

Xiao X, Kroemer A, Gao W, et al. (2008) OX40/OX40L costimulation affects induction of Foxp3+ regulatory T cells in part by expanding memory T cells in vivo. J Immunol;181:3193–201.

Xu, S.; Koski, G. K. ; Maeurer, M.; et al. (2003). Rapid high efficiency sensitization of CD8+ T cells to tumor antigens by dendritic cells leads to enhanced functional avidity and direct tumor recognition through an IL-12-dependent mechanism. J Immunol 171:2251–2261.

Yao, Z.; Liu, Y.; Jones, J.; Strober, S. (2009). Differences in Bcl-2 expression by T-cell subsets alter their balance after in vivo irradiation to favor CD4+Bcl-2hi NKT cells. Eur J Immunol;39(3):763–775.

Zhang, B.; Bowerman, N. A., Salama, J.K., et al. (2007). Induced sensitization of tumor stroma leads to eradication of established cancer by T cells. J Exp Med 204:49–55.

Zou W. (2006) . Regulatory T cells, tumour immunity and immunotherapy. Nature Reviews. Immunology 6:295–307.

6

Induction Therapy in Renal Transplant Recipients

Cheguevara Afaneh, Meredith J. Aull, Sandip Kapur and David B. Leeser
Department of Surgery, Division of Transplant Surgery
New York-Presbyterian Hospital- Weill Cornell Medical College, New York, NY
USA

1. Introduction

1.1 Historical overview

Renal transplantation remains the most effective treatment modality for end-stage renal disease. The initial results with renal transplantation were plagued with significant perioperative morbidity and high rates of immunological events. At the time, the transplant physician's armamentarium consisted of glucocorticoids and azathioprine. As modifications and improvements in surgical technique reduced morbidity, immunological events remained formidable foes to the transplant physician. Significant efforts were undertaken to elucidate the components and mechanisms of these immunological events, ultimately leading to the discovery of lymphocytes as the primary culprits in acute rejection. Early preclinical trials demonstrated that lymphocyte-specific antibodies could be induced in animal models by injecting them with lymphocytes. The serum could then be isolated and re-injected in other animals to decrease the lymphocyte count. Thus, these experiments lead to the earliest forms of antilymphocyte antibody formulations, including antithymocyte globulin, antilymphocyte serum, and antilymphocyte globulin (Bishop et al., 1975; Cosimi et al., 1976). These initial medications had little specificity and broad effects, but their potent ability to treat acute rejection episodes led to their widespread use in the 1970's (Cosimi, 1981a).

The extensive use of these formulations exposed their various drawbacks. Because of nonspecific binding, cross-reactivity with various hematopoietic cells revealed dose-limiting side effects including thrombocytopenia, anemia, and neutropenia (Henricsson et al., 1977; Rosenberg, 1975). Additionally, the method of preparation was not standardized, thus leading to dosing variations. Because these formulations were typically made in rabbits or horses, the proteins had potential antigenic properties leading to the development of serum sickness, cytokine release syndrome, or even anaphylaxis (Niblack et al., 1987; Prin Mathieu et al., 1997; Tatum et al., 1984).

The development of specific, monoclonal antibodies by Kohler and Milstein circumvented many of the drawbacks of polyclonal formulations, including lack of specificity and variability in preparation (Kohler & Milstein, 1975). Muromonab, or OKT3, was the first monoclonal antibody prepared from mouse, which is specific for cluster of differentiation 3 (CD3) (Cosimi et al, 1981b). OKT3 was effective at specifically depleting T cells from the circulation, and became widely used as a valuable tool to combat acute rejection episodes (Ortho Multicenter Transplant Study Group, 1985; Ponticelli et al., 1987). Nevertheless, these monoclonal formulations still maintained some of the similar side effect profile of the polyclonal formulations, including cytokine release syndrome and human antigenic response to animal proteins, which lead to limited dosing in some patients (Jaffers et al., 1986).

The 1980's marked an important era in transplantation with new advances in genetic engineering. Monoclonal antibodies became more sophisticated, targeting specific T cell populations and allowing blockade of T cell activation, such as the interleukin-2 receptor (IL-2R) or CD25 (Vincenti et al., 1997). Moreover, the ability to avoid antigenic proteins by encoding genetic sequences of DNA binding sites of animal proteins onto human antibodies led to the development of chimeric monoclonal antibodies (Boulianne et al., 1984; Jones et al., 1986; Morrison et al., 1984). Using these techniques, soluble fusion proteins can be formed by merging nonantibody receptors with the Fc portion of antibodies.

1.2 Antibodies

Comprehension of the structure and function of antibodies is critical to understanding the efficacy of antibody induction therapy. Antibodies are composed of two identical heavy chains (either μ, γ, α, ε, or δ) and two identical light chains (either κ or λ). The heavy and light chain portions create two identical antigen binding sites (Fab fragment) which are held together by the common region, termed the Fc portion (Capra & Edmundson, 1977). The type of heavy chain differentiates the immunoglobulin type as IgM, IgG, IgA, IgE, and IgD. In clinical transplantation, the IgG molecule is typically utilized, as it's readily produced and structurally feasible to manipulate with ease (Fig. 1).

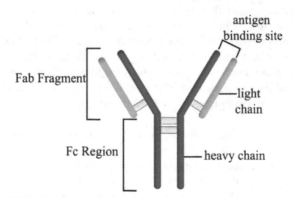

Fig. 1. Basic antibody structure. Depicted is a standard IgG molecule. The heavy chains are colored in blue, while the light chains are colored in green. The yellow lines signify the disulfide bonds

Antibodies are present on the surface of B cells. Upon secretion into the serum, antibodies are able to neutralize circulating antigens. Antibodies maintain their effector functions irrespective of species, which make them useful in early studies of antibody therapies in transplantation. Antibodies are capable of various functions, including mimicking activating ligands of receptors and serving as receptor inhibitors by blocking the ligand binding site

(Tite et al., 1986; Wong et al., 1990). In some instances, antibody binding can lead to both activation and inhibition by inducing surface molecule internalization, whereby the molecule is removed from the surface of the cell (Kerr & Atkins, 1989). This results in a negligible net effect. A major limitation of antibody use is the inability to directly bind intracellular molecules.

Antibodies have the ability to deplete target cells through two fundamental mechanisms. First, antibodies have the capability to activate the complement system resulting in complement-mediated lysis of target cells. Second, certain cells with Fc region receptors have the ability to phagocytose cells covered with antibodies through a mechanism termed antibody-dependent cellular cytotoxicity (ADCC)(Fig.2). The efficacy with which this occurs depends upon the Fab fragment and the Fc region (Ferrant et al., 2004). It is important to note that cells which have significantly matured, or memory cells, are somewhat resistant to antibody-dependent depletion mechanisms, possibly due to increased expression of antiapoptotic or complement regulatory genes (Pearl et al, 2005).

The vast properties of antibodies make them suitable for therapeutic indications. Nevertheless, even minor changes in antibody structure can significantly alter function. Additionally, the interplay of the complement system and ADCC properties further complicates the predicted function of various antibody-depleting therapies.

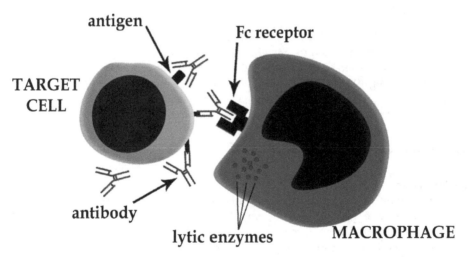

Fig. 2. Antibody-dependent cellular cytotoxicity (ADCC). The Fc receptor on the machrophage is used to bind the constant Fc portion of antibodies to facilitate engulfment of cells coated with antibodies

1.3 Clinical classification of induction agents

Induction immunosuppressive medications can be classified into two groups: depleting agents and non-depleting agents. The categorization is based on the ability of the medication to target specific antigens or cells, leading to a decrease in the total expression or cell count. Most depleting agents are relatively potent with potential for toxicity with prolonged administration. Non-depleting agents are generally well-tolerated. Depleting agents are also used for severe or refractory cases of acute rejection and have proven to be more effective than glucocorticoids in treating episodes of acute rejection (Webster et al., 2006). In addition, the use of induction agents has decreased the rates of acute rejection in the first 6 months compared to no induction therapy (Szczech et al., 1997). Although these short-term benefits appear promising, long-term outcomes, including patient and graft survival rates, have not been shown to be altered by the use of induction therapy. This is possibly related to the effects of long-term maintenance immunosuppressive therapy or patient co-morbidities.

The overall success of a transplanted renal allograft is contingent on both surgical prowess and the use of potent immunosuppressive medications. Although induction therapy has not affected surgical morbidity, the rate of allograft thrombosis has been shown to be reduced in children with the use of induction agents (Humar et al., 2001; Singh et al., 1997). However, not all medications used are FDA-approved for induction therapy. Moreover, it is important to note that these medications are not without definite risks, including serious infectious complications and the development of post-transplant lymphoproliferative disorder (PTLD), which has been well-described with the use of OKT3 and maintenance immunosuppression (Bustami et al., 2004; Jamil et al., 1999). Because of the effects of depleting agents on T cells, appropriate prophylactic therapies should be administered to all transplant recipients. Duration of therapy is typically contingent on the donor and recipient immunological history. Thus, tailoring the immunosuppressive regimen to each patient is critical to avoiding complications.

In 1995 induction therapy was used in less than half of all kidney transplants in the United States, while 10 years later, approximately 70% of all kidney transplant recipients received induction therapy (Meier-Kriesche et al., 2006). Given the availability of various potent, specific induction agents in modern transplantation, the clinical dilemma lies in selecting the most appropriate agent for a given patient, taking into account co-morbidities, donor quality, immunological status, and planned maintenance therapy.

2. Depleting agents

2.1 Antithymocyte globulin
2.1.1 Mechanism

Various polyclonal depleting agents are available; however, this discussion will focus on rabbit antithymocyte globulin (rATG). In rATG, the polyclonal heterologous antibody formulation is produced from immunizing rabbits with human thymocytes, which serve as the immunogens (Fig. 3) (Hardinger, 2006). The rabbit serum is then gathered and purified to remove antibodies with potentially detrimental effects and only the IgG isotypes are collected. Despite these purification techniques, it is possible that the majority of antibodies in these formulations serve no therapeutic purpose (Bonnefoy-Berard et al., 1991). When administered to humans, the rATG antibody formulations bind all antigens that the rabbits were exposed to during the immunization process.

Rabbit ATG binds multiple T cell surface antigens and receptors involved in antigen recognition, adhesion and costimulation. These include CD2, CD3, CD4, CD5, CD8, CD28, CD45, and CD40L. In addition, rATG may also bind non-T cell molecules such as CD16, CD20, CD56, and the major histocompatibility molecules (class I and II) (Bonnefoy-Berard et al., 1991; Hardinger, 2006). The depleting effect of rATG occurs within 24 hours of administration and can persist with a prolonged serum half-life of several weeks (Bunn et al., 1996; Guttmann et al., 1997). The effects of lymphocyte depletion are persists for years following administration, as evidenced by selectively low CD4[+] T cell counts (Brennan et al., 1999; Hardinger et al., 2004).

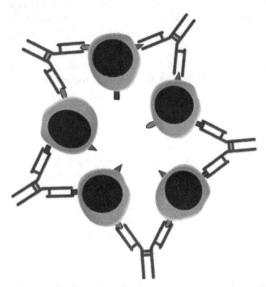

Fig. 3. Polyclonal antibodies. Polyclonal antibodies are non-specific and bind multiple antigens as shown in the figure

2.1.2 Applications
Rabbit ATG has been approved for use as an induction agent and for the treatment of acute rejection in Europe since 1984 (IMTIX-SangStat, 2003). However, in the United States, rATG is indicated only for the treatment of acute rejection (as of 1998). Nevertheless, it is routinely administered as induction therapy in many centers in the United States. Early studies demonstrated an increased risk of infectious complications and post-transplant malignancy when administered in conjunction with cyclosporine (Merion et al., 1984). With a better understanding of PTLD, improved infectious prophylaxis protocols, and experience using lower doses of rATG, the use of rATG as an induction agent has increased.

The most effective use of rATG depends on timing of administration. Ideally, the first dose should be given before the vascular anastomosis at the time of transplantation (typical dose 1.5mg/kg/dose for a total of 4.5 to 7.5 mg/kg). This may minimize ischemia-reperfusion injury and potentially prevent the development of delayed graft function (Shoskes & Halloran, 1996). Delayed graft function is known to portend poorer outcomes in kidney transplant recipients, thus rATG has been used in patients at higher risk of developing this delayed graft function, including recipients of donation after cardiac death donors, and recipients of extended criteria donors (Beiras-Fernandez et al., 2006; Cecka et al., 1993; Shield et al., 1997). It is also administered in patients at higher risk of developing acute rejection in the perioperative period, such as retransplants and patients who may have prolonged avoidance of calcineurin inhibitors as well as to minimize maintenance therapies such as facilitating early corticosteroid withdrawl (Schaffer et al., 2003; Shield et al., 1997).

The use of rATG to treat severe or refractory acute cellular rejection episodes has been well-established. Refractory acute cellular rejection is defined as failure to respond to 3 consecutive days of bolus methylprednisolone (i.e. 500 mg per day) treatment. rATG is superior to glucocorticoids in treating acute cellular rejection episodes. Compared to other polyclonal antibody formulations, rATG has proven to be superior in reversing steroid-resistant rejection and prolonging rejection-free events (Gaber et al., 1998). Patient or graft survival, however, have not been shown to be affected. Given the potency of rATG, it is typically used as supplemental agent to corticosteroids for the treatment of severe or refractory episodes of acute rejection. Additionally, recurrent episodes of acute rejection may be treated with multiple courses of rATG as long as preformed antirabbit antibodies are not present (Bock et al., 1995).

2.1.3 Adverse effects

Patients treated with rATG may experience a variety of side effects. It has been associated with a phenomenon called cytokine release syndrome (Fig. 4), which is common to many polyclonal antibody formulations. Patients may experience mild flu-like symptoms, such as fever, chills, nausea, urticaria, rash, and headache (Guttmann et al., 1997). This occurs as a result of increased production of tumor necrosis factor-α, IL-1, and IL-6 from antibody binding to cell surface receptors and ensuing cell lysis (Debets et al., 1989; Guttmann et al., 1997; Hardinger, 2006). Premedication with corticosteroids, antipyretics, and antihistamines can prevent and/or treat the flu-like symptoms that can occur in a subset of kidney transplant recipients. In some cases, patients may develop more severe shock-like reactions, such as dyspnea, severe hypotension, pulmonary edema, or even anaphylaxis. Although patients frequently experience the mild flu-like symptoms and not the more severe reactions, recipient co-morbid conditions, such as cardiac or pulmonary disease, should be considered when selecting rATG as an induction agent. Serum sickness has also been associated with rATG administration in up to 7-10% of patients (Buchler et al., 2003; Mourad et al., 2001).

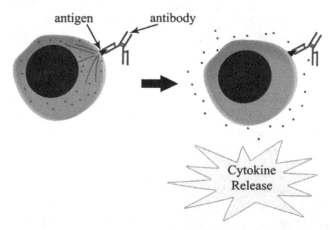

Fig. 4. Antibody activation and cytokine release. Antibodies can bind antigens resulting in activation of the cell and cytokine release as illustrated in the figure

Hematological adverse events may occur, including leucopenia and thrombocytopenia. It is important to monitor white blood cell, lymphocyte, and platelet counts for patients receiving rATG. Not surprisingly, these events may lead to an increase in infectious complications, including cytomegalovirus (CMV), herpes simplex virus, Epstein-Barr virus (EBV), and varicella (Abott et al., 2002; Gourishankar et al., 2004).

2.2 Muromonab (OKT3)
2.2.1 Mechanism
Muromonab, or OKT3, is a monoclonal antibody. It is an IgG2 mouse antibody known to bind the epsilon component of human CD3. The CD3 complex is a T cell receptor intimately involved in T cell signaling and activation via a calcineurin-dependent pathway (Ortho Multicenter Transplant Study Group, 1985). Once the antibody binds the target cell, complement is activated leading to cell lysis and ADCC (Vallhonrat et al., 1999). By this method, most T cells are effectively removed from the peripheral circulation. However, the T cell binding also results in T cell activation before clearance, leading to systemic cytokine release. When OKT3 binds the T cell receptor, the CD3 complex is internalized (Fig. 5) to prevent further activation by persistent antigen presence (Chatenoud et al., 1990). Effectively, T cells that fail to be cleared are unable to be activated by the CD3 complex.

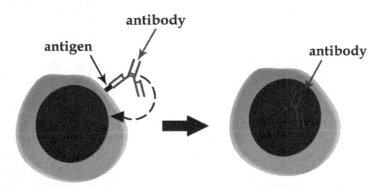

Fig. 5. Internalization of an antibody. This figure is an example of internalization of the antigen-antibody complex after activation to prevent further stimulation by persistently low level of antibody in the peripheral circulation (i.e. OKT3 binding)

2.2.2 Applications
Early studies demonstrated the efficacy of OKT3 as an induction agent in kidney transplantation in conjunction with maintenance immunosuppression (Debure et al., 1988; Norman et al., 1988; Vigeral et al., 1986). Efficacy relies on serum availability, thus once administration of OKT3 ceases, maintenance immunosuppressive therapy is required. Typical dosing is 5 to 10 mg/dose through a peripheral or central line. Premedication with methylprednisolone, acetaminophen, and diphenhydramine can significantly lower the amount of cytokine release associated with first infusion (Chatenoud et al., 1991). Additionally, slower administration rates are helpful in blunting the cytokine response. Dosing can be continued for up to 14 days for a total dose of 70 mg. Patients with

significant sensitization have especially benefitted from OKT3 (Opelz, 1995). In addition, recipients of renal allografts experiencing delayed graft function benefit from OKT3 infusion, as calcineurin inhibitor therapy can be delayed, avoiding added renal toxicity (Benvenisty et al., 1990).

Early studies of OKT3 demonstrated a reduction in acute rejection rates and time to first rejection episodes; however, overall patient and graft survival rates were not changed (Henry et al., 2001; Norman et al., 1993). Its use has been linked to various infectious and malignant morbidities. Aseptic meningitis has also been linked to its use (Martin et al., 2002). Moreover, PTLD rates are significantly increased, especially in EBV negative recipients receiving EBV positive allografts (Thistlethwaite et al., 1988; Cherikh et al., 2003). The significant side effect profile and immunogenicity of OKT3 has lead to a decline in its use as an induction agent.

OKT3 remains an effective treatment for severe episodes of acute cellular rejection, or those refractory to steroid therapy and rATG. In the majority of cases of vigorous rejection, OKT3 has proven efficacious (Cosimi et al., 1981b; Ortho Multicenter Transplant Study Group, 1985; Thistlethwaite et al., 1987). The efficacy of OKT3 is maintained even if prior lymphocyte depleting agents have been used (Ponticelli et al., 1987). However, timing of therapy is important, as a delay in treatment following the 3 days of high-dose methylprednisolone therapy for steroid-resistant acute rejection is associated with decreased success (Tesi et al., 1993). OKT3 has also been used to treat vascular rejection episodes (Banff grade 2 or 3) (Kamath et al., 1997).

2.2.3 Adverse effects

As a monoclonal antibody, OKT3 selectively targets T cells, avoiding the leucopenia and thrombocytopenia associated with rATG. Similar to rATG, OKT3 is associated with cytokine release syndrome. With respect to OKT3, this is more pronounced, especially with the first dose as the T cells may be in a more activated state (i.e. acute cellular rejection). The cytokine release syndrome with OKT3 results in severe flu-like symptoms, including fever, chills, malaise, nausea, vomiting, and even rigors (Thistlethwaite et al., 1988). As vascular permeability increases, patients may experience pulmonary edema, hypotension, and volume overload. If there is renal dysfunction present, patients should undergo hemodialysis prior to first infusion to avoid volume-related complications. Patients should be closely monitored, especially during the initial infusions for cardiac or pulmonary complications.

The utilization of OKT3 is clearly associated with antimouse antibodies in at least 30% of patients, depending on the immunosuppression regimens used at the time (Colvin & Preffer, 1991; Schroeder et al., 1990). The antibodies form against the mouse IgG molecule. If there is antibody formation, OKT3 is typically not reused, although higher doses may overcome this. This can be documented by laboratory evidence of antimouse antibody (Chatenoud et al., 1986; Legendre et al., 1992).

2.3 Alemtuzumab
2.3.1 Mechanism

Alemtuzumab, or Campath-1H, is a monoclonal antibody to rat antihuman CD52 (Fig. 6). It is an IgG1 humanized molecule (Hale et al., 1986). CD52 is present in high abundance on most lymphocytes, including T cell, B cells, and monocytes, but not hematopoietic precursors (Hale, 2001). It effectively depletes T cells, and some B cells and monocytes in the circulation as well as the allograft (Kirk et al., 2003).

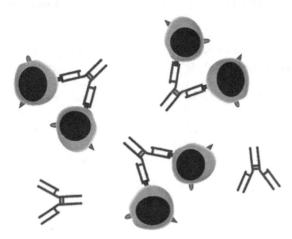

Fig. 6. Monoclonal antibodies. Monoclonal antibodies are specific and bind a single antigen as shown in the figure

2.3.2 Applications

Alemtuzumab has not been approved for use as an induction agent; however, this is a common off-label use. Currently, it is only approved to treat lymphogenous malignancies. As an off-label induction agent, it's been used with various immunosuppression regimens, including steroid-sparing regimens. Effectively, it depletes lymphocytes at the time of transplantation and last for several months to a year before the immune system is reconstituted (Gabardi et al., 2011). Alemtuzumab is given at a dose of 30 mg or 0.3 mg/kg through a peripheral line over 3 hours. Sometimes 2 doses are given, although T cells are expectedly removed within 1 hour of initial administration (Kirk et al., 2003; Pearl et al., 2005).

Alemtuzumab depletes all T cell subsets, but has a predilection for more naïve T cells (Pearl et al., 2005). Memory T cell subsets may not be depleted with this therapy, but these cell types are especially susceptible to calcineurin inhibitors. Because of the prompt and intense depletion, alemtuzumab is especially appealing to use in patients with delayed graft function, as calcineurin inhibitor therapy can be withheld to avoid concomitant calcineurin-induced renal insults.

Early studies of alemtuzumab demonstrated its efficacy as a treatment therapy for acute rejection; however, it was associated with significant infectious morbidity and mortality (Hale et al., 1986). Patients were significantly over-immunosuppressed, especially on a triple maintenance therapy. More recent literature has been small studies or anecdotal data (Clatworthy et al., 2009; Csapo et al., 2005; Jirasiritham et al., 2010). Because its efficacy is greatest against naïve T cells, its use in sensitized patients may-be limited.

In a recent study, alemtuzumab was prospectively compared to basiliximab and rATG as an induction agent in patients on a steroid-sparing immunosuppressive regimen (Hanaway et al., 2011). Alemtuzumab demonstrated lower short-term rates of acute rejection compared to basiliximab in patients at low-risk of developing acute rejection. At 3-years, however, the rates of acute rejection were no different between alemtuzumab and rATG. Additionally, patients receiving alemtuzumab did not experience an increased incidence of adverse events.

2.3.3 Adverse effects
Similar to other depleting agents (rATG and OKT3), alemtuzumab is also associated with cytokine release syndrome, albeit to a lesser extent. If properly premedicated with methylprednisolone, acetaminophen, and diphenhydramine, the cytokine release is blunted. Urticaria and rash manifestations are common, while anaphylaxis and hypotension have also been reported. It has not been associated with antibody formation, as in the case of OKT3. It has been linked to the development of autoimmune thyroiditis in patients treated with alemtuzumab for multiple sclerosis (Coles et al., 1999). This has also been reported in a renal transplant recipient treated with alemetuzumab (Kirk et al., 2006).

3. Non-depleting agents

3.1 Basiliximab
3.1.1 Mechanism
Basiliximab is a chimeric mouse-human monoclonal IgG1 antibody to CD25. CD25 is the α-subunit of the IL-2 receptor, which is a binding site of IL-2. Basiliximab inhibition of IL-2 binding occurs through steric hindrance (Fig.7). In this case, the effect is not depletional, but rather, preventative of early T cell activation (Gabardi et al., 2011).

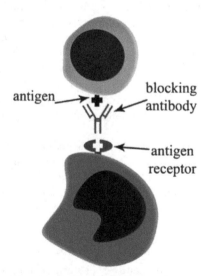

Fig. 7. Antibody blockade. In this figure the antibody functions by blocking the antigen from binding to the receptor

3.1.2 Applications
Basiliximab's biological bias for naïve T cells has limited its role to an induction agent. One dose is typically administered on the day of transplant as well as one dose on postoperative

day 4 (20 mg per dose) through a peripheral line. Its use has been associated with decreased rates of acute cellular rejection compared to no formal induction agent (besides methylprednisolone) on triple or double drug immunosuppression regimens (Kahan et al., 1999; Nashan et al., 1997). Additional studies comparing basiliximab induction to polyclonal antibody depleting induction agents in the setting of triple maintenance immunosuppression regimens have shown similar outcomes, including acute rejection rates and delayed graft function (Lebranchu et al., 2002; Mourad et al., 2004). Basiliximab induction has also been used in steroid avoidance immunosuppression regimens (Afaneh et al., 2010). In the setting of monotherapy or calcineurin inhibitor free regimens, basiliximab has not been shown to be useful (Parrott et al., 2005; Vincenti et al., 2001). In some instances of excellent allograft human leukocyte antigen (HLA)-matching (i.e. 2-haplotype matches), it's been used as an effective induction agent with steroid-sparing immunosuppressive regimens (Afaneh et al., 2010). Given the relatively mild side effect profile, basiliximab is well-tolerated in all patients, even those with significant cardiac or pulmonary co-morbidities. It has no role in the treatment of acute rejection episodes as a rescue agent.

3.1.3 Adverse effects

Because of the mechanism of action of basiliximab, the side effect profile is relatively mild (Kahan et al., 1999; Nashan et al., 1997). Cytokine release syndrome does not occur, as T cells are not activated or stimulated. The most serious adverse event is hypersensitivity, which is rare (<1%)(Gabardi et al., 2011). There is no increased risk of infectious complications or PTLD compared to no induction therapy (Cherikh et al., 2003).

3.2 Daclizumab
3.2.1 Mechanism

Similar to basiliximab, daclizumab is an antagonist to CD25; however, it is a humanized IgG1 antibody. The CD25 molecule was the first humanized monoclonal antibody to be successfully targeted in the field of transplantation (Kirkman et al., 1991). The mechanism of action of daclizumab essentially duplicates that of other IL-2 receptor antagonists.

3.2.2 Applications

Like basiliximab, daclizumab has been shown to decrease the incidence of acute cellular rejection when administered as an induction agent (Hershberger et al., 2005; Nashan et al., 1999). Given the favorable side effect profile, it is tolerated well in recipients, irrespective of co-morbid conditions. The main disadvantage of daclizumab, as compared to basiliximab, is that it is more costly and requires repeated administrations (Gabardi et al., 2011). Because the demand for the medication has been relatively low, it has been discontinued by the manufacturer. It has no role as a rescue agent for acute rejection.

3.2.3 Adverse effects

The side effect profile is similar to that of basiliximab and generally favorable. Cytokine release is not typically associated with this agent (Hershberger et al., 2005; Nashan et al., 1999). Like other IL-2 receptor antagonists, the risk of PTLD is not significantly increased with use (Cherikh et al., 2003).

4. Desensitizing agents

4.1 Rituximab
4.1.1 Mechanism
Rituximab is a monoclonal chimeric antibody to the CD20 molecule. CD20 is a glycoprotein on the cell surface of circulating, mature B cells. Rituximab effectively depletes CD20[+] cells from the circulation by inducing apoptosis (Deans et al., 2002). These cells are precursors to antibody-producing plasma cells, and their role in transplantation is only partially characterized. They may play a role in acute rejection, as B cells can act as antigen-presenting cells.

4.1.2 Applications
Rituximab is approved for use in various lymphomas, leukemias, PTLD, and rheumatoid arthritis (Gabardi et al., 2011; Grillo-Lopez et al., 1999). Peripheral veins can be used for administration and dosing is dependent on the indication. A recent study examining the role of rituximab as an induction agent found no benefit compared to placebo (Tyden et al., 2009). However, it does play a role as a desensitizing agent in patients with preformed donor specific antibodies (DSA), in conjunction with total plasmapheresis and/or intravenous immunoglobulin (IVIG)(Fuchinoue et al., 2011; Sonnenday et al., 2004). Additionally, it has been used to aid in transplanting across blood group barriers in donor recipient pairs and in patients with positive crossmatches following antibody elimination. Rituximab is increasingly being used to treat episodes of vascular rejection and antibody-mediated rejections (Y.T. Becker et al., 2006; Fehr et al., 2009). Finally, rituximab is a proven and effective agent in the treatment of PTLD (Svoboda et al., 2006). Administration does not replace immunosuppression reduction or chemotherapy, but rather supplements the other modalities.

4.1.3 Adverse effects
Rituximab is generally well-tolerated with minimal side effects. Anaphylaxis remains a theoretical concern, as is the case with most agents. Reports on infectious complications related to rituximab have been variable (Grim et al., 2007; Kamar et al., 2010; Nishida et al., 2009). In some instances there was no difference in bacterial, viral, or fungal infections in kidney transplant recipients treated with rituximab, however, this remains controversial.

4.2 Bortezomib
4.2.1 Mechanism
Bortezomib is a proteasomal inhibitor that causes apoptosis of plasma cells. It binds the 26S subunit of the proteasome (Bonvini et al., 2007). Proteasome inhibition ultimately leads to apoptosis during mitosis. Bortezomib selectively causes apoptosis in CD138[+] plasma cells (Perry et al., 2009). Additionally, Bortezomib may block T cell cycling and decrease the number of circulating B cells by reducing bone marrow levels of IL-6 (San Miguel et al., 2008).

4.2.2 Applications
Bortezomib has not been approved for use in kidney transplantation; however, it has been used in sensitized patients (Perry et al., 2009). Bortezomib has been successfully used to decrease DSA levels, which may play a role in acute antibody-mediated rejection (AMR)

(Trivedi et al., 2009). Furthermore, in vivo data has demonstrated a decrease in the percentage of bone marrow plasma cells, antibody production, and allospecificities of plasma cells in bone marrow aspirates of patients treated with bortezomib i in the setting of AMR (Perry et al., 2009).

4.2.3 Adverse events
Bortezomib has been associated with various side effects. Although gastrointestinal side effects are the most common, peripheral neuropathy has also been reported, especially in patients with a pre-existing history of neuropathy (Bonvini et al., 2007). Moreover, myelosuppression and shingles has been reported.

4.3 Intravenous Immunoglobulin (IVIG)
4.3.1 Mechanism
Intravenous immunoglobulin, or IVIG, is pooled polyclonal antibodies from different human donors. These are high-dose human IgG fractions with a wide range of specificities. These are non-T cell specific formulations and have no specific cell targets (Jordan et al., 2011). It is able to bind activated complement components or even inhibit complement activation (Jordan et al., 2009). IVIG may also modulate the alloimmune response by binding to the Fc receptor of antigen-presenting cells, effectively quelling the alloimmune response (Kazatchkine & Kaveri, 2001).

4.3.2 Applications
Despite the inability to deplete T cells, IVIG is an effective treatment of acute cellular rejection. Early studies showed that IVIG was as effective as OKT3 in reversing steroid-resistant acute rejection episodes (Casadei et al., 2001). In the setting of antibody-mediated rejection, IVIG has been shown to be beneficial when used in conjunction with plasmapheresis and/or rituximab (Lefaucher et al., 2009; Shehata et al., 2010). As a desensitization agent alone, no study has demonstrated a clear benefit (Pisani et al., 1999; Shehata et al., 2010). Definitive reduction of antibody was not shown and a survival advantage was not evident.

4.3.3 Adverse effects
The side-effect profile of IVIG increases with dosing. High-dose IVIG is associated with more infusion-related complications, such as headache, thrombotic incidents, hemolysis, bronchospasms, osmotic nephropathy, or even aseptic meningitis (Jordan et al., 2011; Kahwaji et al., 2009). Sucrose-based and high osmolality products have a higher risk of developing osmotic nephropathy as opposed to other preparation. Nevertheless, it is typically well-tolerated, especially at lower doses and most patients report only headache.

5. Experimental agents

5.1 Siplizumab (MEDI-507)
Originally described as BTI-322, siplizumab is a monoclonal humanized antibody to CD2. It is an IgG1k molecule derived from rat (Pruett et al., 2009). CD2, or lymphocyte function-associated antigen-2 (LFA-2), is an important T cell adhesion molecule that binds to CD58, or LFA-3. This is a transmembrane signal transduction molecule that facilitates T cell

receptor binding. Early studies examined the use of siplizumab as an induction agent and treatment modality for acute rejection in solid organ transplantation as well as graft-versus-host disease (Pruett et al., 2009; Squifflet et al., 1997). The first human study of siplizumab demonstrated the safety and feasibility in kidney transplantation, as compared to placebo; however, current endeavors are focused on investigating its use in nonmyeloablative conditioning regimens to achieve mixed chimerism (Kawai et al., 2008; Pruett et al., 2009; Spitzer et al., 2003). In addition, it is being investigated for the treatment of plaque psoriasis (Langley et al., 2010).

5.2 Alefacept

Alefaept is a dimeric fusion protein (Fig.8) constituted from LFA-3 and the human Fc portion of IgG1. Studies have demonstrated inhibition of T cell proliferation and depletion of effector memory T cells (Ellis & Krueger, 2001; Gordon et al., 2003). Currently, alefacept is approved to treat plaque psoriasis. Preclinical studies in nonhuman primates have demonstrated a survival benefit of alefacept, when used in conjunction with costimulatory blockade, but not alone; however in human trials have never shown a benefit (Weaver et al., 2009).

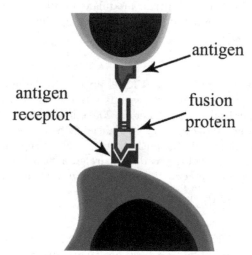

Fig. 8. Mimicry. In this figure, the antibody is fused with a protein structural similar to the intended antigen, which can serve as activating or inhibitory

5.3 Costimulatory blockade
5.3.1 Abatacept

Abatacept is a recombinant cytotoxic T-lymphocyte antigen 4 (CTLA4) fused with the Fc portion of IgG1 (Lenschow et al., 1992; Turka et al., 1992). Animal models demonstrated its ability to delay or even prevent the onset of allograft rejection, which is comparable to basiliximab and some polyclonal antibody therapies (Kirk et al., 1997; Lenschow et al., 1992; Turka et al., 1992). It has been approved for treatment of rheumatoid arthiritis (Genovese et al., 2005; Nogid & Pham, 2006). Further investigations of this medication are not currently under development.

5.3.2 Belatacept

Belatacept is the improved version of abatacept, providing selective blockade of T cell activation as a fusion protein. Two amino acids have been changed to improve dissociation rates when binding to CD80 and CD86 (Vincenti et al., 2005, 2010). In the phase II trial comparing belatacept to cyclosporine, acute rejection rates were similar, while allograft function was significantly improved in patients receiving belatacept (Vincenti et al., 2005). In the phase III trial of kidney transplantation, patients receiving belatacept experienced improved allograft function at 12 months; however, acute rejection rates and severity of acute rejection episodes were significantly higher in the belatacept arm of the study. Additionally, the incidence of PTLD was greater in patients receiving belatacept (Vincenti et al., 2010). An additional study investigating the efficacy of belatacept in kidney transplantation of extended criteria donors demonstrated similar results, with a predilection towards central nervous system (CNS) forms of PTLD (Durrbach et al., 2010). The novelty of costimulation blockade is the ability to avoid calcineurin inhibitors, especially in allografts at increased risk of delayed graft function. Belatacept has recently been approved for the prophylaxis of organ rejection in adult patients receiving a kidney transplant, in combination with basiliximab induction, mycophenolate mofetil, and corticosteroids (Bristol-Myers Squibb Company 2011). Current recommendations include using it only in patients who are EBV seropositive; however, patients should be monitored for an increased risk of infectious complications and Progressive Multifocal Leukoencephalopathy.

5.3.3 CD7 antagonism

SDZCHH380 is a monoclonal antibody targeting CD7. This IgG1 chimeric mouse antibody was initially studied in kidney transplantation (Lazarovits et al., 1993; Sharma et al., 1997). The CD7 molecule is expressed on T cells and natural killer cells during early differentiation, functioning as a costimulatory molecule. Early studies of SDZCHH380 as an induction agent in kidney transplantation demonstrated comparable short and long-term outcomes to OKT3 induction (Sharma et al., 1997). Despite favorable results up to 4 years following administration, further investigative endeavors were not pursued in solid organ transplantation.

5.3.4 T cell receptor antagonism

T10B9, or Medi-500, is a monoclonal antibody to the T cell receptor. Specifically, this is a murine IgMκ molecule to the αβ heterodimer region of the CD3 complex (Brown et al., 1996; Waid et al., 1992, 2009). Because it does not bind directly to the Fc receptor, there is reduced immune stimulation and occurrence of cytokine release syndrome. The end result is T cell depletion. Early studies demonstrated the efficacy of this agent as induction therapy and a treatment modality for acute rejection in solid organ transplantation, as compared to OKT3 (Waid et al., 1997a, 1997b). However, given the efficacy of similar humanized monoclonal antibodies, further investigations in solid organ transplantation were not pursued.

6. Special considerations

6.1 High risk donor kidneys & recipients

Marginal donor kidneys are defined as expanded criteria donors (ECD) or donation after cardiac death donors (DCD). These allografts are at higher risk of developing delayed graft function, which has been shown to decrease overall allograft survival and increase the incidence of acute rejection (Deroure et al., 2010; Rudich et al., 2002). There was a large prospective, international, randomized controlled trial examining the efficacy of rATG versus basiliximab in patients at high risk of delayed graft function (Brennan et al., 2006). Patients were maintained on a cyclosporine-based triple drug immunosuppression regimen and eligibility criteria included ECD or DCD allografts, standard criteria donors (SCD) with greater than 24 hours of cold ischemia time, repeat transplants, panel-reactive antibody value exceeding 20% before transplantation, donors with acute tubular necrosis (ATN), recipient black race, or one or more HLA mismatches. The incidence of delayed graft function was not significantly different between patients receiving rATG and basiliximab induction. However, the incidence of biopsy-proven acute rejection was significantly lower in patients receiving rATG. Additionally, severe rejection episodes requiring antibody therapy were less frequent in the rATG group. Interestingly, the overall incidence of infection was significantly lower in the basiliximab group, yet the incidence of CMV was lower in the rATG group.

6.2 Sensitization & incompatibility

Sensitization to HLA antigen typically occurs as a result of blood transfusions, pregnancy, or previous transplantation (Marfo et al., 2011). These patients are more likely develop circulating DSA and have a positive cross-match during transplantation evaluation. Sensitized patients wait considerable longer on the deceased donor waitlist.

Various modalities have been developed to combat sensitization. Antibodies can be removed by plasmapheresis and immunoadsorption techniques; however anti-HLA antibodies generally rebound and return to baseline (Hakim et al., 1990). As discussed earlier, rituximab has also been used with varying success, as B cells recovery occurs 6 to 12 months following administration. Bortezomib has been used in sensitized patients (Perry et al., 2009). Recently, a new medication called eculizumab has emerged as a humanized monoclonal antibody to complement component 5 (C5) to mediate complement-mediated injury, which may have potential in desensitization protocols (Larrea et al., 2010). IVIG has also been used in sensitized patients to acutely decrease PRA levels, especially in ABO-incompatible patients. Finally, splenectomy has also been used in desensitization protocols of ABO-incompatible patients (Kaplan et al., 2007).

Despite these numerous combinations of these therapies with acceptable short-term outcomes, intermediate-term outcomes have been modest at best. Some have reported graft survival rates at 3 years to be 78% (Haririan et al., 2009) and 4-year graft survival of only 66% (Lefaucher et al., 2007). Additionally, higher rates of clinical and subclinical antibody-mediated rejection have been reported (Haas et al, 2007; Loupy et al., 2009).

6.3 Older recipients

Several considerations should be examined when choosing induction therapy in older recipients. Older patients may have lower rates of acute rejection as a result of diminished immune activity (B.N. Becker 1996; Friedman et al., 2004). There is also a higher rate of infectious complications as well as malignancies (Meier-Kriesche et al., 2001; Stratta et al., 2008). Thus, less intense induction and immunosuppression appear sufficient. However, if significant HLA-mismatch is present, higher rates of acute rejection have been described (Frei et al., 2008; Fritsche et al., 2003; Giessing et al., 2003). Nevertheless, the safety profile of

IL-2 receptor antibodies in patients with considerable comorbidities, such as the older recipients, may be preferred.

7. Acknowledgements

The authors gratefully acknowledge the expert assistance of Ms. Johanna Martin in creating all figures depicted in the chapter.

8. References

Abott, K.C.; Hypolite, I.O.; Viola, R., et al. (2002). Hospitalizations for cytomegalovirus disease after renal transplantation in the United States. *Ann Epidemiol*, Vol.12, No.6, (August 2002), pp. 402-409, ISSN 1047-2797.

Afaneh, C.; Halpern, J.; Cheng, E., et al. (2010). Steroid avoidance in two-haplotype-matched living donor renal transplants with basiliximab induction therapy. *Transplant Proc*, Vol.42, No.10, (December 2010), pp. 4526-9, ISSN 0041-1345.

Becker, B.N.; Ismail, N.; Becker, Y.T., et al. (1996). Renal transplantation in the older end stage renal disease patient. *Semin Nephrol*, Vol.16, No.4, (July 2006), pp. 353-62, ISSN 0720-9295.

Becker, Y.T.; Samaniego-Picota, M., & Sollinger, H.W. (2006). The emerging role of rituximab in organ transplantation. *Transpl Int*, Vol.19, No.8, (August 2006), pp. 621-8, ISSN 0934-0874.

Beiras-Fernandez, A.; Chappell, D.; Hammer, C., et al. (2006). Influence of polyclonal anti-thymocyte globulins upon ischemia reperfusion injury in a non-human primate model. *Transpl Immunol*, Vol.15, No.4, (April 2006), pp. 273-9, ISSN 0966-3274.

Benvenisty, A.I.; Cohen, D.; Stegall, M.D., et al. (1990). Improved results using OKT3 as induction immunosuppression in renal allograft recipients with delayed graft function. *Transplantation*, Vol.49, No.2, (February 1990), pp. 321-7, ISSN 0041-1337.

Bishop, G.; Cosimi, A.B.; Voynow, N.K., et al. (1975). Effect of immunosuppressive therapy for renal allografts on the number of circulating sheep red blood cells rosetting cells. *Transplantation*, Vol.20, No.2, (Augusut 1975), pp. 123-9, ISSN 0041-1337.

Bock, H.A.; Gallati, H.; Zurcher, R.M., et al. (1995). A randomized prospecitve trial of prophylactic immunosuppression with ATG-Fresenius versus OKT3 after renal transplantation. *Transplantation*, Vol.59, No.6, (March 1995), pp. 830-40, ISSN 0041-1337.

Bonnefoy-Berard, N.; Vincent, C., & Revillard, J. (1991). Antibodies against the functional leukocyte surface molecules in polyclonal antilymphocyte and antithymocyte globulins. *Transplantation*, Vol.51, No.3, (March 1991), pp. 669-73, ISSN 0041-1337.

Bonvini, P.; Zorzi, E.; Basso, G., et al. (2007). Bortezomib-mediated 26S proteasome inhibition causes cell-cycle arrest and induces apoptosis in CD-30+ anaplastic large cell lymphoma. *Leukemia*, Vol.21, No.4 (April 2007), pp. 838–42, ISSN 0887-6924.

Boulianne, G.L.; Hozumi, N.; Shulman, M.J., et al. (1984). Production of functional chimaeric mouse/human antibody. *Nature*, Vol.312, No.5995, (December 1984), pp. 643-6, ISSN 0028-0836.

Brennan, D.C.; Flavin, K.; Lowell, J.A., et al. (1999). A randomized,double-blinded comparison of thymoglobulin versus Atgam for induction immunosuppressive therapy in adult renal transplant recipients. *Transplantation*, Vol.67, No.7, (April 1999), pp. 1011-8, ISSN 0041-1337.

Brennan, D.C.; Daller, J.A.; Lake, K.D., et al. (2006). Rabbit antithymocyte globulin versus basiliximab in renal transplantation. *N Engl J Med*, Vol.355, No.19, (November 2006), pp. 1967-77, ISSN 0028-4793.

Bristol-Myers Squibb Company. (2011). Nulojix® (belatacept) prescribing information. Princeton, New Jersey, USA; (2011).

Brown, S.A.; Lucas, B.A.; Waid, T.H., et al. (1996). T10B9 (MEDI-500) mediated immunosuppression: studies on the mechanism of action. *Clin Transplant*, Vol.10, No.6, (December 1996), pp. 607-13, ISSN 0902-0063.

Buchler, M.; Hurault de Ligny, B.; Madec, C., et al. (2003). Induction therapy by anti-thymocyte globulin (rabbit) in renal transplantation: a 1-yr follow-up of safety and efficacy. *Clin Transplant*, Vol.17, No.6, (December 2003), pp. 539-45, ISSN 0902-0063.

Bunn, D.; Lea, C.K.; Bevan, D.J., et al. (1996). The pharmacokinetics of anti-thymocyte globulin (ATG) following intravenous infusion in man. *Clin Nephrol*, Vol.45, No.1, (January 1996), pp. 29-32, ISSN 0301-0430.

Bustami, R.T.; Ojo, A.O.; Wolfe, R.A., et al. (2004). Immunosuppression and the risk of post-transplant malignancy among cadaveric first kidney transplant recipients. *Am J Transplant*, Vol.4, No.1, (January 2004), pp. 87-93, ISSN 1600-6135.

Capra, J.D., & Edmundson, A.B. (1977). The antibody combining site. *Sci Am*, Vol.236, No.1, (January 1977), pp. 50-9, ISSN 0036-8733.

Casadei, D.H.; del C Rial, M.; Opelz, G., et al. (2001). A randomized and prospective study comparing treatment with high-dose intravenous immunoglobulin with monoclonal antibodies for rescue of kidney grafts with steroid-resistant rejection. *Transplantation*, Vol.71, No.1, (January 2001), pp. 53-8, ISSN 0041-1337.

Cecka, J.M.; Gjertson, D., & Terasaki, P. (1993). Do prophylactic antilymphocyte globulins (ALG and OKT3) improve renal transplant in recipient and donor high-risk groups? *Transplant Proc*, Vol.25, No.1, (February 1993), pp. 548-9, ISSN 0041-1345.

Chatenoud, L.; Jonker, M.; Villemain, F., et al. (1986). The human immune response to the OKT3 monoclonal antibody is oligoclonal. *Science*, Vol.232, No.4756), (June 1986), pp. 1406-8, ISSN 0036-8075.

Chatenoud, L.; Ferran, C.; Legendre, C., et al. (1990). In vivo cell activation following OKT3 administration: systemic cytokine release and modulation by corticosteroids. *Transplantation*, Vol.49, No.4, (April 1990), pp. 697-702, ISSN 0041-1337.

Chatenoud, L.; Legendre, C.; Ferran, C., et al. (1991). Corticosteroid inhibition of the OKT3-induced cytokine-related syndrome- dosage and kinetics prerequisites. *Transplantation*, Vol.51, No.2, (February 1991), pp. 334-8, ISSN 0041-1337.

Cherikh, W.S.; Kauffman, H.M.; McBride, M.A., et al. (2003). Association of the type of induction immunosuppression with posttransplant lymphoproliferative disorder, graft survival, and patient survival after primary kidney transplantation. *Transplantation*, Vol.76, No.9, (Novemeber 2003), pp. 1289-93, ISSN 0041-1337.

Clatworthy, M.R.; Friend, P.J.; Calne, R.Y., et al. (2009). Alemtuzumab (CAMPATH-1H) for the treatment of acute rejection in kidney transplant recipients: long-term follow-up. *Transplantation*, Vol.87, No.7, (April 2009), pp. 1092-5, ISSN 0041-1337.

Coles, A.J.; Wing, M.; Smith, S., et al. (1999). Pulsed monoclonal antibody treatment and autoimmune thyroid disease in multiple sclerosis. *Lancet*, Vol.354, No.9191, (Novemeber 1999), pp. 1691-5, ISSN 0140-6736.

Colvin, R.B., & Preffer, F.I. (1991). Laboratory monitoring of therapy with OKT3 and other murine monoclonal antibodies. *Clin Lab Med*, Vol.11, No.3, (September 1991), pp. 693-714, ISSN 0272-2712.

Cosimi, A.B.; Wortis, H.H.; Delmonico, F.L., et al. (1976). Randomized clinical trial of antilthymocyte globulin in cadaver renal allograft recipients: importance of T cell monitoring. *Surgery*, Vol.80, No.2, (August 1976), pp. 155-63, ISSN 0039-6060.

Cosimi, A.B. (1981a). The clinical value of antilymphocyte antibodies. *Transplant Proc*, Vol.13, No.1, (March 1981), pp. 462-8, ISSN 0041-1345.

Cosimi, A.B.; Burton, R.C.; Colvin, R.B., et al. (1981b). Treatment of acute renal allograft rejection with OKT3 monoclonal antibody. *Transplantation*, Vol.32, No.6, (December 1981), pp. 535-9, ISSN 0041-1337.

Csapo, Z.; Benavides-Viveros, C.; Podder, H., et al. (2005). Campath-1H as rescue therapy for the treatment of acute rejection in kidney transplant patients. *Transplant Proc*, Vol.37, No.5, (June 2005), pp. 2032-6, ISSN 0041-1345.

Deans, J.P.; Li, H.; Polyak, M.J., et al. (2002). CD20-mediated apoptosis: signaling through lipid rafts. *Immunology*, Vol.107, No.2, (October 2002), pp. 176-82, ISSN 0019-2805.

Debets, J.M.H.; Leunissen, K.M.L.; van Hooff, H.J., et al. (1989). Evidene of involvement of tumor necrosis factor in adverse reactions during treatment of kidney allograft rejection with antithymocyte globulin. *Transplantation*, Vol.47, No.3, (March 1989), pp. 487-92, ISSN 0041-1337.

Debure, A.; Chekoff, N.; Chatenoud, L., et al. (1988). One-month prophylactic use of OKT3 in cadaver kidney transplant recipients. *Transplantation*, Vol.45, No.3, (March 1988), pp. 546-53, ISSN 0041-1337.

Deroure, B.; Kamar, N.; Depreneuf, H., et al. (2010). Expanding the criteria of renal kidneys for transplantation: use of donors with acute renal failure. *Nephrol Dial Transplant*, Vol.25, No.6, (June 2010), pp. 1980-6, ISSN 0931-0509.

Durrbach, A.; Pestana, J.M.; Pearson, T., et al. (2010). A phase III study of belatacept versus cyclosporine in kidney transplants from extended criteria donors (BENEFIT-EXT study). *Am J Transplant*, Vol.10, No.3, (March 2010), pp. 547-57, ISSN 1600-6135.

Ellis, C.N.; Krueger, G.G. & Alefacept Clinical Study Group. (2001). Treatment of chronic plaque psoriasis by selective targeting of memory effector T lymphocytes. *N Engl J Med*, Vol.345, No.4, (July 2001), pp. 248-55, ISSN 0028-4793.

Fehr, T.; Rüsi, B.; Fischer, A., et al. (2009). Rituximab and intravenous immunoglobulin treatment of chronic antibody-mediated kidney allograft rejection. *Transplantation*, Vol.87, No.12, (June 2009), pp. 1837-41, ISSN 0041-1337.

Ferrant, J.L.; Benjamin, C.D.; Cutler, A.H., et al. (2004). The contribution of the Fc effector mechanisms in the efficacy of anti-CD154 immunotherapy depends on the nature of the immune challenge. *Int Immunol*, Vol.16, No.11, (Novemeber 2004), pp. 1583-94, ISSN 0953-8178.

Frei, U.; Noeldeke, J.; Machold-Fabrizii, V., et al. (2008). Prospective age-matching in elderly kidney transplant recipients – a 5-year analysis of the Eurotransplant Senior Program. *Am J Transplant*, Vol.8, No.1, (January 2007), pp. 50-7, ISSN 1600-6135.

Friedman, A.L.; Goker, O.; Kalish, M.A., et al. (2004). Renal transplant recipients over aged 60 have diminished immune activity and a low risk of rejection. *Int Urol Nephrol*, Vol.36, No.3, (2004), pp. 451-6, ISSN 0301-1623.

Fritsche, L.; Horstrup, J.; Budde, K., et al. (2003). Old-for-old kidney allocation allows successful expansion of the donor and recipient pool. *Am J Transplant*, Vol.3, No.11, (November 2003), pp. 1434-9, ISSN 1600-6135.

Fuchinoue, S.; Ishii, Y.; Sawada, T., et al. (2011). The 5-year outcome of ABO-incompatible kidney transplantation with rituximab induction. *Transplantation*, Vol.91, No.18, (April 2011), pp. 853-7, ISSN 0041-1337.

Gabardi, S.; Martin, S.T.; Roberts, K.L., et al. (2011). Induction immunosuppressive therapies in renal transplantation. *Am J Health Syst Pharm*, Vol.68, No.3, (February 2011), pp. 211-8, ISSN 1079-2082.

Gaber, A.O.; First, M.R.; Tesi, R.J., et al. (1998). Results of the double-blind, randomized, multicenter, phase III clinical trial of Thymoglobulin versus Atgam in the treatment of acute graft rejection episodes after renal transplantation. *Transplantation*, Vol.66, No.1, (July 1998), pp. 29-37, ISSN 0041-1337.

Genovese, M.C.; Becker, J.C.; Schiff, M., et al. (2005). Abatacept for rheumatoid arthritis refractory to tumor necrosis alpha inhibition. *N Engl J Med*, Vol.353, No.11, pp. 1114-23, ISSN 0028-4793.

Genzyme Corporation. (2005).. Thymoglobulin (rabbit antithymocyte globulin) prescribing information. Cambridge, MA; 2005.

Giessing, M.; Budde, K.; Fritsche, L., et al. (2003). 'Old-for-old' cadaveric renal transplantation: surgical findings, perioperative complications and outcome. *Eur Urol*, Vol.44, No.6, (December 2003), pp. 701-8, ISSN 0302-2838.

Gordon, K.B.; Vaishnaw, A.K.; O'Gorman, J., et al. (2003). Treatment of psoriasis with alefacept: correlation of clinical improvement with reductions of memory T-cell counts. *Arch Dermatol*, Vol.139, No.12, (December 2003), pp. 1563-70, ISSN 0003-987X.

Gourishankar, S.; McDermid, J.C.; Jhangri, G.S., et al. (2004). Herpes zoster infection following solid organ transplantation: incidence, risk factors and outomes in the current immunosuppressive era. *Am J Transplant*, Vol.4, No.1, (January 2004), pp. 108-15, ISSN 1600-6135.

Grillo-Lopez, A.J.; White, C.A.; Varns, C., et al. (1999). Overview of the clinical development of rituximab: first monoclonal antibody approved for the treatment of lymphoma. *Semin Oncol*, Vol.26, No.5, (October 1999), pp. 66-73, ISSN 0093-7754.

Grim, S.A.; Pham, T.; Thielke, J., et al. (2007). Infectious complications associated with the use of rituximab for ABO-incompatible and positive cross-match renal transplant recipients. *Clin Transplant*, Vol.21, No.5, (September 2007), pp. 628-32, ISSN 0902-0063.

Guttmann, R.D.; Caudrelier, P.; Alberici, G., et al. (1997). Pharmacokinetics, foreign protein immune response, cytokine release, and lymphocyte subsets in patients receiving thymoglobuline and immunosuppression. *Transplant Proc*, Vol.29, No.7A, pp. 24S-6, ISSN 0041-1345.

Haas, M.; Montgomery, R.A.; Segev, D.L., et al. (2007). Subclinical acute antibody-mediated rejection in positive crossmatch renal allografts. *Am J Transplant*, Vol.7, No.3, (January 2007), pp. 576-85, ISSN 1600-6135.

Hakim, R.M.; Milford, E.; Himmelfarb, J., et al. (1990). Extracorporeal removal of anti-HLA antibodies in transplant candidates. *Am J Kidney Dis*, Vol.16, No.5, (November 1990), pp. 423-31, ISSN 0272-6386.

Hale, G.; Waldmann, H.; Friend, P., et al. (1986). Pilot study of CAMPATH-1, a rat monoclonal antibody that fixes human complement, as an immunosuppressant in organ transplantation. *Transplantation*, Vol.42, No.3, (September 1986), pp. 308-11, ISSN 0041-1337.

Hale, G. (2001). The CD52 antigen and development of the CAMPATH antibodies. *Cytotherapy*, Vol.3, No.3, (2001), pp. 137-43, ISSN 1465-3249.

Hanaway, M.J.; Woodle, E.S.; Mulgaonkar, S., et al. (2011). Alemtuzumab induction in renal transplantation. *N Engl J Med*, Vol. 364, No.20, (May 2011), pp. 1909-19, ISSN 0028-4793.

Hardinger, K.L.; Schnitzler, M.A.; Miller, B., et al. (2004). Five–year follow up of thymoglobulin versus ATGAM induction in adult renal transplantation. *Transplantation* 2004; 78: 136, ISSN 0041-1337.

Hardinger, K.L. (2006). Rabbit antithymocyte globulin induction therapy in adult renal transplantation. *Pharmacotherpay*, Vol.26, No.12, (December 2006), pp. 1771-83, ISSN 0277-0008.

Haririan, A.; Nogueira, J.; Kukuruga, D., et al. (2009). Positive cross-match living donor kidney transplantation: Longer-term outcomes. *Am J Transplant*, Vol.9, No.3, (February 2009), pp. 536-42, ISSN 1600-6135.

Henricsson, A.; Husberg, B., & Bergentz, S.E. (1977). The mechanism behind the effect of ALG on platelets in vivo. *Clin Exp Immunol*, Vol.29, No.3, (September 1977), pp. 515-22, ISSN 0009-9104.

Henry, M.L.; Pelletier, R.P.; Elkhammas, E.A., et al. (2001). A randomized prospective trial of OKT3 induction in the current immunosuppression era. *Clin Transplant*, Vol.15, No.6, (December 2001), pp. 410-4, ISSN 0902-0063.

Hershberger, R.E.; Starling, R.C.; Eisen, H.J., et al. (2005). Daclizumab to prevent rejection after cardiac transplantation. *N Engl J Med*, Vol.352, No.26, (June 2005), pp. 2705-13, ISSN 0028-4793.

Humar, A.; Ramcharan, T.; Denny, R., et al. (2001). Are wound complications after a kidney transplant more common with modern immunosuppression? *Transplantation*, Vol.72, No.12, (December 2001), pp. 1920-3, ISSN 0041-1337.

IMTIX–SangStat. (2003). Thymoglobuline (rabbit antithymocyte globulin) prescribing information. Lyon, France; 2003.

Jaffers, G.J.; Fuller, T.C.; Cosimi, A.B., et al. (1986). Monoclonal antibody therapy: anti-idiotype and non-anti-idiotype antibodies to OKT3 arising despite intense immunosuppression. *Transplantation*, Vol.41, No.5, (May 1986), pp. 572-8, ISSN 0041-1337.

Jamil, B.; Nicholls, K.; Becker, G.J., et al. (1999). Impact of acute rejection therapy on infections and malignancies in renal transplant recipients. *Transplantation*, Vol.68, No.10, (November 1999), pp. 1597-603, ISSN 0041-1337.

Jirasiritham, S.; Khunprakant, R.; Techawathanawanna, N., et al. Treatment of simultaneous acute antibody-mediated rejection and acute cellular rejection with alemtuzumab in kidney transplantation: a case report. *Transplant Proc*, Vol.42, No.3, (April 2010), pp. 987-9, ISSN 0041-1345.

Jones, P.T.; Dear, P.H.; Foote, et al. (1986). Replacing the complementarity-determining regions in human antibody with those from a mouse. *Nature*, Vol.321, No.6069, (May 1986), pp. 522-5, ISSN 0028-0836.

Jordan, S.C.; Toyoda, M., & Vo, A.A. (2009). Intravenous immunoglobulin a natural regulator of immunity and inflammation. *Transplantation*, Vol.88, No.1, (July 2009), pp. 1-6, ISSN 0041-1337.

Jordan, S.C.; Toyoda, M.; Kahwaji, J., et al. (2011). Clinical Aspects of Intravenous Immunoglobulin Use in Solid Organ Transplant Recipients. *Am J Transplant*, Vol.11, No.2, (January 2011), pp. 196-202, ISSN 1600-6135.

Kahan, B.D.; Rajagopalan, P.R. & Hall, M. (1999). Reduction of the occurrence of acute cellular rejection among renal allograft recipients treated with basiliximab, a chimeric anti-interleukin-2-receptor monoclonal antibody. *Transplantation*, Vol.67, No.2, pp. 276-84, ISSN 0041-1337.

Kahwaji, J.; Barker, E.; Pepkowitz, S., et al. (2009). Acute hemolysis after high dose IVIG therapy in highly HLA sensitized patients. *Clin J Am Soc Nephrol*, Vol.4, No.12, (October 2009), pp. 1993-7, ISSN 1555-9041.

Kamar, N.; Milioto, O.; Puissant-Lubrano, B., et al. (2010). Incidence and predictive factors for infectious disease after rituximab therapy in kidney-transplant patients. *Am J Transplant*, Vol.10, No.1, (July 2009), pp. 89-98, ISSN 1600-6135.

Kamath, S.; Dean, D.; Peddi, V.R., et al. (1997). Efficacy of OKT3 as primary therapy for histologically confirmed acute renal allograft rejection. *Transplantation*, Vol.64, No.10, (November 1997), pp. 1428-32, ISSN 0041-1337.

Kaplan, B.; Gangemi, A.; Thielke, J., et al. (2007). Successful rescue of refractory severe antibody mediated rejection with splenectomy. *Transplantion*, Vol.83, No.1, (January 2007), pp. 99-100, ISSN 0041-1337.

Kawai, T.; Cosimi, A.B.; Spitzer, T.R., et al. (2008). HLA-mismatched renal transplantation without maintenance immunosuppression. *N Engl J Med*, Vol.358, No..4, (January 2008), pp. 353-61, ISSN 0028-4793.

Kazatchkine, M.D. & Kaveri, S.V. (2001). Immunomodulation of autoimmune and inflammatory disease with intravenous immune globulin. *N Engl J Med*, Vol.345, No.10, (September 2001), pp. 747-55, ISSN 0028-4793.

Kerr, P.G. & Atkins, R.C. (1989). The effects of OKT3 therapy on infiltrating lymphocytes in rejecting renal allografts. *Transplantation*, Vol.48, No.1, (July 1989), pp. 33-6, ISSN 0041-1337.

Kirk, A.D.; Harlan, D.M.; Armstrong, N.N., et al. (1997). CTLA4-Ig and anti-CD40 ligand prevent renal allograft rejection in primates. *Proc Natl Acad Sci U S A*, Vol.94, No.16, (August 1997), pp. 8789-94, ISSN 0027-8424.

Kirk, A.D.; Hale, D.A.; Mannon, R.B., et al. (2003). Results from a human renal allograft tolerance trial evaluating the humanized CD52-specific monoclonal antibody alemtuzumab (CAMPATH-1H). *Transplantation*, Vol.76, No.1, (July 2003), pp. 120-9, ISSN 0041-1337.

Kirk, A.D.; Hale, D.A.; Swanson, S.J., et al. (2006). Autoimmune thyroid disease after renal transplantation using depletional induction with alemtuzumab. *Am J Transplant*, Vol.6, No.5, (May 2006), pp. 1084-5, ISSN 1600-6135.

Kirkman, R.L.; Shapiro, M.E.; Carpenter, C.B., et al. (1991). A randomized prospective trial of anti-Tac monoclonal antibody in human renal transplantation. *Transplantation*, Vol.51, No.1, (January 1991), pp. 107-13, ISSN 0041-1337.

Kohler, G. & Milstein, C. (1975). Continuous cultures of fused cells secreting antibody of predefined specificity. *Nature*, Vol.256, No.5517, (August 1975), pp. 495-7, ISSN 0028-0836.

Langley, R.G.; Papp, K.; Bissonnette, R., et al. (2010). Safety profile of intravenous and subcutaneous siplizumab, an anti-CD2 monoclonal antibody, for the treatment of plaque psoriasis: results of two randomized, double-blind, placebo-controlled studies. *Int J Dermatol*, Vol.49, No.7, (July 2010), pp. 818-28, ISSN 0011-9059.

Larrea, C.F.; Cofan, F.; Oppenheimer, F., et al. (2010). Efficacy of eculizumab in the treatment of recurrent atypical hemolytic-uremic syndrome after renal transplantation. *Transplantation*, Vol.89, No.7, (April 2010), pp. 903-4, ISSN 0041-1337.

Lazarovits, A.I.; Rochon, J.; Banks, L., et al. (1993). Human mouse chimeric CD7 monoclonal antibody for the prophylaxis of kidney transplant rejection. *J Immunol*, Vol.150, No.11, (June 1993), pp. 5163-74, ISSN 0022-1767.

Lebranchu, Y.; Bridoux, F.; Buchler, M., et al. (2002). Immunoprophylaxis with basiliximab compared with antithymocyte globulin in renal transplant patients receiving MMF-containing triple therapy. *Am J Transplant*, Vol.2, No.1, pp. 48-56, ISSN 1600-6135.

Lefaucheur, C.; Nochy, D.; Hill, G.S., et al. (2007). Determinants of poor graft outcome in patients with antibody-mediated acute rejection. *Am J Transplant*, Vol.7, No.4, (April 2007), pp. 832-41, ISSN 1600-6135.

Lefaucheur, C.; Nochy, D.; Andrade, J., et al. (2009). Comparison of combination plasmapheresis/IVIG/Anti-CD20 versus high dose IVIG in the treatment of antibody-mediated rejection. *Am J Transplant*, Vol.9, No.5, (May 2009), pp. 1099-107, ISSN 1600-6135.

Legendre, C.; Kreis, H.; Bach, J., et al. (1992). Prediction of successful allograft rejection retreatment with OKT3. *Transplantation*, Vol.53, No.1, (January 1992), pp. 87-90, ISSN 0041-1337.

Lenschow, D.J.; Zeng, Y.; Thistlethwaite, J.R., et al. (1992). Long-term survival of xenogeneic pancreatic islet grafts induced with CTLA4Ig. *Science*, Vol.257, No.5071, (August 1992), pp. 789-92, ISSN 0036-8075.

Loupy, A.; Suberbielle-Boissel, C.; Hill, G.S., et al. (2009). Outcome of subclinical antibody-mediated rejection in kidney transplant recipients with preformed donor-specific antibodies. *Am J Transplant*, Vol.9, No.11, (September 2009), pp. 2561-70, ISSN 1600-6135.

Marfo, K.; Lu, A.; Ling, M., et al. (2011). Desensitization protocols and their outcome. *Clin J Am Soc Nephrol*, Vol.6, No.4, (March 2011), pp. 922-36, ISSN 1555-9041.

Martin, M.A.; Massanari, M.; Nghiem, D.D., et al. (1988). Nosocomial aseptic meningitis associated with administration of OKT3. *JAMA*, Vol.259, No.13, (April 1988), pp. 2002-5, ISSN 0002-9955.

Meier-Kriesche, H.U.; Ojo, A.O.; Hanson, J.A., & Kaplan, B. (2001). Exponentially increased risk of infectious death in older renal transplant recipients. *Kidney Int*, Vol.59, No.4, (April 2001), pp. 1539-43, ISSN 0085-2538.

Meier-Kriesche, H.U.; Li, S.; Gruessner, R.W., et al. (2006). Immunosuppression: evolution in practice and trends, 1994-2004. *Am J Transplant*, Vol.6, No.5, (2006), pp. 1111-31, ISSN 1600-6135.

Merion, R.; White, D.J.; Thiru, S., et al. (1984). Cyclosporine: five years experience in cadaveric renal transplantation. *N Engl J Med*, Vol.310, No.3, (January 1984), pp. 148-54, ISSN 0028-4793.

Morrison, S.L.; Johnson, M.J.; Herzenberg, L.A., et al. (1984). Chimeric human antibody molecules: mouse antigen-binding domains with human constant region domains. *Proc Natl Acad Sci U S A*, Vol.81, No.21, (November 1984), pp. 6851-5, ISSN 0027-8424.

Mourad, G.; Garrigue, V.; Squifflet, J.P., et al. (2001). Induction versus noninduction in renal transplant recipients with tacrolimus-based immunosuppression. *Transplantation*, Vol.72, No.6, (September 2001), pp. 1050-5, ISSN 0041-1337.

Mourad, G.; Rostaing, L.; Legendre, C., et al. (2004). Sequential protocols using basiliximab versus antithymocyte globulins in renal-transplant patients receiving mycophenolate mofetil and steroids. *Transplantation*, Vol.78, No.4, (August 2004), pp. 584-90, ISSN 0041-1337.

Nashan, B.; Moore, R.; Amlot, P., et al. (1997). Randomized trial of basiliximab versus placebo for control of acute cellular rejection in renal allograft recipients. CHIB201 International Study Group. *Lancet*, Vol.350, No.9086, (October 1997), pp. 1193-8, ISSN 0140-6736.

Nashan, B.; Light, S.; Hardie, I.R., et al. (1999). Reduction of acute renal allograft rejection by daclizumab. *Transplantation*, Vol.67, No.1, (January 1999), pp. 110-5, ISSN 0041-1337.

Niblack, G.; Johnson, K.; Williams, T., et al. (1987). Antibody formation following administration of antilymphocyte serum. *Transplant Proc*, Vol.19, No.1, (February 1987), pp. 1896-7, ISSN 0041-1345.

Nishida, H.; Ishida, H.; Tanaka, T., et al. (2009). Cytomegalovirus infection following renal transplantation in patients administered low-dose rituximab induction therapy, *Transpl Int*, Vol.22, No.10, (July 2009), pp. 961-9, ISSN 0934-0874.

Nogid, A. & Pham, D.Q. (2006). Role of abatacept in the management of rheumatoid arthritis.*Clin Ther*, Vol.28, No.11, (November 2006), pp. 1764-78, ISSN 0149-2918.

Norman, D.J.; Shield, C.F. III; Barry, J., et al. (1988). Early use of OKT3 monoclonal antibody in renal transplantation to prevent acute rejection. *Am J Kidney Dis*, Vol.11, No.2, (February 1988), pp. 107-10, ISSN 0272-6386.

Norman, D.J.; Kahana, L.; Stuart, F.P. Jr., et al. (1993). A randomized clinical trial of induction therapy with OKT3 in kidney transplantation. *Transplantation*, Vol.55, No.1, (January 1993), pp. 44-50, ISSN 0041-1337.

Opelz, G. (1995). Efficacy of rejection prophylaxis with OKT3 in renal transplantation. Collaborative Transplant Study. *Transplantation*, Vol.60, No.11, (December 1995), pp. 1220-4, ISSN 0041-1337.

Ortho Multicenter Transplant Study Group. (1985). A randomized clinical trial of OKT3 monoclonal antibody for acute rejection of cadaveric renal transplants. *N Engl J Med*, Vol. 313, No.6, (August 1985), pp. 337-42, ISSN 0028-4793.

Parrott, N.R.; Hammad, A.Q.; Watson, C.J., et al. (2005). Multicenter, randomized study of the effectiveness of basiliximab in avoiding addition of steroids to cyclosporine a monotherapy in renal transplant recipients. *Transplantation*, Vol.79, No.3, (February 2005), pp. 344-8, ISSN 0041-1337.

Pearl, J.P.; Parris, J.; Hale, D.A., et al. (2005). Immunocompetent T-cells with a memory-like phenotype are the dominant cell type following antibody-mediated T-cell depletion. *Am J Transplant*, Vol.5, No.3, (March 2005), pp. 465-74, ISSN 1600-6135.

Perry, D.K.; Burns, J.M.; Pollinger, H.S., et al. (2009). Proteasome inhibition causes apoptosis of normal human plasma cells preventing alloantibody production. *Am J Transplant*, Vol.9, No.1, (January 2009), pp. 201-9, ISSN 1600-6135.

Pisani, B.A.; Mullen, G.M.; Malinowska, K., et al. (1999). Plasma- pheresis with intravenous immunoglobulin G is effective in patients with elevated panel reactive antibody prior to cardiac transplantation. *J Heart Lung Transplant*, Vol.18, No.7, (July 1999), pp. 701-6, ISSN 1053-2498.

Ponticelli, C.; Rivolta, E.; Tarantino, A., et al. (1987). Treatment of severe rejection of kidney transplant with OKT3.PAN. *Transplant Proc*, Vol.1, No.1, (February 1987), pp. 1908-9, ISSN 0041-1345.

Prin Mathieu, C.; Renoult, E.; Kennel De March, A., et al. (1997). Serum anti-rabiit and anti-horse IgG, IgA, and IgM in kidney transplant recipients. *Nephrol Dial Transplant*, Vol.12, No.10, (October 1997), pp. 2133-9, ISSN 0931-0509.

Pruett, T.L.; McGory, R.W.; Wright, F.H., et al. (2009). Safety profile, pharmacokinetics, and pharmacodynamics of siplizumab, a humanized anti-CD2 monoclonal antibody, in renal allograft recipients. *Transplant Proc*, Vol.41, No.9, (November 2009), pp. 3655-61, ISSN 0041-1345.

Rosenberg, J.C.; Lekas, N.; Lysz, K., et al. (1975). Effect of antithymocyte globulin and other immune reactants on human platelets. *Surgery*, Vol.77, No.4, (April 1975), pp. 520-9, ISSN 0039-6060.

Rudich, S.M.; Kaplan, B.; Magee, J.C., et al. (2002). Renal transplantations performed using non-heart-beating organ donors: going back to the future? *Transplantation*, Vol.74, No.12, (December 2002), pp. 1715-20, ISSN 0041-1337.

San Miguel, J.F.; Schlag, R.; Khuageva, N.K., et al. (2008). Bortezomib plus melphalan and prednisone for initial treatment of multiple myeloma. *N Engl J Med*, Vol.359, No.9, (August 2008), pp. 906-17, ISSN 0028-4793.

Schaffer, D.; Langone, A.; Nylander, W.A., et al. (2003). A pilot protocol of a calcineurin-inhibitor free regimen of kidney transplant recipients of marginal donor kidneys or with delayed graft function. *Clin Transplant*, Vol.17, No.9, (2003), pp. 31-4, ISSN 0902-0063.

Schroeder, T.J.; First, M.R.; Mansour, M.E., et al. (1990). Antimurine antibody formation following OKT3 therapy. *Transplantation*, Vol.49, No.1, pp. 48-51, ISSN 0041-1337.

Sharma, L.C.; Muirhead, N., & Lazarovits, A.I. (1997). Human mouse chimeric CD7 monoclonal antibody (SDZCHH380) for the prophylaxis of kidney transplant rejection: analysis beyond 4 years. *Transplant Proc*, Vol.29, No.1-2, (February 1997), pp. 323-4, ISSN 0041-1345.

Shehata, N.; Palda, V.; Meyer, R., et al. (2010). The use of immunoglobulin therapy for patients undergoing solid organ transplantation: an evidence -based practice guideline. *Transf Med Rev*, Vol.24, No.1, (January 2010), pp. S7-27, ISSN 0887-7963.

Shield, C.F.; Edwards, E.B.; Davies, D.B., et al. (1997). Antilymphocyte induction therapy in cadaver renal transplantation. *Transplantation*, Vol.63, No.9, (May 1997), pp. 125763 ISSN 0041-1337.

Shoskes, D.A. & Halloran, P.F. (1996). Delayed graft function in renal transplantation: etiology, management and long-term significance. *J Urol*, Vol.155, No.6, (June 1996), pp. 1831-40, ISSN 0022-5347.

Singh, A.; Stablein, D., & Tejani, A. (1997). Risk factors for vascular thrombosis in pediatric renal transplantation: a special report of the North American Pediatric Renal Transplant Cooperative Study. *Transplantation*, Vol.63, No.9, (May 1997), pp. 1263-7, ISSN 0041-1337.

Sonnenday, C.J.; Warren, D.S.; Cooper, M., et al. (2004). Plasmapheresis, CMV, hyperimmune globulin, and anti-CD20 allow ABO-incompatible renal transplantation without splenectomy. *Am J Transplant*, Vol.4, No.8, (August 2004), pp. 1315-22, ISSN 1600-6135.

Spitzer, T.R.; McAfee, S.L.; Dey, B.R., et al. (2003). Nonmyeloablative haploidentical stem-cell transplantation using anti-CD2 monoclonal antibody (MEDI-507)-based conditioning for refractory hematologic malignancies. *Transplantation*, Vol.75, No.10, (May 2003), pp. 1748-51, ISSN 0041-1337.

Squifflet, J.P.; Besse, T.; Malaise, J., et al. (1997). BTI-322 for induction therapy after renal transplantation: a randomized study. *Transplant Proc*, Vol.29, No.1-2, (February 1997), pp. 317-9, ISSN 0041-1345.

Stratta, P.; Morellini, V.; Musetti, C., et al. (2008). Malignancy after kidney transplantation: results of 400 patients from a single center. *Clin Transplant*, Vol.22, No.4, (February 2008), pp. 424-7, ISSN 0902-0063.

Svoboda, J.; Kotloff, R., & Tsai, D.E. (2006). Management of patients with post-transplant lymphoproliferative disorder: the role of rituximab. *Transpl Int*, Vol.19, No.4, (April 2006), pp. 259-69, ISSN 0934-0874.

Szczech, L.A.; Berlin, J.A.; Aradhye, S., et al. (1997). Effect of anti-lymphocyte induction therapy on renal allograft survival: a meta-analysis. *J Am Soc Nephrol*, Vol.8, No.11, (November 1997), pp. 1771-7, ISSN 1046-6673.

Tatum, A.H.; Bollinger, R.R., & Sanfilippo, F. (1984). Rapid serological diagnosis of serum sickness from antilymphocyte globulin therapy using enzyme immunoassay. *Transplantation*, Vol.38, No.6, (December 1984), pp. 582-6, ISSN 0041-1337.

Tesi, R.J.; Elkhammas, E.A.; Henry, M.L., et al. (1993). OKT3 for primary therapy of the first rejection episode in kidney transplants. *Transplantation*, Vol.55, No.5, (May 1993), pp. 1023-9, ISSN 0041-1337.

Thistlethwaite, J.R. Jr; Gaber, A.O.; Haag, B.W., et al. (1987). OKT3 treatment of steroid-resistant renal allograft rejection. *Transplantation*, Vol.43, No.2, (February 1987), pp. 176-84, ISSN 0041-1337.

Thistlethwaite, J.R. Jr; Stuart, J.K.; Mayes, J.T., et al. (1988). Complications and monitoring of OKT3 therapy. *Am J Kidney Dis*, Vol.11, No.2, (February 1988), pp. 112-9, ISSN 0272-6386.

Tite, J.P.; Sloan, A.; Janeway, C.J. (1986). The role of L3T4 in T cell activation: L3T4 may be both an Ia-binding protein and a receptor that transduces a negative signal. *J Mol Cell Immunol*, Vol.2, No.4, (1986), pp. 179-90, ISSN 0724-6803.

Trivedi, H.L.; Terasaki, P.I.; Feroz, A., et al. (2009). Abrogation of anti-HLA antibodies via proteasome inhibition. *Transplantation*, Vol.87, No.10, (May 2009), pp.1555-61, ISSN 0041-1337.

Turka, L.A.; Linsley, P.S.; Lin, H., et al. (1992). T-cell activation by the CD28 ligand B7 is required for cardiac allograft rejection in vivo. *Proc Natl Acad Sci U S A*, Vol.89, No.22, (November 1992), pp. 11102-5, ISSN 0027-8424.

Tyden, G.; Genberg, H.; Tollemar, J., et al. (2009). A randomized, double-blind, placebo-controlled, study of single-dose rituximab as induction in renal transplantation. *TransplantationI*, Vol.87, No.9, (May 2009), pp. 1325-9, ISSN 0041-1337.

Vallhonrat, H.; Williams, W.W.; Cosimi, A.B., et al. (1999). In vivo generation of C4b, Bb, iC3b, and SC5b-9 after OKT3 administration in kidney and lung transplant recipients. *Transplantation*, Vol.67, No.2, (January 1999), pp. 253-8, ISSN 0041-1337.

Vigeral, P.; Chkoff, N.; Chatenoud, L., et al. (1986). Prophylactic use of OKT3 monoclonal antibody in cadaveric kidney recipients: utilization of OKT3 as the sole immunosuppressive agent. *Transplantation*, Vol.41, No.6, (June 1986), pp. 730-3, ISSN 0041-1337.

Vincenti, F.; Lantz, M.; Birnbaum, J., et al. (1997). A phase I trial of humanized anti-interleukin 2 receptor antibody in renal transplantation. *Transplantation*, Vol.63, No.1, (January 1997), pp. 33-8, ISSN 0041-1337.

Vincenti, F.; Ramos, E.; Brattstrom, C., et al. (2001). Multicenter trial exploring calcineurin inhibitors avoidance in renal transplantation. *Transplantation*, Vol.71, No.9, (May 2011), pp. 1282-7, ISSN 0041-1337.

Vincenti, F.; Larsen, C.; Durrbach, A., et al. (2005). Costimulation blockade with belatacept in renal transplantation. *N Engl J Med*, Vol.353, No.8, (August 2005), pp. 770-81, ISSN 0028-4793.

Vincenti, F.; Charpentier, B.; Vanrenterghem, Y., et al. (2010). A phase III study of belatacept-based immunosuppression regimens versus cyclosporine in renal transplant recipients (BENEFIT study). *Am J Transplant*, Vol.10, No.3, (March 2010), pp. 535-46, ISSN 1600-6135.

Waid, T.H.; Lucas, B.A.; Thompson, J.S., et al. (1992). Treatment of acute cellular rejection with T10B9.1A-31 or OKT3 in renal allograft recipients. *Transplantation*, Vol.53, No.1, (January 1992), pp. 80-6, ISSN 0041-1337.

Waid, T.H.; Lucas, B.A.; Thompson, J.S, et al. (1997a). Treatment of renal allograft rejection with T10B9.1A-31 or OKT3: Final analysis of a phase 2 clinical trial. *Transplantation*, Vol.64, No.2, (July 1997), pp. 274-81, ISSN 0041-1337.

Waid, T.H.; Thompson, J.S.; McKeown, J.W., et al. (1997b). Induction immunotherapy in heart transplantation with T10B9.1A-31: a phase I study. *J Heart Lung Transplant*, Vol.16, No.9, (September 1997), pp. 913-6, ISSN 1053-2498.

Waid, T.H.; Thompson, J.S.; Siemionow, M., et al. (2009). T10B9 monoclonal antibody: a short-acting nonstimulating monoclonal antibody that spares gammadelta T-cells and treats and prevents cellular rejection. *Drug Des Devel Ther*, Vol.3, (Septemeber 2009), pp. 205-12 ISSN 1177-8881.

Weaver, T.A.; Charafeddine, A.H.; Agarwal, A., et al. (2009). Alefacept promotes co-stimulation blockade based allograft survival in nonhuman primates. *Nat Med*, Vol.15, No.7, (July 2009), pp. 746-9, ISSN 1078-8956.

Webster, A; Pankhurst, T.; Rinaldi, F., et al. (2006). Polyclonal and monoclonal antibodies for treating acute rejection episodes in kidney transplant recipients. *Cochrane Database Syst Rev*, Vol.19, No.2, (April 2006), pp. CD004756, ISSN 1469-493X.

Wong, J.T.; Eylath, A.A.; Ghobrial, I., et al. (1990). The mechanism of anti-CD3 monoclonal antibodies: mediation of cytolysis by inter-T cell bridging. *Transplantation*, Vol.50, No.4, (October 1990), pp. 683-9, ISSN 0041-1337.

7

The Role of Cyclosporine A in the Treatment of Prosthetic Vascular Graft Infections with the Use of Arterial Homografts

Artur Pupka and Tomasz Płonek
Wroclaw Medical University
Poland

1. Introduction

Infections of prosthetic grafts in vascular surgery are the cause of many serious postoperative complications including death (Bahnini et al.,1991; Callow,1996; Wilson,2001; Yeager&Porter,1992). Encouraging results were obtained when cold-preserved fresh arterial homografts and other biologic grafts were used to replace infected prosthetic grafts (Chiesa et al.,1998, 2002). Cooling down the grafts only to 4°C allows preservation of the arterial endothelium. However, the endothelium is immunogenic, and thus immunosuppression is needed (Cerilli et al.,1985; Methe et al.,2007; Paul et al.,1985; Pober et al.,1984). Moreover, organ donors should be selected with respect to histocompatibility and blood group types (Gabriel et al.,2002; Mirelli et al.,1998, 1999; Scolari et al.,1998). Experimental studies show that immunosuppressive treatment is helpful after the implantation of cold-preserved fresh arterial homografts (Azuma et al.,1999; Gabriel&Fandrich,2002). On the other hand, there is a concern that immunosuppressive drugs can exacerbate the infection. There are no clinical studies examining the need to use immunosuppression after the transplantation of fresh arterial homografts in prosthetic graft infections (Mirelli et al.,1999). We assumed that administration of Cyclosporine A with a concomitant antibiotic therapy may improve the viability of the fresh arterial homografts and improve the patients' condition.

One of the diagnostic methods used to detect infections in vascular surgery is scintigraphy with the use of Technetium-99m labeled leucocytes. Leucocytes migrate and accumulate in the infected area allowing for the area of accumulation to be estimated (Plissonnier et al.,1995). Objective monitoring of the infection after an arterial graft implantation facilitates the decision of choosing the right treatment, especially for patients treated with immunosuppressive drugs.

The aim of our study was to assess the influence of Cyclosporine A administration on the outcome of patients who underwent fresh arterial homograft transplantation in the treatment of prosthetic graft infections.

2. Materials and methods

2.1 Study design

We carried out a prospective, non-randomized observational study. 79 patients were admitted to our clinic between March 2001 and January 2009 due to a prosthetic graft infection. In all cases we observed infection of the prosthetic graft with purulent fistulas, fluid spaces around the prostheses and bleeding from the vascular anastomoses. All patients that could not wait for the fresh arterial homograft had the prosthesis replaced with a silver coated prosthesis (27 patients). 52 patients who could wait for the arterial homograft were put on a waiting list and were treated with antibiotics and local disinfectants until they had the infected prosthesis replaced with an arterial homograft. According to the protocol approved by the Ethics Committee of the University of Medicine of Wroclaw, patients decided whether they wanted to take Cyclosporine A after obtaining detailed information about the possible benefits and risks of taking this medication.   We defined early and late postoperative periods as ≤30 days and >30days respectively. The patients were divided into 2 groups: Group 1 – consisting of 26 patients who received 1-3 mg/kg of Cyclosporine A per day with dose adjustments to maintain a serum concentration of 120-140 mg/ml and group 2 - consisting of 26 patients who were treated without immunosuppressive drugs (Table 1). All patients with positive cross-match were assigned to group 1 (3 patients).

Characteristics of homograft recipients	Group 1 (N=26)	Group 2 (N=26)
Age (years, mean+-SD)	42-68 (57±1)	50-71 (59±5)
Male	25	24
Female	1	2
Additional illnesses		
Diabetes	8 (30%)	8 (31%)
Ischemic heart disease	15 (58%)	14 (54%)
Renal failure	4 (15%)	4 (15%)
Leg necrosis	7 (27%)	6 (23%)
Graft-duodenal fistula	6 (23%)	5 (19%)

Table 1. Characteristics of homografts recipients

In each case, the infection was confirmed with Duplex- Doppler Ultrasound, CT and scintigpraphy using Technetium-99m labeled leucocytes. The patients received antibiotics (vancomycin, ciprofloxacin, imipenem) according to the antibiogram, usually for a period of up to 30 days after the operation.

All of the homografts were evaluated before the implantation using scanning electron microscopy. In each case, the examination revealed a non-damaged arterial wall and the presence of the endothelium.

Immunological characteristics of patients qualified for an arterial transplantation		
Homograft	Group 1 (N=26)	Group 2 (N=26)
ABO compatibility	26 (100%)	26 (100%)
Negative cross-match	23 (88%)	26 (100%)
Number of incompatibilities in HLA (average+-SD)	3.7±1.8	3.7±1.5
Negative virological examination in donor	26 (100%)	26 (100%)
Time of graft's preservation (hrs, average+-SD)	6-24 (15.2±4.8)	8-22 (14.4±4.9)

Table 2. Immunological characteristics of patients qualified for an arterial transplantation

2.2 Patients
2.2.1 Group 1
The administration of Cyclosporine A (Sandimmun®; Novartis Pharma GmbH) began intraoperatively after revascularization. In this group, 21 Y-shaped, 4 ilio-femoral and 1 aorto-femoral cold-preserved fresh arterial grafts were implanted. The time of simple hypothermia preservation of aortic allografts did not exceed 24 hours. 3 patients from this group had slightly positive cross-match results with the donors' lymphocytes. Microbiological cultures from the specimens from the groin, retroperitoneal space and the infected prosthesis revealed MRSA (24 patients; 92 %), *Staphylococcus epidermidis* (10; 38%) and *Pseudomonas aeruginosa* (7; 27%) infections.

2.2.2 Group 2
In group 2, 22 bifurcated and 4 ilio-femoral arterial allografts were implanted. The time of homograft preservation did not exceed 22 hours. Bacteriological cultures confirmed the infection with MRSA (21 patients; 81%), *S.epidermidis* (9; 35%) and *P.aeruginosa* (5; 19%).

2.3 Homografts
There was no statistical difference in tissue histocompatibility between both groups (Table 2). Arterial homografts were collected from dead donors with a confirmed brain death. During this procedure, a fragment of an artery was taken for a microbiological and microscopic evaluation. Homografts were preserved in the UW (University of Wisconsin) fluid. Just before the operation, the tissues surrounding the allograft were removed and smaller arterial branches were tied up using monofilament sutures.

2.4 Methods
The postoperative treatment (the course of infection and the effects of the therapy), was monitored using scintigraphy. Before and after the operation, computed tomography (CT), duplex-doppler ultrasound, and in some cases, angiography were performed. Microbiological examination, tissue histocompatibility (A and B locus from class I HLA and D locus from class II HLA), ABO compatibility and cross-matches were carried out in every patient. The activity of CD3+, CD4+ and CD8+ lymphocytes was measured before and after the vascular procedure on the 1st, 3rd, 7th day, and in the 1st, 3rd, 6th, 12th, 18th and 24th month after the operation. Virological and serological examinations were performed in each donor (anty-HIV, HBs-Ag, anty-HBc, anty-HCV, anty-EBV, Hbe-Ag, anty-CMV, VDRL test).
The primary endpoint was the recurrence of infection confirmed by clinical and laboratory examinations or by scintigraphy. Secondary endpoints were early and late postoperative mortality and morbidity, amputations, graft patency, rupture of the graft and presence of the graft aneurysm.

2.5 Statistical analysis
Statistical analysis was performed with the use of Statistica 9,0 software. The results were analyzed by parametrical and non-parametrical tests such as chi-square, chi-square analysis of variance (ANOVA) and the U test of Mann-Whitney. Statistical significance was assumed at p<0.05.

2.6 Ethical approval for research

The protocol of this study was approved by the Ethics Committee of the University of Medicine of Wroclaw.

3. Results

52 patients were enrolled into the study. The mean ± standard deviation (SD) follow-up was 23.3 ± 6.1 months in group 1 and 19.2 ± 10.7 months in group 2. A long-term follow up was completed for 15 patients from group 1 and 14 from group 2.

3.1 Postoperative morbidity and mortality
3.1.1 Postoperative mortality

In group 1, one (4%) patient with an aorto-duodenal fistula died 14 days after the operation due to septic shock and one (4%) died 11 months after the operation due to a cerebrovascular accident. In group 2, four (15%) patients died in the early postoperative period. Two patients (8%) died due to a graft-duodenal fistula on the 5th and 19th postoperative day, one (4%) in the course of septic shock (3rd day) and one (4%) due to myocardial infarction (7th day). Two (8%) patients died in the late postoperative period due to rupture of the allograft (4th and 5th postoperative month) (Table 3, Fig.1). The mortality was higher in group 2 (23%) than in group 1 (8%), but this difference failed to reach statistical significance (p>0.05).

Postoperative mortality	Group 1 (N=26)	Group 2 (N=26)
Early<30 days		
Septic shock	1 (4%)	1 (4%)
Graft-duodenal fistula	-	2 (8%)
Myocardial infarction	-	1 (4%)
	1 (4%)	**4 (15%)**
Late>30 days		
Rupture of graft	-	2 (8%)
Cerebrovascular accident	1 (4%)	-
	1 (4%)	**2 (8%)**

Table 3. Postoperative mortality

3.1.2 Postoperative morbidity

In the group treated with cyclosporine, three (12%) early complications (graft thrombosis, wound dehiscene with evisceration, a hematoma in the inquinal area) and three (12%) late complications (symptoms of bowel ischemia, lower extremity ischemia, tibial arteries occlusion) were observed. Graft aneurysms or late thrombosis of the transplanted artery were not detected in this group. In the group treated without immunosuppression, there were no early complications and 9 (35%) late complications (MRSA inferction of the homograft, 5 cases of homograft aneurysms of which 3 ruptured and 3 femoral amputations due to graft thrombosis) (Table 4). The incidence of late postoperative complications was statistically greater in group 2 than in group 1 (p=0.030). There was no statistically significant difference between group 1 and 2 in the occurrence of early postoperative complications and in the number of both early and late complications.

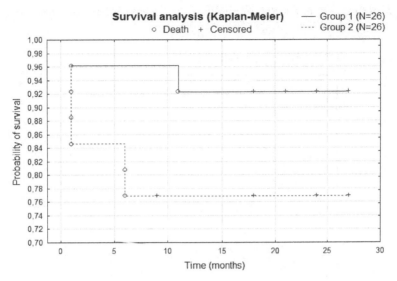

Fig. 1. Kapalan-Meier survival analysis of the patients

Postoperative morbidity	Group 1 (N=26)	Group 2 (N=26)
Early<30 days		
Infection of postoperative wound	1 (4%)	-
Graft thrombosis	1 (4%)	-
Hematoma	1 (4%)	-
	3 (12%)	**0 (0%)**
Late>30 days		
Graft infection	-	1 (4%)
Graft thrombosis - amputation	-	3 (12%)
Low extremity ischemia	2 (8%)	-
Graft aneurysm	-	2 (8%)
Symptoms of bowel ischemia	1 (4%)	-
Rupture of graft	-	3 (12%)
	3 (12%)	**9 (35%)**

Table 4. Postoperative morbidity

3.2 Laboratory and radiological examinations

In both groups, laboratory and radiological examinations confirmed the regression of the infection after the arterial graft implantation. Acute phase proteins were within normal range. The ultrasound examination showed no evidence of fluid spaces around the homografts. Scintigraphy revealed the statistically significant (p=0.011) decrease of accumulation of the Tc-99m labeled leucocytes around the allograft in both groups during the whole observation period of 27 months. The biggest drop in the area of accumulated leucocytes was in the 6th postoperative month in both groups. The rate of the decrease was slightly greater in the group without immunosuppression, but this difference did not reach statistical significance.

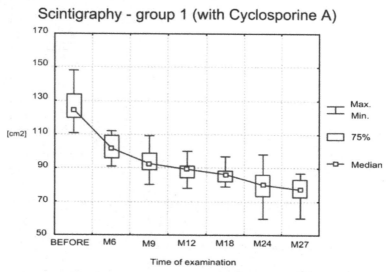

Fig. 2. The reduction of the area of accumulation of Tc99-labelled lymphocytes in patients from group 1 (with Cyclosporine A)

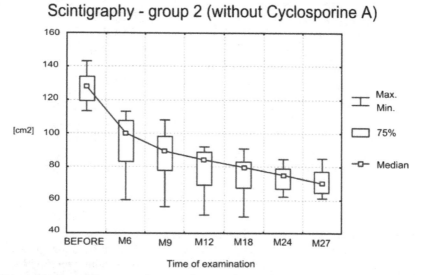

Fig. 3. The reduction of the area of accumulation of Tc99-labelled lymphocytes in patients from group 2 (without Cyclosporine A)

The total reduction of the area of accumulation of the Tc-99m labeled leucocytes during the postoperative period was 35% in group 1 and 44% in group 2 (Fig. 2,3). The statistically significant (p=0.016) difference between both groups in the area of accumulation was observed 18 months after the operation, and it was bigger in group 2.

When there was an increase or no decrease of the leucocytes accumulation, antibiotics were administered according to the antibiogram. This took place 4 times in group 1 (15%) and 3 times in group 2 (12%). The antibacterial treatment resulted in the reduction of the leucocytes accumulation and there were no further clinical signs of reinfection.

3.3 The activity of CD3+, CD4+ and CD8+ lymphocytes in blood

The analysis of the immunological response in both examined groups revealed an increase in the activity of CD3+ and CD4+ lymphocytes and a decrease in the activity of CD8+ lymphocytes. The increase in activity of CD3+ lymphocytes in group 1 was observed from the first postoperative day and it was statistically significant (p=0.04). The increase in activity of CD3+ lymphocytes was greater in group 2 than in group 1, and reached its maximal value on the 7th postoperative day (Fig.4,5). This difference in activity was also statistically significant (p=0.038). Statistical differences in CD3+ lymphocyte activity between both groups began in the sixth postoperative month and lasted until the 24th month (p=0.027).

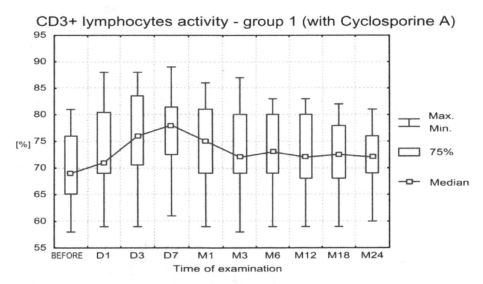

Fig. 4. The CD3+ lymphocytes' activity in patients from group 1 (with Cyclosporine)

The increase in activity of CD4+ lymphocytes was larger in group 2 than in group 1 (Fig. 6,7). The change in activity of CD4+ lymphocytes in both groups was statistically significant (p=0.035). The maximum activity was noted on the 7th postoperative day. A statistically significant difference in activity of CD4+ lymphocytes between both groups was seen on the first day (p=0.032) and in the third month after the arterial graft implantation (p=0.041).

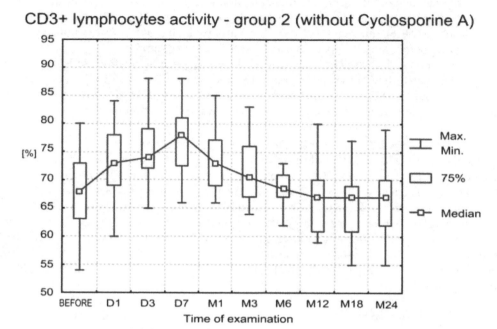

Fig. 5. The CD3+ lymphocytes' activity in patients from group 2 (without Cyclosporine)

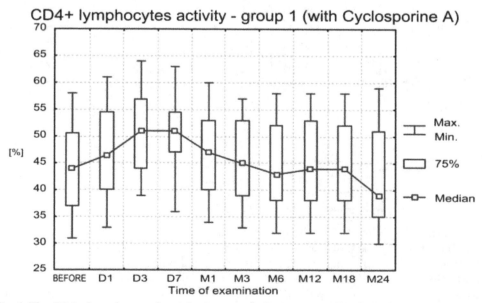

Fig. 6. The CD4+ lymphocytes' activity in patients from group 1 (with Cyclosporine)

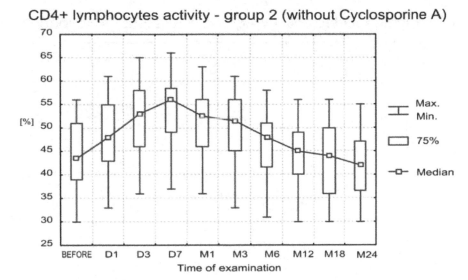

Fig. 7. The CD4+ lymphocytes' activity in patients from group 2 (without Cyclosporine)

The decrease in activity of CD8+ lymphocytes was at its maximum on the 7th day in group 1 and in the 1st month in group 2 after the operation (Fig. 8,9). This decrease was statistically significant ($p=0.02$) in both examined groups. The difference in activity of these leucocytes between group 1 and 2 was statistically significant ($p=0.016$) in the 18th month of the observation and was greater in group 2.

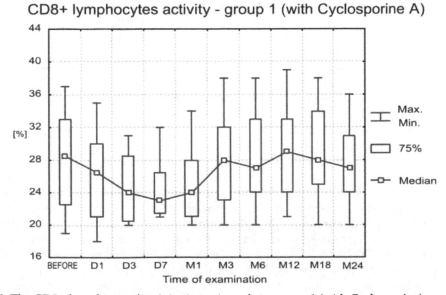

Fig. 8. The CD8+ lymphocytes' activity in patients from group 1 (with Cyclosporine)

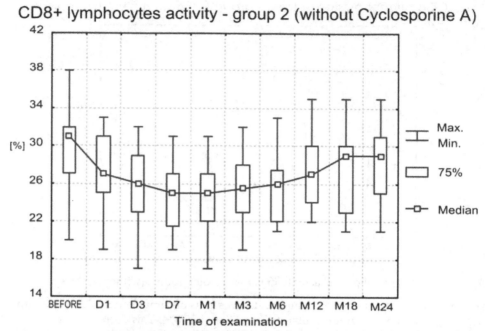

Fig. 9. The CD8+ lymphocytes' activity in patients from group 2 (without Cyclosporine)

3.4 Scanning electron microscopy

Scanning electron microscopy examinations were performed in two patients. One patient from group 1 and another one from group 2 had the arterial homografts removed due to late postoperative complications. The tissue specimens were prepared in the usual manner and assessed by an experienced histologist.

9 months after the transplantation, we collected a fragment of the ilio-femoral homograft from a patient from group 2, who had the transplanted artery removed due to an MRSA infection and rupture of the graft. Scanning electron microscopy (SEM) revealed a complete destruction of the homograft's wall - absence of the endothelium, single, damaged cells and cell fragments of the medial membrane (Fig.11).

We collected a fragment of the artery from a patient from group 1, who was operated on 13 months after the homograft implantation due to an arterial embolism. SEM showed the presence of the endothelial cells (which were mechanically detached), the intimal wall with thickened elastic lamina, a large amount of elastic and collagen fibres, fibrin inclusions, active myoblasts and myofibroblasts (Fig.10). The above mentioned patient stopped taking prescribed immunosuppressive drugs and was admitted to the hospital 12 months after the previous embolectomy. He suffered from lower extremity ischemia in the course of an arterial homograft embolism. Thrombectomy was carried out but this procedure did not improve the blood supply to the leg. Consequently, an amputation was performed. During this operation, a fragment of the arterial homograft's wall was collected. SEM revealed the absence of endothelial cells and the presence of cell apoptosis.

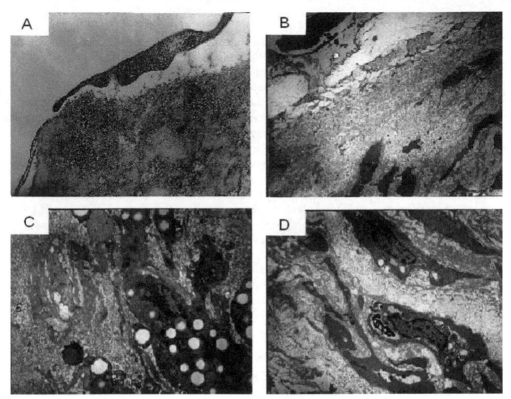

Fig. 10. Scanning electron microscope image - homograft with immunosuppression. A) Endothelial cells. B) Thickened elastic lamina of the intimal wall. C) Active myofibroblasts fagocyting lipids. D) Active myofibroblasts producing collagen

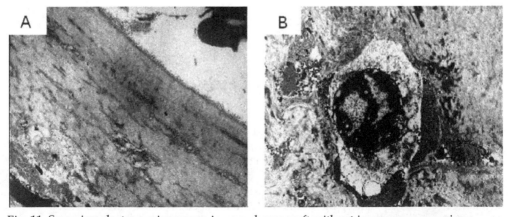

Fig. 11. Scanning electron microscope image - homograft without immunosuppression. A) Absence of endothelium. B) Apoptosis

4. Discussion

The infections of synthetic prostheses in our study were classified as third degree, according to the Szilagy scale, and fifth degree according to the Samson scale (Samson et al.,1988; Szilagyi et al.,1972). The replacement of the infected prosthesis with an arterial allograft was a reasonable solution in these life threatening conditions. We chose cold-preserved fresh arterial homografts because we believed the deep-freeze method was more likely to decrease long-term viability of the arterial wall and less likely to cause the degradation of the endothelium (Bujan et al.,2000; Desgranges et al.,1998; Manaa et al.,2003; Pascual et al.,2001, 2002; Vischjager et al., 1996a, 1996b).

Some scientists claim that the arterial homograft is characterized by low immunogenity and maintain that the graft rejection process is inconsiderable and does not cause an impaired functioning and survivability of the graft (Mirelli et al.,1998, 1999). This is why some vascular surgery centers transplant the arteries without the selection of ABO and HLA compatible donors. There are also numerous research studies showing that the usage of fresh arterial homografts with a preserved endothelium is associated with the immunological response of the graft recipient. This suggests the importance of the selection of donors of the same blood type and similar HLA histocompatibility when fresh arterial allografts are to be used (Chiesa et al.,1998; da Gama et al.,1994; Mirelli et al.,1998, 1999; Prager et al.,2002). We believe that in life threatening infections, the transplantation of the artery despite a slightly positive cross-match is acceptable. In this situation, the usage of immunosuppressive drugs is reasonable. However, we agree that the ABO compatibility is essential (Bracale et al.,1999; Chiesa et al.,1998; Prager et al.,2002).

Clinical trials show that there are changes in an arterial homograft's wall typical for a chronic rejection process (Allaire et al.,1994; Bandyk et al.,2001; Mirelli et al.,1999; Ruotolo et al.,1997). Immunosuppressive treatment can help to stop the degradation of the arterial wall and prolong its viability (Vischjager et al.,1996a, 1996b). However, there is still a question of whether or not to use these drugs in the presence of the infection.

Prolonged functioning of the arterial graft in patients treated with the immunosuppressive drugs was confirmed in some experimental trails (Deaton et al.,1992; Miller et al.,1993; Vermassen et al.,1991; Vischjager et al.,1996). In his experimental trial, Azuma et al. observed that lack or discontinuation of the intake of immunosuppressive medications caused the degradation of the arterial graft's wall and loss of the endothelial cells (Azuma et al.,1999). It was also proven that insufficient dosages of these drugs caused an impaired functioning of the transplanted artery (Gabriel et al.,2002; Geerling et al.,1994; Stoltenberg et al.,1995).

In our study, the increase in activity of CD3+ and CD4+ lymphocytes and the decrease in activity of CD8+ lymphocytes (probably caused by the increase of the infiltration of the homograft's wall by these cells) in transplanted patients suggest arterial allograft's antigenicity.A larger decrease in CD3+ and CD4+ lymphocyte activity and a smaller decrease in CD8+ lymphocyte activity were observed in patients treated with Cyclosporine A than in those treated without immunosuppression. We assume that this was caused by the reduced immunological response of T helper lymphocytes (CD4+) and a smaller infiltration of the allograft by cytotoxic lymphocytes (CD8+). We also believe that this mechanism could help to keep the arterial wall undamaged (Mirelli et al.,1998, 1999).

One month of an antibiotic therapy and the replacement of the infected prosthesis with an arterial homograft lead to the remission of the infection despite the immunosuppressive treatment in almost all patients. This was confirmed with radiological examinations, mainly scintigraphy, using Technetium-99m labeled leucocytes. The maintenance of a small accumulation of the labeled leucocytes around the homograft can be regarded as a chronic reaction against the foreign tissue. We stopped administering the antibiotics according to the scintigraphy results. Prolonged antibiotic and cyclosporine A therapy did not cause any complications associated with decreased immunity. We assume that the application of immunosuppressive drugs reduced the immunological response of the patients against transplanted grafts.

In patients who received immunosuppressive drugs no graft aneurysms were observed compared to 5 cases (19%) of this complication in patients without this therapy. Cyclosporine A may have helped to stop the degradation process of the arterial wall and thus prevented its aneurismal dilatation. The number of cases of postoperative infections was even smaller in those who received immunosuppressive medications. Our study suggests that profits from reasonable immunosuppression outweigh the risk of potential infection in patients with an arterial homograft implanted due to infection of a vascular prosthesis.

5. Conclusions

We believe that Cyclosporine A helped to stop the processes of damaging the graft's wall. Patients treated with this drug had fewer late postoperative complications. Our study suggests that cyclosporine A can be used in patients with an infection of a synthetic vascular prosthesis, undergoing the implantation of a fresh arterial allograft. We found out that fresh arterial homografts may be immunogenic in an extent which leads to its chronic rejection by the patient's immunological system. The results support the hypothesis that Cyclosporine A may prevent the autoimmunologic response of the patient and reduce the risk of damaging the arterial homograft.

Our study was carried out on a relatively small group of patients and it could be the reason why some of the differences between both examined groups of patients failed to reach statistical significance. Therefore, a multicentre randomized trial is needed to definitively establish the role of immunosuppression in the treatment of prosthetic vascular graft infections with the use of arterial homografts.

6. References

Allaire, E., Guettier, C., Bruneval, P., Plissonnier, D.&Michel, J. B. (1994). Cell-free arterial grafts: morphologic characteristics of aortic isografts, allografts, and xenografts in rats. *J Vasc Surg*, 19, 3, (Mar), 446-456, 0741-5214 (Print)

Azuma, N., Sasajima, T.&Kubo, Y. (1999). Immunosuppression with FK506 in rat arterial allografts: fate of allogeneic endothelial cells. *J Vasc Surg*, 29, 4, (Apr), 694-702, 0741-5214 (Print)

Bahnini, A., Ruotolo, C., Koskas, F.&Kieffer, E. (1991). In situ fresh allograft replacement of an infected aortic prosthetic graft: eighteen months' follow-up. *J Vasc Surg*, 14, 1, (Jul), 98-102, 0741-5214 (Print)

Bandyk, D. F., Novotney, M. L., Back, M. R., Johnson, B. L.&Schmacht, D. C. (2001). Expanded application of in situ replacement for prosthetic graft infection. *J Vasc Surg*, 34, 3, (Sep), 411-419; discussion 419-420, 0741-5214 (Print)

Bracale, G. C., Porcellini, M., Bernardo, B., Bauleo, A.&Capasso, R. (1999). Arterial homografts in the management of infected axillofemoral prosthetic grafts. *J Cardiovasc Surg (Torino)*, 40, 2, (Apr), 271-274, 0021-9509 (Print)

Bujan, J., Pascual, G., Garcia-Honduvilla, N., Gimeno, M. J., Jurado, F., Carrera-San Martin, A.&Bellon, J. M. (2000). Rapid thawing increases the fragility of the cryopreserved arterial wall. *Eur J Vasc Endovasc Surg*, 20, 1, (Jul), 13-20, 1078-5884 (Print)

Callow, A. D. (1996). Arterial homografts. *Eur J Vasc Endovasc Surg*, 12, 3, (Oct), 272-281, 1078-5884 (Print)

Cerilli, J., Brasile, L., Galouzis, T., Lempert, N.&Clarke, J. (1985). The vascular endothelial cell antigen system. *Transplantation*, 39, 3, (Mar), 286-289, 0041-1337 (Print)

Chiesa, R., Astore, D., Piccolo, G., Melissano, G., Jannello, A., Frigerio, D., Agrifoglio, G., Bonalumi, F., Corsi, G., Costantini Brancadoro, S., Novali, C., Locati, P., Odero, A., Pirrelli, S., Cugnasca, M., Biglioli, P., Sala, A., Polvani, G., Guarino, A., Biasi, G. M., Mingazzini, P., Scalamogna, M., Mantero, S., Spina, G., Prestipino, F.&et al. (1998). Fresh and cryopreserved arterial homografts in the treatment of prosthetic graft infections: experience of the Italian Collaborative Vascular Homograft Group. *Ann Vasc Surg*, 12, 5, (Sep), 457-462, 0890-5096 (Print)

Chiesa, R., Astore, D., Frigerio, S., Garriboli, L., Piccolo, G., Castellano, R., Scalamogna, M., Odero, A., Pirrelli, S., Biasi, G., Mingazzini, P., Biglioli, P., Polvani, G., Guarino, A., Agrifoglio, G., Tori, A.&Spina, G. (2002). Vascular prosthetic graft infection: epidemiology, bacteriology, pathogenesis and treatment. *Acta Chir Belg*, 102, 4, (Aug), 238-247, 0001-5458 (Print)

da Gama, A. D., Sarmento, C., Vieira, T.&do Carmo, G. X. (1994). The use of arterial allografts for vascular reconstruction in patients receiving immunosuppression for organ transplantation. *J Vasc Surg*, 20, 2, (Aug), 271-278, 0741-5214 (Print)

Deaton, D. W., Stephens, J. K., Karp, R. B., Gamliel, H., Rocco, F., Perelman, M. J., Liddicoat, J. R., Glick, D. B.&Watkins, C. W. (1992). Evaluation of cryopreserved allograft venous conduits in dogs. *J Thorac Cardiovasc Surg*, 103, 1, (Jan), 153-162, 0022-5223 (Print)

Desgranges, P., Beaujan, F., Brunet, S., Cavillon, A., Qvarfordt, P., Melliere, D.&Becquemin, J. P. (1998). Cryopreserved arterial allografts used for the treatment of infected vascular grafts. *Ann Vasc Surg*, 12, 6, (Nov), 583-588, 0890-5096 (Print)

Gabriel, M.&Fandrich, F. (2002). Estimation of graft arteriosclerosis after allogeneic fresh and cryopreserved aortic transplantation in the rat. *Transplant Proc*, 34, 2, (Mar), 711-712, 0041-1345 (Print)

Gabriel, M., Kostrzewa, A.&Sobieska, M. (2002). Immune response after cryopreserved aortic allograft replacement for major vascular infection. *Transplant Proc*, 34, 2, (Mar), 713-714, 0041-1345 (Print)

Geerling, R. A., de Bruin, R. W., Scheringa, M., Bonthuis, F., Jeekel, J., Ijzermans, J. N.&Marquet, R. L. (1994). Suppression of acute rejection prevents graft arteriosclerosis after allogeneic aorta transplantation in the rat. *Transplantation*, 58, 11, (Dec 15), 1258-1263, 0041-1337 (Print)

Manaa, J., Sraieb, T., Khayat, O., Ben Romdhane, N., Hamida, J.&Amor, A. (2003). [The effect of cryopreservation on the structural and functional properties of human vascular allografts]. *Tunis Med*, 81 Suppl 8, 645-651, 0041-4131 (Print)

Methe, H., Hess, S.&Edelman, E. R. (2007). Endothelial immunogenicity--a matter of matrix microarchitecture. *Thromb Haemost*, 98, 2, (Aug), 278-282, 0340-6245 (Print)

Miller, V. M., Bergman, R. T., Gloviczki, P.&Brockbank, K. G. (1993). Cryopreserved venous allografts: effects of immunosuppression and antiplatelet therapy on patency and function. *J Vasc Surg*, 18, 2, (Aug), 216-226, 0741-5214 (Print)

Mirelli, M., Nanni-Costa, A., Scolari, M. P., Iannelli, S., Buscaroli, A., Ridolfi, L., Petrini, F., Stella, A., DeSanctis, L., Borgnino, L. C., Stefoni, S., D'Addato, M.&Bonomini, V. (1998). Mismatch-specific anti-HLA antibody production following aorta transplants. *Transpl Int*, 11 Suppl 1, S444-447, 0934-0874 (Print)

Mirelli, M., Stella, A., Faggioli, G. L., Scolari, M. P., Iannelli, S., Freyrie, A., Buscaroli, A., De Santis, L., Resta, F., Bonomini, V.&D'Addato, M. (1999). Immune response following fresh arterial homograft replacement for aortoiliac graft infection. *Eur J Vasc Endovasc Surg*, 18, 5, (Nov), 424-429, 1078-5884 (Print)

Pascual, G., Garcia-Honduvilla, N., Rodriguez, M., Turegano, F., Bujan, J.&Bellon, J. M. (2001). Effect of the thawing process on cryopreserved arteries. *Ann Vasc Surg*, 15, 6, (Nov), 619-627, 0890-5096 (Print)

Pascual, G., Jurado, F., Rodriguez, M., Corrales, C., Lopez-Hervas, P., Bellon, J. M.&Bujan, J. (2002). The use of ischaemic vessels as prostheses or tissue engineering scaffolds after cryopreservation. *Eur J Vasc Endovasc Surg*, 24, 1, (Jul), 23-30, 1078-5884 (Print)

Paul, L. C., Baldwin, W. M., 3rd&van Es, L. A. (1985). Vascular endothelial alloantigens in renal transplantation. *Transplantation*, 40, 2, (Aug), 117-123, 0041-1337 (Print)

Plissonnier, D., Nochy, D., Poncet, P., Mandet, C., Hinglais, N., Bariety, J.&Michel, J. B. (1995). Sequential immunological targeting of chronic experimental arterial allograft. *Transplantation*, 60, 5, (Sep 15), 414-424, 0041-1337 (Print)

Pober, J. S., Gimbrone, M. A., Jr., Collins, T., Cotran, R. S., Ault, K. A., Fiers, W., Krensky, A. M., Clayberger, C., Reiss, C. S.&Burakoff, S. J. (1984). Interactions of T lymphocytes with human vascular endothelial cells: role of endothelial cells surface antigens. *Immunobiology*, 168, 3-5, (Dec), 483-494, 0171-2985 (Print)

Prager, M., Holzenbein, T., Aslim, E., Domenig, C., Muhlbacher, F.&Kretschmer, G. (2002). Fresh arterial homograft transplantation: a novel concept for critical limb ischaemia. *Eur J Vasc Endovasc Surg*, 24, 4, (Oct), 314-321, 1078-5884 (Print)

Ruotolo, C., Plissonnier, D., Bahnini, A., Koskas, F.&Kieffer, E. (1997). In situ arterial allografts: a new treatment for aortic prosthetic infection. *Eur J Vasc Endovasc Surg*, 14 Suppl A, (Dec), 102-107, 1078-5884 (Print)

Samson, R. H., Veith, F. J., Janko, G. S., Gupta, S. K.&Scher, L. A. (1988). A modified classification and approach to the management of infections involving peripheral arterial prosthetic grafts. *J Vasc Surg*, 8, 2, (Aug), 147-153, 0741-5214 (Print)

Scolari, M. P., De Sanctis, L. B., Iannelli, S., Bonomini, V., D'Addato, M., Stella, A.&Mirelli, M. (1998). Aorta transplantation in man: clinical and immunological studies. *Int J Artif Organs*, 21, 8, (Aug), 483-488, 0391-3988 (Print)

Stoltenberg, R. L., Geraghty, J., Steele, D. M., Kennedy, E., Hullett, D. A.&Sollinger, H. W. (1995). Inhibition of intimal hyperplasia in rat aortic allografts with cyclosporine. *Transplantation*, 60, 9, (Nov 15), 993-998, 0041-1337 (Print)

Szilagyi, D. E., Smith, R. F., Elliott, J. P.&Vrandecic, M. P. (1972). Infection in arterial reconstruction with synthetic grafts. *Ann Surg*, 176, 3, (Sep), 321-333, 0003-4932 (Print)

Vermassen, F., Degrieck, N., De Kock, L., Goubeau, J., Van Landuyt, K., Noens, L.&Derom, F. (1991). Immunosuppressive treatment of venous allografts. *Eur J Vasc Surg*, 5, 6, (Dec), 669-675, 0950-821X (Print)

Vischjager, M., Van Gulik, T. M., De Kleine, R. H., Van Marle, J., Pfaffendorf, M., Klopper, P. J.&Jacobs, M. J. (1996). Experimental arterial allografting under low and therapeutic dosages of cyclosporine for immunosuppression. *Transplantation*, 61, 8, (Apr 27), 1138-1142, 0041-1337 (Print)

Vischjager, M., Van Gulik, T. M., Van Marle, J., Pfaffendorf, M.&Jacobs, M. J. (1996). Function of cryopreserved arterial allografts under immunosuppressive protection with cyclosporine A. *J Vasc Surg*, 24, 5, (Nov), 876-882, 0741-5214 (Print)

Wilson, S. E. (2001). New alternatives in management of the infected vascular prosthesis. *Surg Infect (Larchmt)*, 2, 2, (Summer), 171-175; discussion 175-177, 1096-2964 (Print)

Yeager, R. A.&Porter, J. M. (1992). Arterial and prosthetic graft infection. *Ann Vasc Surg*, 6, 5, (Sep), 485-491, 0890-5096 (Print)

8

HIV/AIDS Associated Malignant Disorders: Role of Highly Active Antiretroviral Therapy

Angel Mayor, Yelitza Ruiz, Diana Fernández and Robert Hunter-Mellado
Retrovirus Research Center, Universidad Central del Caribe School of Medicine, Bayamón
Puerto Rico

1. Introduction

Persons infected with the human immunodeficiency virus (HIV) have an elevated risk for the development of Cancer. Some of the malignant processes are intrinsic to the immunological impact of the HIV infection; others are more often related to the risk scenarios associated to the viral inoculum and subsequent development of the infection. In general terms, malignant transformation is fundamentally caused by genetic alterations to individual cells, which allow the presence of the disorganized autonomous growth of cells and the development of properties associated to the survival of the cancer cells. Properties associated to successful growth of the cancer include the capacity for relative autonomous growth, evasion of the normal regulatory process present within bodies, capacity of tissue invasion, spread to other organs and disruption of the normal organ homeostasis. Predisposing conditions that lead to an increased risk for the malignant transformation include chronic inflammatory states, congenital or acquired genetic mutations, autoimmune diseases, and exposure to environmental factors. The presence of HIV infection, particularly in the context of a deteriorated immune system is associated to an increased risk for the development of Kaposi's sarcoma, high-grade non-Hodgkin's lymphomas, central nervous system lymphoma and invasive uterine cervical cancer. Collectively these entities may be the initial manifestation of HIV infection and are intimately associated to the deteriorated immune system associated to the infection. As such they are considered AIDS defining conditions. The spectrum of HIV associated malignant disorders also includes non-AIDS defining cancers. Non-AIDS defining malignancies are often seen in patients who are at younger age than usual, are associated to a more aggressive behavior and tend to be diagnosed at a more advanced stage. The most common non-AIDS defining malignancies include Hodgkin's lymphomas, non-small cell lung cancer, head and neck cancer, ano-genital cancer, hepatic cancer and possibly multiple myeloma. The role of the HIV virus in triggering the malignant transformation of cells appears to be a direct effect by promoting cancer growth, and indirect in others by disrupting the human regulatory symbiosis provided by the immune system. The introduction of multiple spectrum antiretroviral therapy (ART) and the availability of highly active antiretroviral therapy (HAART) have caused a dramatic improvement in the immunological function of infected subjects with an associated increment in the overall survival of these patients. The use of HAART has been intimately associated to a dramatic decrease in not only AIDS defining opportunistic infections but in some of the AIDS defining tumors particularly Kaposi's sarcoma and non

Hodgkin's lymphomas. Nevertheless changes in the incidence of invasive cervical carcinoma and non-AIDS defining cancers have not been so remarkable. HIV infection has become a chronic condition associated to a longer lifespan of patients and the introduction of an evolving list of co-morbid conditions, including cancer. Under this scenario, understanding the trends on cancer development in this population of patients has become of marked importance, since they represent the next boundary that is limiting the survival of the HIV infected patient. In this chapter we describe the changing trends in the incidence of malignant disorders which affect the HIV infected patients with a particular emphasis on the role of HAART in the expression of these malignant conditions (Bedimo et al, 2004; Bonne et al., 2008; Bower et al, 2006; Caceres et al., 2010; Crum-Clanflone et al, 2009; Engels et al., 2008; Gurlich et al., 2002; Long et al., 2008;Mitsuyasy et al., 2011; Newcomb-Fernandez et al., 2003; Patel et al., 2008; Simard et al., 2010) .

2. Cancer

Hereditary or acquired genetic mutations, autoimmune disorders, and exposure to certain environmental agents may singly or in a combined synergistic fashion, predispose to the development of neoplasms. The role of HIV in inducing the malignant transformation of cells appears to be an indirect effect by disrupting the human immune regulatory process. Immunological deficiency induced by HIV causes a progressive impairment of the cellular immunity responsible for the control of viral growth and the immune recognition against virus-infected or altered cells in the different stages of malignant transformation. HIV induced cytokine deregulation disrupts the host's capacity to control oncogenic viral reactivation and replication, ultimately increasing the risk for malignant transformation. Oncogenic viruses, including the Ebstein-Barr virus (EBV), human herpesvirus 8 (HHV 8), certain subtypes of the human papilloma virus, hepatitis B virus (HBV), and hepatitis C virus (HCV) have all been causally related to the increasing prevalence of cancer development in these patients. In addition the presence of certain risky lifestyle behaviors often present in the HIV infected patients such as smoking, alcohol use, use of illegal drugs and sexual promiscuity may contribute and accelerate the risk of malignant transformation in these subjects. HIV associated severe immunosuppression may be interrupted or partially restored with the use of ART. Improvement or partial restoration of the cell-mediated immunity and the suppression of the HIV viral load will not only improve the patients' immunological status but will improve the overall clinical status with an improvement in overall survival. An increment in the survival of the HIV infected patient leads to an aging patient cohort with a higher likelihood of oncogenic viruses exposure. These elements alter the clinical course of the HIV infection with the development of new morbidity patterns such as altered toxicity profiles of medications, development of metabolic disorders, long lasting co-infections (including HPV, HHV, HCV, HBV and EBV), development of an increased risk of cardiovascular diseases and non-AIDS defining neoplasms. Even though, for many of the tumors described in this chapter, there are no specific prevention guidelines, other than the need to diagnose early and institute therapy as early as possible.

2.1 AIDS defining malignances

Kaposi's sarcoma, high-grade non-Hodgkin's lymphomas, including the high-grade immunoblastic or diffuse large cell lymphoma, the small noncleaved (Burkitt, Burkitt-like or non-Burkitt) lymphoma, primary central nervous system lymphoma (PCNSL), and invasive cervical cancer are neoplasms included as AIDS defining conditions. With the introduction of HAART the spectrum of these cancers has changed, with a dramatic reduction in the incidence of Kaposi's sarcoma and non-Hodgkin's lymphomas. However, the impact of HAART in the invasive cervical cancer had not been significant. It is relevant to mention that in spite of HAART, the risk for AIDS defining cancers continues to be significantly higher as compared to the non HIV infected general population (Simard et al., 2010).

2.1.1 Kaposi's sarcoma

Kaposi's sarcoma is an angio-proliferative disease characterized by tumors composed of new blood vessel (angiogenesis), endothelial spindle cell growth, inflammatory cell infiltration and edema. Kaposi's sarcoma is classified in four epidemiologic variants: the classic, the African endemic, the iatrogenic, and the epidemic AIDS-related. The clinical manifestation of this sarcoma in patients with AIDS is variable but usually presents as a multiple, small, innocuous pigmented cutaneous or oral-pharyngeal lesions. These may grow and spread causing symptom-producing visceral disease. Alternatively it may develop in a multifocal fashion in several sites at the same time. In both cases it may result in a life-threatening process with the need of aggressive therapy.

2.1.1.1 Pathophysiology

The pathogenesis of the condition was clarified in 1994 when human herpes virus-8 (HHV-8) also known as Kaposi's sarcoma -associated herpes virus (KSHV) was described and detected in all forms of Kaposi's sarcoma. HHV-8 is a transmissible DNA virus with a seroprevalence in the United States between 1%-5%. The pathogenesis of AIDS related Kaposi's sarcoma is multifactorial and includes HHV-8 infection, HIV induced cytokine malfunction, and stimulation transactivating transduction (TAT) protein by HIV. HHV-8 is an oncogenic virus transmitted both sexually and through body fluids such as saliva and blood, which encodes a cell protein involved in signal transduction, cell cycle regulation and inhibition of apoptosis. HHV-8 is critical in the pathogenesis of this AIDS related sarcoma, but by itself is not sufficient to cause the cancer. The risk of this cancer is directly related to the degree of immune suppression in the host and can remain in a latent phase for many years. The interaction between HIV-TAT protein and the immune suppressed state of the host allows the activation of the virus resulting in an abnormal inflammatory response and the promotion of angiogenesis by inducing lymphatic reprogramming of the vascular endothelium.

2.1.1.2 Clinical manifestation and diagnosis

The clinical presentation of Kaposi's sarcoma ranges from irregular reddish discrete lesions to violaceous or brown nodules, macules, patches, or plaques. The lesions are usually painless, do not blanch under pressure and may be associated with edema, lymph node or visceral involvement. Pathologic confirmation is required to establish a diagnosis of Kaposi's sarcoma since bacillary angiomatosis can mimic this malignancy even for the seasoned clinician. The lesions may occur in any part of the body, including the face, chest, oral mucosa, penis or scrotum, rectum, and conjunctiva. The oral cavity can be extensively involved resulting in airway obstruction. The gastrointestinal tract is a common site of the disease. These lesions are often asymptomatic but can be associated with abdominal pain, gastro-intestinal bleeding, diarrhea, abdominal cramps, and weight loss. Visceral involvement occurs in over 50% of the cases. Pulmonary involvement is the second most common extra-cutaneous location and may present with life threatening manifestations. Pulmonary involvement is often associated with obstructive respiratory symptoms, hemoptysis and chest pain. The clinical course of this sarcoma is variable with the presence of slowly progressive lesions over the course of many years, or it may have a rapid progression over a course of weeks or months. The external appearance of the cutaneous lesions may lead to emotional distress and stigmatization. The use of corticosteroid therapy has been associated with the induction or exacerbation of this cancer in the context of the HIV infected individual (Bellan et al, 2003; Dezube, 2007).

2.1.1.3 Therapy

The decision to institute therapy needs to consider the extent, location and rate of tumor growth as well as the patient's symptoms, and immune system condition. Optimization of HAART therapy is critical in all patients with Kaposi's sarcoma since this tumor is intrinsically linked to the degree of immunosuppression and the fact that up to 91% of lesions regress with HAART. Immune reconstitution is a primordial therapeutic goal in every patient. For limited skin lesions, the application of topical therapy with liquid nitrogen, vinblastine or retinoic acid may be appropriate. External beam radiotherapy is also an option in certain cases. Interferon-α is an immunomodulator with antiviral and anti-angiogenic effect that has been used with some success in patients with the cutanous form of the disease. Its widespread use has been hampered by its toxicity profile, which is often moderate to severe in nature. For patients with edema, extensive mucocutaneous disease, or symptomatic pulmonary or gastrointestinal involvement, the administration of systemic chemotherapy is recommended. Several single agent drugs are active in this AIDS related sarcoma. These include vincristine, vinblastine, etoposide, anthracyclines, bleomycin and taxol with an overall response rate of 76%. The administration of combination chemotherapy has been utilized since early 1991 for rapidly progressive mucocutaneous or visceral disease. The most common drug combination has been doxorubicin, bleomycin and vincristine (ABV) or bleomycin and vincristine (BV). The use of liposomal anthracyclines is currently considered the optimal first line therapy for the treatment of advanced Kaposi's sarcoma. This single agent therapy has been reported to have similar or improved response rates to other drugs but less toxicity. Paclitaxel (taxol) is the most recent introduction to the systemic chemotherapeutic agents available for these patients. Its use is often prescribed as second line therapy for patients with refractory disease. The response rate with paclitaxel is between 59-71%. Additional drugs that have variable rate of success in this disease include inhibitors of angiogenesis such as thalidomide, inhibitors of tyrosine kinase or mammalian rapamycin pathways such as imatinib and sunitinib. The response rate after standard chemotherapy is usually very good, but they tend to be short lasting. The high incidence of opportunistic infections associated to the administration of chemotherapy along with the chemotherapy associated cytopenias, are major issues in the management of these patients (Berretta et al, 2003; Dezube, 2007).

2.1.1.4 Epidemiology

Kaposi's sarcoma is a rare condition in the HIV negative population; however, it is the most common malignancy associated with HIV infection. This cancer had been more often detected in HIV-positive persons with more advanced immunosuppression (CD4+ T lymphocyte counts of <200 cells/μL), and especially in men who have sex with men (MSM). Among MSM the transition of the HHV-8 is predominately by deep kissing. In these individuals the HHV-8 prevalence that is associated with their number of homosexual partners is considerably greater when compare to the other HIV risk behavior groups. The probability of developing Kaposi's sarcoma in HIV infected persons who are infected with HHV-8 is significantly high. The overall incidence of this cancer was as high as 20% among patients with AIDS before the advent of effective ART. However the incidence decreases dramatically since the introduction of HAART and remains low (Bedimo et al., 2004). The HIV/AIDS Cancer Match Study of 263.254 AIDS cases followed in 15 States of the United States between 1980 and 2008 reveals a significant reduction of this sarcoma incidence of 80% (RR, 0.2: 95% CI, 0.2%-0,2%) in the HAART era (Simard et al, 2010). This study concord with previous studies performed in United States and Puerto Rican's HIV cohorts that reported a significant reduction in the incidence or prevalence of this cancer after the antiretroviral therapies era (Engel et al., 2008; Crum-Cianflone et al., 2009; Mayor et al., 2008b). Despite the significant incidence reduction of Kaposi's sarcoma the risk of this cancer in HIV infected persons remains significantly elevated in the HAART era, when compare to the general population (Simard et al., 2010; Engels et al., 2008; Patel et al., 2008).

2.1.1.5 Prevention

Routine screening for HHV-8 by PCR or serologic testing is not indicated for HIV-infected persons. It has been advocated that HAART therapy will reduce the incidence of Kaposi's sarcoma by improving the immunological state and preventing tumor growth. Thus opportune antiretroviral therapy is an effective preventive strategy for patients who qualify.

2.1.2 Non Hodgkin's lymphoma

Non-Hodgkin's lymphomas represent a diverse group of malignant conditions of the immune system. These tumors are 60-100 times more common in the HIV infected patient as compared to the general population. There are three histological subtypes that are responsible for the majority of non-Hodgkin's lymphomas diagnosed in HIV patients and they include small non-cleaved lymphomas (Burkitts and non Burkitts like), high grade large cell, and the immunoblastic lymphomas, commonly present with the brain as primary site. With the institution of HAART the incidence of lymphomas in these patients has decreased but the decrement is much less as compared to the other AIDS defining conditions. The risk of developing non-Hodgkin's lymphomas has decreased from 1,226 to 306 per 100,000 person years after the introduction of HARRT (Simard et al., 2010). However, the prevalence of these lymphomas in HIV persons after HAART remains high when compare to HIV negative population (Engels et al., 2008; Simard et al., 2010; Bierman et al., 2004; Doweiko, 2007b).

2.1.2.1 Pathophysiology

The pathogenesis of AIDS related non-Hodgkin's lymphomas are fundamentally related to repeated stimulation and proliferation of B cells in the setting of a T–cell immunodeficiency. This results in the loss of immune surveillance and the continued proliferation of aberrant B cell clones. Etiologic agents implicated in the abnormal B cell proliferative response include HIV, Ebstein Barr virus and other infections. The presence of HIV induces the expression of cytokines (IL-6, IL-10 and TNF-α), which also contribute to B cell activation and proliferation. The process of B cell expansion results in lymph node enlargement and is usually accompanied by polyclonal hypergammaglobulinemia. The enhanced proliferative response of B cells increases the opportunity of genetic error, which may result in the dysregulation of suppressor genes (p53) and/or activation of proto-oncogenes (c-myc, BCL-6 or ras). The majority of AIDS-related non-Hodgkin's lymphomas (75%) carry alterations in at least one proto-oncogene and more than 90% have alterations in at least one of the suppression genes. The presence of activation cytokines such as IL-6 and IL-10 contribute to the chronic B cell stimulation resulting in continued growth. Specifically, IL-6 activity that increases early in the course of HIV infection is predictive of the likelihood of lymphoma developing over time. IL10 is an autocrine growth factor for lymphoma and an inhibitor of cellular immune response. Elevated levels of IL-10 are associated to a worse prognosis in AIDS related non-Hodgkin's lymphomas (Bellan et al, 2003; Doweiko, 2007b).

2.1.2.2 Clinical manifestation and diagnosis

The presence of constitutional symptoms (fever, weight loss and night sweats) is seen in 80-90% of patients with AIDS-related non-Hodgkin's lymphomas. It is vital to exclude the presence of opportunistic infections in these patients prior to instituting antineoplastic therapy. Most patients initially present with advanced stage of lymphoma with 80% presenting as a stage IV. Common sites of extra-nodal involvement include central nervous system (30%), gastrointestinal tract (25%), bone marrow (25%) and liver (17%). Nevertheless any site of the body may be involved with AIDS-related non-Hodgkin's lymphomas including the rectum, soft tissue, oral cavity, lungs and heart. Bone marrow and leptomeningeal involvement are more often associated with small, non cleaved (Burkitt-like) lymphoma. Patients with gastrointestinal involvement may present with pain, weight loss, bleeding, obstruction and perforation in 40% of the cases. The prognosis of this group of patients tends to be better; they respond very well to therapy and have a longer survival. Patients with primary central nervous system lymphoma often present with focal neurologic deficits, seizures, and or altered mental status. A diagnosis of non-Hodgkin's lymphomas requires histological confirmation by biopsy with immunephenotypic and molecular rearrangement studies. A complete staging evaluation must be done once a diagnosis is made utilizing body imaging studies of the brain, bone marrow aspiration and biopsy, liver function studies and spinal fluids analysis if clinically indicated. The presence of Ebstein Barr virus DNA in cerebrospinal fluid by polymerase chain reaction is a high specific and sensitive diagnosis criterion for primary central nervous system lymphoma.

The majority of in HIV related non-Hodgkin's lymphomas are associated with one of three histological subtypes mentioned above. The presence of small non-cleaved lymphomas (Burkitts and non Burkitts like) accounts for 40% of them and is usually seen in patients with a higher CD4 counts than other types. They often express an abnormal p53 and c-myc or ras oncogenes. The high-grade large cell histology is seen in 40% of patients and is associated with an abnormal expression of BCL-6 in 40% of the cases. One of the particular presentations of this histology is primary effusion lymphoma. Primary effusion lymphoma occurs as a late manifestation of HIV infection and has a poor clinical outcome and a shorter 6 months survival as compared to other sites of this histology. This high-grade lymphoma originates in the pleura, pericardium, peritoneum, serosal surface or rarely in the meninges. The etiologic cause of this lymphoma is related to herpes virus-8 infection of the tumor clone. A previous history of Kaposi sarcoma increases the risk of developing primary effusion lymphoma, and often genomic material containing the imprint of KSHV/HHV8 genes is found in the malignant clone of cells. The remaining 30% of AIDS-related non-Hodgkin's lymphomas are inmunoblastic plasmocytoid lymphomas and are considered to be related to EBV infection. The most important presentation of this histology is the primary central nervous system lymphoma, which accounts for 20% of all AIDS related lymphomas. This histology is seen in advanced stage AIDS with CD4 cell counts below 30 cells/mm, and they rarely occur outside the brain. The incidence of primary central nervous system lymphoma has decreased with the introduction of HAART but remains a disease with poor outcome. This type of lymphomas is the second most common brain space-occupying lesion in patients with AIDS after toxoplasmosis. The most common location for primary central nervous system lymphomas is cerebral hemispheres, following by basal ganglia, cerebellum, and brain stem, with less than 10% involving posterior fossa. Unlike primary central nervous system lymphoma in the general population, these tumors can have ring-enhancement due to their rapid growth. The tumors usually measure at least 3 cm and may present with central necrosis. Management of this primary lymphoma consists of radiation therapy, the use of corticosteroids and alkylating agents. This therapy will increase length of survival but they rarely induce lasting remissions (Bierman et al., 2004; Doweiko, 2007b).

2.1.2.3 Treatment

The mainstay of therapy for patients with AIDS related non-Hodgkin's lymphomas are systemic chemotherapy. The common used regimens include R-CHOP, m-BACOP, EPOCH although no regimen appears superior to the other. System prophylaxis with intrathecal cytarabine (ARA-C 50 mg) or methotrexate (10-12 mg) every week for four weeks has been shown to reduce central nervous system relapse in the high risk group of patients. The major complication of chemotherapy is myelosuppression with its associated morbidities. Several studies have shown that co-administration with hematopoietic growth factors may enhance the chemotherapy toleration. In addition, prophylaxis with trimethropim/sulfa, azithromycin, fluconazole, ciprofloxacin, and valgancyclovir can reduce the risk of infection during intensive chemotherapy regimen. Refractory or relapse systemic lymphomas have a very poor prognosis with no satisfactory second line therapy available. An important factor in the management of AIDS related non-Hodgkin's lymphomas is the use of HAART to reduce the viral load and enhance the immune system management of the malignant clone.

2.1.2.4 Epidemiology

In the United States, 3% of the AIDS cases present with lymphoma. The major risk factors include older age, magnitude and duration of the immunosuppression, no prior HAART use or insufficient immunologic or virologic response to HAART. The types of risky practices associated to HIV infections are not associated to the presence of lymphoma. AIDS related non-Hodgkin's lymphomas are seen more frequent in men than in women and is seen more often in whites than in blacks. The standardized incidence rate of AIDS associated lymphoma is significantly higher than in the general population (Grulich et al., 2007). Most of the AIDS related non-Hodgkin's lymphomas (75%) have advanced HIV disease, however 25 % of patients develop the disease when the viral load is undetectable. Different studies had reported a significant reduction in the incidence of these lymphomas with the availability of effective antiretroviral therapies, particularly HAART (Bedimo et al., 2004). For example the HIV/AIDS Cancer Match Study of Simard et al, reported a 70% decline in their incidence (RR, 0.3: 95% CI, 0.2%-0.3%) as compared to the pre-HAART era (Simard, et al., 2010). The study found significant reduction in the diffuse large B cell and in the CNS Hodgkin's lymphomas NHL, but no differences were seen in the Burkitt-like histological lymphomas. Similar findings were documented in the other United States and Puerto Rican AIDS cohorts (Engels et al., 2008; Mayor et al., 2008b). Despite this significant reduction, non-Hodgkin's lymphomas risk remained significantly higher in HIV infected persons after HAART when compared to the general population as reported by Patle et al, Simard et al. and Engels et al.

2.1.2.5 Prevention

The risk of developing non-Hodgkin's lymphoma is directly proportional to the disruption of the immune system. The appropriate and opportune use of antiretroviral therapy (HAART) is necessary to reduce this risk. There are no specific prevention guidelines, other than the need to diagnose early and institute therapy as early as possible.

2.1.3 Invasive cervical cancer

Cervical cancer is a malignant proliferation of the squamous epithelium of the ectocervix causing squamous cell carcinoma. Malignant proliferation of the glandular lining of the endocervix carries histology of adenocarcinoma. More than 95% of cervical tumors have squamous cell histology and infection with the Human papilloma virus (HPV) is a necessary factor for the malignant transformation in the majority of these patients. Several subtypes of the HPV have delineated as responsible for the development of cervical dysplasia, which represents the usual histological antecedent to invasive tumors of the ectocervix. A higher incidence of HPV-related dysplasia, more advanced stages of cervical dysplasia and refractoriness to standard therapy is characteristic of this disease in females who also have HIV infection. The similarities in risk profiles and transmission modes between HIV and HPV explain the common and widespread presence of HPV in this group of patients. The higher risk of developing cervical dysplasia in HIV infected women initially promoted the inclusion of cervical cancer as one of the AIDS defining condition in 1993. The presence of HIV associated immunosuppression contributes to an impaired HPV clearance, facilitating progression of early stage to more advanced forms of dysplasia. The role of HIV in the ultimate transformation to cervical carcinoma is not so clearly defined. Cervical cancer is a tumor, which can be prevented and clearly curable if diagnosed at an early stage. Aggressive prevention strategies have significantly decreased the incidence and prevalence of this tumor in developed countries (Molpus &Jone, 2004; Powrie & Cu-Uvin, 2007).

2.1.3.1 Pathophysiology

The majority of squamous cell carcinomas of the cervix are preceded by a premalignant epithelial dysplasia known as cervical intraepithelial neoplasia and squamous intraepithelial lesions. These lesions slowly progress to the invasive form of cervical cancer. HPV infection has an important role in the genesis of this dysplasia and in the progression to an invasive state. This is in large part due to the chronic inflammatory insult induced by this oncogenic virus. HPV infection is the most common sexually transmitted infection in the US with an increasing prevalence seen among HIV infected individuals. HPV Types 16, 18, and 31 are the major virus associated with cervical cancer. Type 16 is more frequently associated with squamous cell histology and type 18 with adenocarcinoma. Other factors associated to the increase incidence of the cervical cancer in these patients include, the use of tobacco, younger age of first intercourse, higher number of sexual partners, immunosuppression, multiple pregnancies, use of hormonal medications, and to a lesser degree family antecedents (Molpus &Jone, 2004; Powrie & Cu-Uvin, 2007).

2.1.3.2 Clinical manifestation and diagnosis

Cervical cancer is asymptomatic in its early stage and is most often seen in patients over the age of 30 years. As the cancer progresses some patients may present with non-menstrual vaginal bleeding, post coital bleeding, postmenopausal bleeding, pain during the sexual intercourse or abnormal vaginal discharges. With more advanced stages of the cancer, the presence of back and pelvic pain, bowel and bladder malfunction, lymph nodes enlargement or urinary obstruction may be present. Cervical intraepithelial neoplasia (CIN) also knows as cervical dysplasia, and invasive stage cancer is diagnosed by histological changes, usually based on cytologic examination of the cervical cells. The Pap smear cervical cytology is the established screening test to evaluate for dysplasia or cancer. A single Pap smear has a sensitivity of 50% and a specificity of 81% when compared to a biopsy of the area. Consecutive Pap smears increase the sensitivity to 99%. In situations where the Pap smears suggests an intraepithelial lesion or the presence of carcinoma, a colposcopy and directed biopsy is usually diagnostic. Any suspicious visible lesion in this anatomic area requires a biopsy.

2.1.3.3 Therapy

The management of cervical dysplasia among HIV-infected patients does not differ from the general guidelines used for the general population. Observation without specific intervention is usually recommended for low degree of cervical dysplasia (CIN 1) unless the lesion persists over a period of 18-24 month. If the lesions evolve to a more advanced degree of dysplasia, or if there is poor adherence to routine monitoring, immediate intervention is necessary. Conventional therapies used for treatment of CIN 2 or 3 dysplasia stage include cryotherapy, laser therapy, cone biopsy, and a loop electrosurgical excision procedure (LEEP). In patients with CIN 1 that have not been treated with one of the outlined interventions, Pap smears or colposcopy should be repeated every 4-6 months to monitor for persistence or progression of lesions. Recurrence rates of 40%-60% after therapy has been reported among HIV-1 infected women undergoing these procedures. Very early stage of cervical cancer with a depth of invasion of less than 3 mm can be treated with hysterectomy or cervical conization. Lager tumors require radical hysterectomy with pelvic lymphadenectomy or pelvic radiation therapy. For advanced stages, therapy with radiation or cisplatin-based chemotherapy is indicated in a palliative or neo-adjuvant basis. Since recurrence of CIN and cervical cancer after conventional therapy is increased in the HIV-infected populations, these patients need careful and repeated follow up examinations with frequent cytologic screening and colposcopic examination if necessary.

2.1.3.4 Epidemiology

Cervical carcinoma is the second most common cause of cancer related mortality in the world. The prevalence of this tumor is much higher in countries in which primary and secondary prevention strategies are not fully implemented. It is estimated that over 12,800 new cases are diagnosed annually in the United States with an associated yearly mortality of 4,600 patients. With the introduction of cervical cytologic screening, the incidence of invasive cancer and mortality associated to this condition has decreased dramatically. Nevertheless the incidence of cervical carcinoma in HIV infected women (16 per 100.000 women) continues to be higher than in the general women population (7 per 100,000) in United States for the year 2004. Contrary to the other AIDS defining malignancies; the incidence of cervical cancer incidence has not changed (RR, 0.8: 95%CI (0.5-1.2) with the introduction of HAART (Bedimo et al.,2004). The standardized incidence ratio (SIR) of cervical cancer continues to be significantly higher in HIV infected females when compared to the general female population (Simard et al., 2010; Engels et al., 2008; Patel et al., 2008). The immunosuppressive effects of the HIV appear to have a lesser role in the pathogenesis of this tumor as compared to the oncogenic effects of HPV. The oncogenic effects of HPV are not interrupted with HAART, limiting the impact of antiretroviral therapy on the overall incidence of cervical cancer in this population of patients. Nevertheless continued immunosupression is associated to a more aggressive disease once invasive carcinoma is present.

2.1.3.5 Prevention

Primary and secondary prevention are essential in order to reduce the incidence of invasive cervical carcinoma in HIV infected women. Early detection of dysplastic changes in the cervical cells and the use of the recently available HPV vaccine are preventive methods directed to reduce the incidence of invasive cancer. HIV infected women need to have a Pap smear on initial evaluation and six months after the initial evaluation. If both tests are negative then follow up exams every year is suggested. If there is cervical dysplasia, a history of a cervical lesion or if the patient is positive for HPV, the Pap smear should be repeated every 4 to 6 months. Some Gynecologists advocate the use of HPV DNA assays as a screening modality in HIV infected females to identify women with a higher risk of dysplasia. Other assays to detect the HPV mRNA of E6 or E7 protein are also used with similar reasons. If a Pap smear demonstrates dysplasia or atypia, colposcopic directed biopsy of the cervix is indicated. HPV vaccine is now available for the active immunization against some of the most common HPV oncogenic virus. This vaccine does not immunize against all oncogenic HPV viruses, thus repeated screening through Pap smear continue to be relevant in the immunized patient. HPV vaccine will provide immunization in females prior to the infection, thus the vaccine is recommended prior to sexual activity usually ages of 9 and 26 years. The efficacy of the vaccine in inducing an effective immune response in the HIV infected host is unknown at this time. Educational interventions on cervical cancer along with its relation with HIV and HPV infections need to be reinforced amongst all health workers and patients.

2.2 Non AIDS defining malignancies (HIV-related)

There are several malignancies that are not AIDS defining, which has a higher prevalence amongst HIV infected individuals. These HIV associated malignancies include, Hodgkin's lymphoma, non-small cell lung cancer, head and neck cancer, anal cancer, liver cancer, multiple myeloma, and central nervous system malignances (Engels, et al., 2008; Simard et al, 2010; Nguyen et al,2010). Most of these malignant conditions can be attributed to persistent infection with oncogenic viruses and are not directly associated to the HIV induced immunodeficiency. The enhanced life expectancy of HIV infected patients with the use of HAART has allowed an increased period of vulnerability where the patients can be exposed to oncogenic viruses. An increase in the period of viral latency also accompanies an increase in survival. Nevertheless, the immunological deficiency associated to HIV contributes to the progressive impairment of cellular immunity against oncogenic viruses and virus-infected tumor cells. HIV infection elicits a cytokine deregulation, which disrupts the host capacity to control the reactivation and replication of oncogenic viruses, increasing the risk of malignant transformation.

2.2.1 Hodgkin's lymphoma

Hodgkin lymphoma is one of the most common non-AIDS defining malignancy in HIV positive patients with an incidence which is 18 times more frequent than in the general population. This lymphoma is characterized by the orderly spread of disease from one lymph node group to another and by the present of systemic symptoms. This histology has been associated to intravenous drug use, but the occurrence of this lymphoma is not exclusively restricted to this risk profile. The diagnosis of Hodgkin lymphoma is usually established late in the course of the HIV infection, when patients present a CD4+ T cell count of 300 cells per mm³ or less.

2.2.1.1 Pathophysiology

The histology presentation of Hodgkin lymphoma among HIV positive patients tends to be more unfavorable as compared to the general population. The mixed cellularity and the lymphocyte-depleted histology subtypes are more frequently found in HIV infected persons when compared to the general population. Contrary, the nodular sclerosis type is less frequent in HIV persons. The general population with Hodgkin lymphoma demonstrates tumor with an extensive infiltrate of T lymphocytes as compared with the HIV patient in which the malignant cellular infiltrate is substantially depleted of T lymphocytes. These variations in histology convey a more aggressive course for the Hodgkin lymphoma in HIV infected patient. Epstein Barr virus (EBV) is associated with Hodgkin lymphoma, and may play an important role in the pathogenesis of this disorder since 80%-90% of patients with HIV related Hodgkin lymphoma have EBV genome integrated within Reed-Sternberg cells (RSC). This proportion is higher than the one detected in the general population. The RSCs are the malignant cells seen in Hodgkin lymphoma and their presence is essential for the diagnosis of this disorder. The survival of the RSC depends on the antiapoptotic nuclear factor (NF) κB pathways. The activation of this pathway relies on the recruitment of inflammatory cells to the tumor mileu, which provide essential signals that stimulates the proliferation and inhibits the apoptosis of the RSC. In advanced AIDS stages, the incidence of Hodgkin lymphoma may decrease due to inability of the tumor mileu to recruit lymphocytes and other inflammatory cells essential for the survival of the RSC. The latent expression of EBV-associated transforming protein on the surface of the RSC may also help the proliferation of malignant cells. This latent protein mimics the activated CD40 receptor and allows the constitutive activation of the NF κB pathways, resulting in inhibition of the RSC apoptosis. Thus EBV can potentially promote oncogenesis independent of the availability of inflammatory and activated CD4 T cells. The nodular sclerosing histology appears to be less associated to EBV infection and is more likely to be seen in patients with a higher CD4 cell count. All patients with Hodgkin lymphoma require complete staging with total body imaging studies and bone marrow examinations (Portlock & Yahalom, 2004; Doweiko, 2007b).

2.2.1.2 Clinical manifestation and diagnosis

The clinical manifestations of Hodgkin lymphoma in HIV infected patients differ from the presentation seen in the general population. HIV associated Hodgkin lymphoma is more aggressive in nature, usually presents in advanced stages of the disease with more than 75% having stage III or IV at diagnosis. Liver and spleen involvement is seen in 65% of patients and bone marrow involvement in 50%. More than 80% of these patients present constitutional symptoms such as unexplained fever, night sweats, or significant weight loss. The overall survival of HIV related Hodgkin lymphoma prior to the introduction of HAART was around 18 months. This high mortality was associated to an increased vulnerability of infections after systemic chemotherapy and the short disease free interval often associated with this cancer. The introduction of HAART has improved the survival of patients with HIV related Hodgkin lymphoma, decreasing the incidence of opportunistic infections, and allowing greater tolerance to the antineoplastic drugs.

2.2.1.3 Therapy

The therapy of Hodgkin lymphoma depends of the stage of disease at initial presentation. The therapy of this lymphoma is multidisciplinary in nature with external beam radiation therapy, chemotherapy or a combination of both. Surgical interventions have a limited role. Radiation therapy or chemotherapy is an effective treatment for stage I and II of the Hodgkin lymphoma. For more advanced stages, the use of combination chemotherapy with the ABVD regimen (adriamycin, bleomycin, vinblastine and dacarbazine) along with involved field radiation in selected patients is recommended. A rate of 80% of complete remission is associated with this regimen.

2.2.1.4 Epidemiology

Hodgkin's lymphoma accounts for less than 1% of all the tumors in the US and is more common in men than in women. There are two incidence peaks between the ages of 15 to 34 and in those over the age of 55 years. Hereditary factors, infection with Epstein-Barr virus, and T-lymphocyte immune dysfunction, are associated with this type of cancer. The risk for Hodgkin's lymphoma is significantly higher in the HIV/AIDS population with a standardized incidence rates between 5.6 and 16.2 in relation to the general population (Grulich et al., 2007). This type of lymphoma has a more aggressive debut in HIV infected persons, than in the general population. When evaluating the effect of antiretroviral therapies in the incidence of Hodgkin's lymphoma a great majority of the studies reported a significant increment of this type of cancer in the HIV population after the availability of HAART (Bedimo et al., 2004). Standardized incidence rates of Hodgkin's lymphoma that in the pre HAART era was around 2.0 increased beyond 6.0 in the HAART era (Simard et al, 2010; Engels et al., 2008).

2.2.1.5 Prevention

There are not specific measures to prevent this type of lymphoma.

2.2.2 Lung cancer

Lung cancer is one of the most frequent tumors seen in the general population and is the leading cause of cancer related mortality in the United States. Around 90% of the genesis of this neoplasm is directly associated to the use of tobacco. Passive smokers have a small but significant risk of developing lung cancer when compared to non-smoking population (Miller, 2004). Other risk factors for lung cancer include a genetic predisposition, exposure to environmental toxins, the presence of chronic pulmonary infections, and the presence of an immunosuppressive state. This later risk factor has been confirmed in the organ transplanted populations of patients, which require prolonged use of immunosuppressant therapy (Grulich et al., 2007). The incidence of lung cancer is increased in HIV infected individuals and is often diagnosed in younger age individuals with a history of smoking. The implementation of HAART has not resulted in a significant change in the lung cancer incidence in these patients (Bonnet & Chene, 2008).

2.2.2.1 Pathophysiology

The majority of malignant tumors of the lung originate from the bronchial epithelium. These bronchogenic carcinomas are histologically divided into small cell lung cancers and non-small cell lung cancers. The non-small cell lung cancers are subdivided into adenocarcinoma, squamous cell carcinoma and large cell carcinoma. The adenocarcinoma is the most frequent histological subtype found in HIV infected patients. The presence of small cell lung cancers tends to be less common in HIV infected persons. The management of small cell lung cancers is generally chemotherapy and for early stages of non-small cell lung cancers, the use of surgery or radiotherapy is usually employed. The process of malignant transformation towards lung cancer is associated to a multistep accumulation of genetic mutations, which regulate growth, and apoptosis of the respiratory epithelium. Premalignant lesions including squamous dysplasia and atypical alveolar hyperplasia have been associated with some chromosomal mutations including chromosomes 3p, 2p, and 9p. Bronchogenic carcinomas have been related to alterations in chromosomes 3p, 5q, 9p, 11p, 13q and 17P. The majority of the genetic alterations in these tumors involve deletions of tumor suppressor genes that are essential for the proliferation of tumor cells. Other than genetic mutations, an increase in cellular proliferation may be the result of autocrine growth through factors that include neuropeptide growth factors, insulin like growth factors, transforming growth factor alpha, stem cell growth factor, and heregulins. The precise mechanisms behind the increased incidence of HIV associated lung cancer remains unknown. Immunological damage induced by the virus, pulmonary epithelium damage induced by recurrent infections, the use of tobacco and other drugs are synergistic factors which could contribute to the development of this cancer in the HIV population.

2.2.2.2 Clinical manifestation and diagnosis

Lung cancer is usually asymptomatic when it is detected in its early stages. It is not unusual to have an abnormal routine chest radiograph as the initial test, which leads to the diagnosis. In late stages the presence of pulmonary related symptoms is common. Common symptoms and findings in these patients include cough, changes in frequency and intensity of a chronic cough, hemoptysis, airways obstruction, chest pain, disnea, postobstructive pneumonia, fever and pleural effusion. Symptoms related to direct organ invasion to the heart, great vessels of the upper mediastinum, brain, bone, adrenal glands and liver may be present (Miller, 2004). In metastatic cancer, cervical and supraclavicular lymphadenopathy may be present. HIV associated lung cancer is usually diagnosed in the late stages and as a consequence is associated to a worse prognosis (James, 2006). A diagnosis of lung cancer can be made by examination of sputum cytology or histological evaluation of tissue biopsy. Positron- emission tomography scanning or contrast nodule enhancement CT is occasionally used as a non-invasive alternative to discriminate between a malignant and a non-malignant pulmonary lesion. This technique is associated to a high number of false negative and false positive results.

2.2.2.3 Therapy

Surgery is the most appropriate treatment in non-small cell lung cancer for patients that have potentially resectable disease. It is imperative that patients in whom a pulmonary resection is being considered, the baseline pulmonary function tests are adequate to tolerate the resection and that the general medical condition is optimal to minimize surgical complications. Immunological status is not a very important prognostic variable to preclude surgical cure for these patients. Radiation therapy is also an effective treatment for the non-small cell lung cancer, especially when combined with chemotherapy. In advanced stages of the disease, palliative chemotherapy in the form of cisplatin, carboplatin, paclitaxel, mitomycin, vinca alkaloids, gemcitabine, vinorelbine, ifosfamide and etoside may be used. The therapeutic interventions available for HIV positive patients are similar to their HIV negative counterparts.

2.2.2.4 Epidemiology

Lung cancer is one of the most frequent tumors in the US and is the leading cause of cancer related mortality. In 2007, the incidence in the United States was of 65.5 per 100,000. Lung cancer is the most frequent non- AIDS defining tumor in the HIV infected patient. The standardized incidence ratio (SIR) of this tumor is higher in the HIV infected population, as compared to the general population (Simard et al., 2010; Engels et al., 2008; Bonnet et al., 2008; Patel et al., 2008). The impact of HAART in modifying the incidence of the HIV associated lung cancer is minimal. Engel et al. has reported that the SIR for the lung cancer before and after HAART therapy remains 2.6 in their study cohort (Engels et al., 2006).

2.2.2.5 Prevention

The predominant intervention, which will reduce the incidence and prevalence of lung cancer in the HIV infected population, is the avoidance or reduction in tobacco exposition. It is highly recommended that non-smokers remain free of tobacco and that smokers reduce or cease tobacco use. This recommendation continues to be relevant even in the group in with a diagnosis of lung cancer has been established. In addition HIV infected persons need remain compliant with their HIV therapy in order to reduce the likelihood of recurrent pneumonia and other respiratory complications associated to HIV.

2.2.3 Hepatocelullar carcinoma

Hepatocellular carcinoma is the most common primary liver cancer, with an estimated incidence of 500,000 worldwide cases per year. It is more common in men and more frequently seen between the ages of 50 and 60 years old. Hepatocellular carcinoma is the third leading cause of cancer mortality worldwide. The incidence rates of this carcinoma in United States have historically been lower as compared to other tumors; nevertheless it has doubled in the past decades. In addition the trends of mortality associated to this tumor have increased at a faster rate than most other tumors of the body. Hepatocellular carcinoma often arises in the setting of a damaged liver, as seen in liver cirrhosis. As a consequence the risk factors for hepatic cirrhosis are also risk factors for this cancer. The most common external agents responsible for hepatic cirrhosis include prolonged abuse of alcohol, and chronic infection with the Hepatitis virus type B (HBV) and C (HCV) virus. The coexistence of HIV and HCV infection has been associated to a synergistic damage to the liver leading to a higher incidence of this liver cancer. The incidence of Hepatocellular carcinoma in HIV infected persons has increased with the introduction of HAART. With the growing armamentarium of anti retroviral interventions available for these patients, the survival and quality of life have markedly improved. This survival improvement has permitted re-exposition or continued expositions to drugs, alcohol, tobacco and viral agents, which will compound the extent of liver tissue damage in this high-risk population.

2.2.3.1 Pathophysiology

Hepatocellular carcinoma is an epithelial tumor that arises from the malignant transformation of the hepatocyte. In the majority of patients the tumor originates in the background of a cirrhotic liver suggesting the need of a damaged liver for the malignant transformation to occur. As a consequence all conditions, which lead to hepatic cirrhosis, increase the risk of this carcinoma. The conditions, which are considered risky factors for hepatic cirrhosis, include chronic HBV or HCV infections, chronic alcohol abuse, hemochromatosis, sialohepatitis, certain congenital hepatic disorders, and exposure to hepatotoxic agents. There are exceptional cases in which Hepatocellular carcinoma develops in the absence of liver damage. The exact mechanism for the genesis of this malignancy is uncertain in many of the scenarios described. In patients with chronic HBV infection, the integration of the HBV DNA into the hepatocyte genome produces a significant disturbance in the host tumor suppressor genes and an activation of oncogenes. This leads to a disruption in the cell's cycle, inhibition of the DNA repair mechanisms, and inhibition of hepatocyte apoptosis. These mechanisms contribute to the malignant transformation and tumor proliferation. In chronic HCV infection, immune mediated inflammation is present which results in inhibition of hepatocyte apoptosis. It has been postulated that the co-existence of HBV, HCV and HIV infection produces a significant increment in the risk in developing Hepatocellular carcinoma. These co-infections have also been associated with a reduction in the therapeutic efficacy for HBV and HCV, resulting in continued active co-infection with an augmentation in the incidence and the progression of this neoplasm (Fallon et al., 2006; McDonald et al., 2008).

2.2.3.2 Clinical manifestation and diagnosis

Hepatocelullar carcinoma usually presents with pain in the right upper quadrant of the abdomen, jaundice and hepatomegaly. Constitutional symptoms may include, fever, early satiety, lost of weight and anorexia. Occasionally some patients may present with hepatic function decompensation causing ascites, lower extremity edema, esophageal varices bleeding, acute portal hypertension, and encephalopathy. Laboratory findings related to liver failure may be present including elevated levels of alkaline phosphatase, total bilirubin, ALT or AST. The presences of an elevated α-Fetoprotein or des-gamma carboxyprothrombin are markers for the presence of the liver carcimoma and may be used as measures of tumor growth. Ultra sound (US), three-phase tomography (CT) or magnetic resonance imaging (MRI) is the imaging techniques that suggest the presence of this neoplasm. Histological evaluation of the hepatic mass is often used to confirm the diagnosis. Current guidelines suggest that in the presence of an elevated level of α-Fetorprotein and the presence of a hepatic mass in the context of a cirrhotic liver, a confirmatory biopsy is not necessary. Tissue confirmation is recommended for cases without elevated level of α-Fetorprotein or if the diagnosis remains uncertain (Fallon et al., 2006; McDonald et al., 2008).

2.2.3.3 Therapy

The prognosis of the Hepatocelullar carcinoma is variable and it largely depends whether complete surgical resection of the tumor is possible. Effective surgical interventions are compromised when the primary tumor is large, if there is vascular involvement, if the tumor infiltrates both hepatic lobes, and if there is evidence of metastatic disease. In addition, poor residual hepatic function may prevent hepatic resection. It is estimated that less than 15% of the patients with this cancer are surgical candidates and of these 60% have a tumor recurrence. Additional therapeutic interventions, which may be appropriate, include liver transplantation, hepatic chemoembolization, intratumoral injection of ethanol, and radiofrequency ablation. Hepatic transplantation is performed in patients with Hepatocelullar carcinoma without metastasis, which fulfills the Milan criteria. Systemic therapy with one of the tyrosine kinase receptor inhibitors such as sorafenid or sunitinib may be used. These therapies are not considered curative in nature but will increase survival (Fallon et al., 2006; McDonald et al., 2008).

2.2.3.4 Epidemiology

Hepatocelullar carcinoma is the fourth more common malignant tumor in men and the sixth most common in females in the United States. It is the third leading cause of cancer mortality worldwide. The incidence of Hepatocelullar carcinoma in HIV infected patients is higher than in the general population in great measure related to the common transmission related practices shared between HIV with HBV and HCV. Co-infected patients have been reported to present with more advanced Hepatocelullar carcinoma, and have a higher mortality as compared with patients who are HIV negative. The introduction of HAART has improved the life expectancy among HIV positive individuals but has allowed a greater risk for exposure to additional agents with oncogenic potential. In the HIV/AIDS Cancer Match Study of Simard and collaborators an increment in incidence of Hepatocelullar carcinoma of 90% (RR, 1.9: 95% CI, 0.9%-3.92%) was seen when comparing the pre HAART with the post HAART era (Simard et al., 2010). Other studies have confirmed this evolving increasing trend in the incidence and prevalence of this malignancy across time in different populations (Engels et al., 2008; Mayor et al., 2008b). Furthermore, the standardized incidence ratio (SIR) of Hepatocelullar carcinoma is significantly higher in the HIV infected patient as compared to the general population (Simard et al., 2010).

2.2.3.5 Prevention

The pathogenesis of Hepatocelullar carcinoma is intimately associated to alcohol abuse and chronic infection with HBV and HCV. Primary, secondary and tertiary preventive measures that reduce the risk for exposure to these agents or viruses will directly and indirectly reduce the incidence of this cancer. This is particularly true in the higher risk groups such as those with HIV infection. It has been shown that patients with HIV infection have high-risk practices that predispose them to co-infection with hepatitis A (HAV), HBV, and HCV. In addition alcohol abuse continues to be common practice in these patients. HAV infection carries a predominant fecal-oral viral transmission route that involucrate more commonly men who have sex with men and injecting drug users; HBV infection is predominantly transmitted by percutaneous or mucous contact with infected blood or body fluids including semen and saliva. HIV associated risk groups such as men who have sex with men, high risk heterosexual contact, or injecting drug use are the predominant group with this risk factor. Lastly, HCV infection is transmitted principally by percutaneous contact with infected blood, and this is a relevant issue in HIV patients who are injecting drug use (Samet, 2007) or who received transfusions of unscreened blood. Most patients with acute HBV or HCV infection are asymptomatic and early diagnosis rarely occurs. Approximately 4 % of the HBV mono-infected persons and 20% co-infected with HIV will develop chronic liver disease. Over 80% of HCV infected individuals will eventually develop chronic hepatic disease. In the majority of patients with either infection, the process will remain asymptomatic and undetected many years prior to the onset of liver damage and the development of cancer. All patients infected with HIV should undergo screening testing for HAV, HBV and HCV. In patients who are positive for the HCV serology and in those with unexplained liver disease determination of HCV virus load is suggested. Repeated testing after 4 months of follow up may be required in some cases if the infection was recently adquired. If high risk behaviors persist after an initial negative screening test, repeat testing on an annual basis is recommended. There is no HCV vaccine available. In patients where HBV infection is suspected, determination for the presence of the multiple viral components and antibodies in the serum is recommended. If the surface antigen (HBsAg) and the surface antibody (HBsAb) are negative, then vaccination against the HBV is suggested. This is particularly relevant for the HIV infected individual since the risk for HBV is high in this group. In individuals with detectable HBsAg, detectable HBsAb, or with elevated serum liver enzymes levels, the determination of the HBV viral load needs to be done. Chronic inactive viral infection is determined when the antibodies are positive and the viral load is negative. Both HCV and HBV require opportune therapy in order to minimize the extent of liver damage. HCV chronic infection is treated principally by the combination of peg interferon alpha and Ribavirin. Chronic HBV infection is treated with antiviral agents such as Lamivudine (3TC), Ettricitabine (FTC), Adefovir or Tenofovir. HIV co-infected persons on ART need to be monitored with liver function tests, since concomitant ART could cause liver damage and be responsible for metabolic disorders when used in combination with other medications.

Counseling and educational interventions directed to reduce the risk behavior associated to HBV, HCV and HIV transmission play an important role in Hepatocelullar carcinoma prevention (Center for Disease Control, 2001). One example of an intervention used in our cohort was a multimedia educational intervention, which was validated in Hispanic HIV injecting drug users in Puerto Rico (Mayor el al., 2010). This intervention motivated the participant to abolish their risky behaviors practices when injecting drugs. The Health Belief Model and Social Cognitive Theory were used as theoretical framework to modify the decision making process that led to the avoidance, or reduction of the risk factors relevant for acquiring new HCV infection (Mayor et al., 2008a). We are planning to extend this intervention to patients who are at an early stage of drug addiction in order to capture a larger cohort of patients who have not been infected with HBV or HCV. Counseling and educational interventions regarding alcohol use and abuse is an important approach particularly in the HIV infected person who has a high prevalence of both drug and alcohol use and abuse.

2.2.4 Squamous cell cancer of the anus

Squamous cell carcinoma of the anus is a tumor that originates from the epidermal cells of the hair bearing perianal skin. This tumor may develop outside and beyond the anal verge. The tumor is responsible for 3% of the malignancies of the lower gastrointestinal tract. It is intimately associated to infections with one of the carcinogenic types of HPV. The majority of patients with this tumor had anal intercourse as HIV risk factors, especially in the MSM group (Davis, 2008; Doweiko, 2007a; National Institute of Health, 2011).

2.2.4.1 Pathophysiology

Quite similar in pathogenesis to uterine cervix neoplasias, HPV infection has an important role in the genesis of the anal dysplasia or anal intraepithelial neoplasia (AIN) and its progression to squamous cell cancer. HPV is the most common sexually transmitted infection in the United Sates. The incidence of HPV infection is high and there is evidence of an increasing prevalence of infection in the HIV infected group of patients. HIV associated risk factor of MSM is associated to a high prevalence of anal HPV infection and at higher risk of developing anal cancer. The degree of anal dysplasia is inversely correlated with CD4+ T lymphocyte count, suggesting an important role of the immune system in controlling the impact of HPV infection. With improvement in survival associated to HAART, the latency period for HPV infection has also increased, incrementing the risk of malignant transformation of the dysplastic tissue. Anal squamous cell cancer has a more aggressive presentation and clinical course in HIV infected persons when compared to HIV negative individuals. Other risk factors for the development of anal dysplasia include, heavy cigarette smoking, anal intercourse, and a greater number of lifetime sexual partners. These factors have all been associated to the increasing incidence of the anal cancer in men and in women across the world (Daling et al., 2004).

2.2.4.2 Clinical manifestations and diagnosis

Dysplasia of the squamous epithelium of the anus is a silent condition that becomes symptomatic as it evolves to the malignant stage. Anal carcinoma can induce changes in the intestinal habits, rectal bleeding, rectal itching, rectal irritation or the presence of lumps in the anal area. Low back pain and vaginal symptoms could be also part of the symptoms associated to these processes. In advanced stages the malignant process could ulcerate and infiltrate the anal sphincter muscle, incrementing the magnitude of the symptoms. A disruption of the integrity of the anal mucosa seen in these tumors may predispose to the development of infections in this area. The presence of anal dysplasia and invasive carcinoma require pathologic confirmation. The anal Pap smear is a screening test to evaluate cytologic changes in the anal epithelium in high-risk persons. High-resolution anoscopy (HRA) should be considered if the anal Pap smear shows atypical cytology and should be performed in patients who have low or high grade squamous intraepithelial lesions. Visible lesions should be biopsied to determine the magnitude of the histological changes and to rule out invasive cancer.

2.2.4.3 Therapy

Localized dysplasia requires clinical follow-up with anoscopy and colposcopic biopsy every 4 to 6 months. Lesions can be removed with photocoagulation. Frank carcinoma should be managed with surgical excision or a combination of chemotherapy with concomitant radiotherapy. Chemotherapy with 5-fluorouracil, mitomycin-C, platinum and other analogues has been used with success, particularly for early stage tumors. This modality will preserve anal sphincter function in the majority of patients. More advanced tumors will require an abdomino/perineal tumor resection with the placement of a permanent colostomy.

2.2.4.4 Epidemiology

Prior to the HIV epidemic, the presence of carcinoma of the anus was seen in the older patient, particularly women. With the onset of HIV infection in the community, anal carcinoma is detected in younger patients, and very often associated to HPV infection. Anogenital dysplasia and anal carcinoma are more frequently associated with HPV types 16, 18, 31, 33 and 35. Similar to other tumors influenced by external agents such as viruses, the incidence of anal carcinoma has increased significantly in the HAART era (Simard et al.,

2010; Engels et al., 2008; Long et al., 2008). Simard and coauthors in their United States HIV/AIDS Cancer Matched Study reported a 190% increment in the incidence of anal carcinoma (RR, 2.9: 95% CI, 2.1%-4.0%) in the HAART era when compared to pre HAART era. HAART associated increments in the survival of HIV infected patients will also prolong the HPV carcinogenic effects over the anal epithelium leading to an increased incidence of malignant transformation.

2.2.4.5 Prevention

Although formal guidelines recommending anal Pap smear screening have not been adopted, it is clear that anal cytologic screening for HIV-infected men and women at risk of HPV infection or with anogenital warts is warranted. Follow up exams are mandatory for patients with anal dysplasia, or history of anal cancer. Risk reduction education and intervention in sexual and smoking behaviors could have an indirect effect in the prevention of the anal cancer.

2.2.5 Oral cavity/pharynx cancer

The malignant processes of the cavities of the head and neck have different histological types. In this discussion we are reviewing the data associated to squamous cell carcinoma of the oropharyngeal tract. Other important histologies cancers of the oral cavity and pharynx, such as lymphomas, sarcomas, thyroid tumors and benign tumors are not addressed in this section. The squamous cell carcinomas, which originate in the oral cavity, oropharynx, hypopharynx, and larynx are strongly associated to the use of tobacco. The tobacco may be inhaled in several forms such as cigarettes or cigars, or it may be smokeless such as chewing tobacco or snuff. Tumors localized in the oropharynx may also be vinculated to infection with HPV (Posner, 2004). As anticipated the incidence of oropharyngeal cancer is higher in the HIV infected patient as compared to the general population and the incidence of this tumor is higher in the post HAART era.

2.2.5.1 Pathophysiology

Tobacco use in any form, alcohol consumption, HPV infection, a weakened immune system, micronutrient deficiencies, and poor oral hygiene have all been implicated in the pathogenesis of head and neck neoplasms (Kreimer et al.,2004; Marur et al., 2010; Posner, 2004, National Institute of Health, 2005). Smoking produces a direct exposure of the oral and pharynx mucosa to nicotine and other carcinogenic components of the tobacco, which increase the risk of squamous cell proliferation. Frequent and heavy consumption of alcohol produces local and systemic carcinogenic effect over the mucosa. It is well established the synergism associated between the use of alcohol and tobacco abuse and the risk of head and neck tumors. Infection with HPV types 16 has also been implicated in oropharyngeal tumors. The exact mechanism of HPV associated tumor transformation is unclear. It is postulated that HPV induces the inactivation of tumor suppressor proteins or genes, which promote cell immortality and dedifferentiation. HPV infection is very common and widespread in HIV infected patients. Damage of the HIV individuals' immune integrity may enhance the tissue susceptibility induced by HPV.

2.2.5.2 Clinical manifestations and diagnosis

The clinical manifestation are varied and related to the location and stage of the tumor. Lumps, masses, ulcers may be present in the oral cavity. Problems with swallowing, bleeding or pain may be some of the symptoms. There may be restrictions in the movement of the tongue, or difficulty swallowing certain products. Other manifestations my include, loose tooth, pain in the different bone structures of the face, difficulties with visual acuity, hoarseness, and lymph node enlargement. A diagnosis should be suspected on the basis of the clinical manifestations, physical examination of the head and neck region, endoscopy, computer tomography (CT) scan, magnetic resonance imaging (MRI), positron-emission tomography (PET). Histological confirmation with a needle aspiration and biopsy or excisional biopsy needs to be done. Complete staging of the tumor should follow a histological diagnosis (Posner, 2004).

2.2.5.3 Therapy

The management of these cancers is varied and may include surgery, radiotherapy, chemotherapy, neoadjuvant-chemotherapy, chemo-radiotherapy, and combination-modality interventions. Nutritional support to prevent significant weight loss is important. Associated morbidities such as lung, heart or liver dysfunction need to be identified in order to modify the cancer therapy to be instituted. Speech rehabilitation is occasionally required. Lifelong follow-up is suggested.

2.2.5.4 Epidemiology

Head and neck cancers account for 3 to 5% of all the tumors diagnosed in the United States. It is the sixth most common cancer worldwide. About 40,000 new cases are detected annually. The majority (95%) are squamous cell carcinomas with the oropharynx representing the most common anatomic site (Posner, 2004). These cancers are three times more common in men with a peak incidence over the age of 50 years of age. Approximately 13,000 deaths are attributable each year to these cancers. The patient with HIV infection is at a higher risk for oropharyngeal cancer with a SIR between 2.1 and 5.6 (Grulich et al., 2007; Patel et al., 2008). As with the other HPV related cancers, the impact of HAART in the natural history of these tumors remains unclear. Engels and co-authors have reported a decline in the rates of HIV associated oropharyngeal cancer with the introduction of HAART showing a reduction of the standardized incidence ratio (SIR) from 2.5 to 1.5. Nevertheless the risk of HIV associated head and neck cancer is higher as compared to the general population (Simard et al., 2010; Engels et al., 2008).

2.2.5.5 Prevention

There is no approved test for the early detection of oral cavity/pharynx cancers. Consequently the prevention of these tumors rests on improving the risky behavior patterns of patients. Smoking and alcohol abuse avoidance and cessation are the most important prevention measure for this type of cancer. Up today there is not an effective prevention protocol for HPV in relation to oropharynx cancer. Having a faithful relation with one person, limiting the number of sex partners, having a partner who did not have o had few sex partners, could limit the probability of HPV infection, but not eliminate it.

3. Conclusion

The use of HAART for patients with HIV infection has led to a partial restoration of the immune system prolonging the survival of these patients. The success of this therapy has dramatically altered the natural history and clinical course of infection. HIV/AIDS has become a chronic disease with the co-existence of co-morbid conditions, which have an important effect on the health of these patients. An increased likelihood of exposure to cancer promoters such as oncogenic viruses, increments in the exposure to tobacco and alcohol and continued risky practices have had a major role in the increased risk of developing malignant conditions in these patients. The incidence of most of the AIDS defining malignancies have decreased in large part due to immune restoration present in many patients. However, the incidence of other tumors such as uterine cervical cancers, Hodgkin's lymphoma, certain non-Hodgkins lymphomas, HPV related cancers, lung cancer, and liver cancer have all seen an increase in the HAART era. The synergistic effects of tobacco use, alcohol use, dietary elements and viral co-infections are having an effect in the malignant transformation of tissues in the HIV infected patient. Consequently, an appropriate and opportune management of the HIV infection needs to be supplemented with cancer preventive strategies in this high-risk group of patients. Implementation of recommended cancer screening techniques, educational intervention, and relevant vaccination in the HIV infected populations should decreased the morbidity and mortality rate of HIV associated malignancies. Furthermore, adequate and opportune cancer prevention efforts would be cost effective in the management of this high risk population. Researches into the barriers present, which are obstacles to the implementation of these important prevention techniques, are very relevant and require further evaluation.

4. Acknowledgement

This publication was made possible by the RCMI-NIH Grant number G12RR03035 from the National Center for Research Resources and the NIH Grant number U45RR026139. We would like to thank Christine Miranda for her help in the chapter preparation.

5. References

Bedimo, R., Chen, R. Y., Accortt, N. A., Raper, J. L., Linn, C., Allison, J. J., Dubay, J., Saag, M. S., & Hoesley, C. J. (2004). Trends in AIDS-defining and non-AIDS-defining malignancies among HIV-infected patients: 1982-2002. *Clinical Infectious Diseases*, Vol. 39, No. 1, (November 2004), pp. (1380-1384), ISSN 1058-4838

Bellan, C., De Falco, G., Lazzi, S., & Leoncini L. (2003) Pathologic aspects of AIDS malignancies. Oncogene, Vol.22, No 42, (September 2003), pp. (6639-6645), ISSN 0950-9232

Berretta, M., Cinelli, R., Martellotta, F., Spina, M., Vaccher, E., & Tirelli, U. (2003). Therapies approaches to AIDS-Related malignancies. *Oncogene*, Vol. 22, No 42, (September 2003), pp. (6646-6659), ISSN 0950-9232

Bierman, P. J., Lee Harris, N., & Armitage, J. O. (2004). Non-Hodgkin's lymphomas, In: *Cecil Textbook of Medicine*, Lee Goldman & Dennis Ausiello, pp. (1174-1183), Saunders, ISBN 978-0721696522, United States

Bonnet, F., & Chêne, G. (2008). Evolving epidemiology of malignancies in HIV. *Current Opinion in Oncology*, Vol. 20, No. 1, (September 2008), pp. (534-540), ISSN 1040-8746

Bower, M., Palmieri, C., & Dhillon, T. (2006). AIDS-related malignancies: changing epidemiology and the impact of highly active antiretroviral therapy. *Current Opinion in Infectious Diseases*, Vol. 19, No. 1, (February 2006), pp. (14-19), ISSN 0951-7375

Cáceres, W., Cruz-Amy, M., & Díaz-Meléndez, V. (2010). AIDS-related malignancies: revisited. *Puerto Rico Health Sciences Journal*, Vol. 29, No. 1, (March 2010), pp. (70-75), ISSN 0738-0658

Centers for Disease Control and Prevention (2001). A comprehensive strategy for the prevention and control of Hepatitis C virus infection and its consequences, In: *Centers for Disease Control and Prevention*, June 22, 2011, Available from: http://www.cdc.gov/hepatitis/HCV/Strategy/NatHepCPrevStrategy.htm

Crum-Clanflone, N., Huppler Hullsiek, K., Marconi, V., Weintrob, A., Ganesan, A., Vincent Barthel, R., Fraser, S., Agan, B. K., & Wegner, S. (2009). Trends in the incidence of cancers among HIV-infected persons and the impact of antiretroviral therapy: a 20-year cohort study. *AIDS*, Vol. 23, No. 1, (January 2009), pp. (41-50), ISSN 0269-9370

Daling, J.R., Madeleine, M.M., Johnson, L.G., Schwartz, S.M., Shera, K.A., Wurscher,M.A., Carter, J.J., Porter, P.J., Gallowway, D.A., & McDougall, J.K. (2004). Human papillomavirus, smoking, and sexual practices in the etiology of anal cancer. *Cancer*, Vol. 101, No. 2, (June 2004), pp. (270-280), ISSN 1097-0142

Davis, B. (2007). Men who have sex with men, In: *HIV*, Howard Libman & Harvey J. Makadon, pp. (304-308), American College of Physicians, ISBN 978-1930513730, United States

Dezube, B. J. (2007). Kaposi's sarcoma, In: *HIV*, Howard Libman & Harvey J. Makadon, pp. (271-281), American College of Physicians, ISBN 978-1930513730, United States

Doweiko, J. P. (2007). Anogenital squamous cell cancer, In: *HIV*, Howard Libman & Harvey J. Makadon, pp. (292-294), American College of Physicians, ISBN 978-1930513730, United States

Doweiko, J. P. (2007). HIV-related lymphomas, In: *HIV*, Howard Libman & Harvey J. Makadon, pp. (282-291), American College of Physicians, ISBN 978-1930513730, United States

Engels, E. A., Biggar, R. J., Irene Hall, H., Cross, H., Crutchfield, A., Finch, J. L., Grigg, R., Hylton, T., Pawlish, K. S., McNeel, T. S., & Goedert, J. J. (2008). Cancer risk in people infected with human immunodeficiency virus in the United States. *International Journal of Cancer*, Vol. 123, No. 1, (April 2008), pp. (187-194), ISSN 1097-0215

Engels, E. A., Brock, M. V., Chen, J., Hooker, C. M., Gillison, M., & Moore, R. D. (2006). Elevated incidence of lung cancer among HIV-infected individuals. *Journal of Clinical Oncology*, Vol. 24, No. 9, (March 2006), pp. (1383-1388), ISSN 0732-183X

Fallon, M. (2004). Hepatic tumors, In: *Cecil Textbook of Medicine*, Lee Goldman & Dennis Ausiello, pp. (1222-1225), Saunders, ISBN 978-0721696522, United States

Grulich, A. E., Li, Y., McDonald, A., Correll, P. K. L., Law, M. G., & Kaldor, J. M. (2002). Rates of non-AIDS-defining cancers in people with HIV infection before and after AIDS diagnosis. *AIDS*, Vol. 16, No. 1, (January 2002), pp. (1155-1161), ISSN 0269-9370

Grulich, A. E., van Leeuwen, M. T., Falster, M. O., & Vajdic, C. M. (2007). Incidence of cancers in people with HIV/AIDS compared with immunosuppressed transplant recipients: a meta-analysis. *The Lancet*, Vol. 370, No. 1, (July 2007), pp. (59-67), ISSN 0140-6736

James J. S. (2006). Lung cancer: very high death rate with HIV, huge reduction possible with CT screening for early diagnosis, In: *AIDS Treatment News*, June 22, 2011, Available from: http://www.aidsnews.org/2006/12/lung-cancer.html

Kreimer, A. R., Alberg, A. J., Daniel, R., Gravitt, P. E., Viscidi, R., Garrett, E. S., Shah, K. V., & Gillison, M. L. (2004). Oral human papillomavirus infection in adults is associated with sexual behavior and HIV serostatus. *The Journal of Infectious Diseases*, Vol. 189, No. 4, (February 2004), pp. (686-698), ISSN 0022-1899

Long, J.L., Engels, E.A., Moore, R.D, & Gebo, K.A. (2008). Incidence and outcome of malignancy in the HAART era in an urban cohort of HIV-infected individuals. *AIDS*, Vol. 22, No. 4, (February 2008), pp. (489-496), ISSN 0269-9670

Marur, S., D'Souza, G. D., Westra, W. H., & Forastiere, A. A. (2010). HPV-associated head and neck cancer: a virus-related cancer epidemic. *The Lancet Oncology*, Vol. 11, No. 8, (May 2010), pp. (781-789), ISSN 1470-2045

Mayor, A. M., Fernández, D.M., Colón, H. M., Thomas, J.C., & Hunter-Mellado, R. F. (2010). The effectiveness evaluation of a multimedia Hepatitis C prevention program for HIV infected individuals. *Ethnicity and Disease*, Vol. 20, No. 1, (December 2010), pp. (158-162), ISSN 1049-510X

Mayor, A. M., Fernández, D.M., Colón, H. M., Thomas, J.C., & Hunter-Mellado, R. F. (2008). Feasibility and acceptability of a multimedia Hepatitis C prevention program for Hispanic HIV infected persons. *Ethnicity and Disease*, Vol. 18, No. 2, (April 2008), pp. (195-199), ISSN 1049-510X

Mayor, A. M., Gómez, M. A. Rios-Olivares, E., & Hunter-Mellado, R. F. (2008). AIDS-defining neoplasm prevalence in a cohort of HIV-infected patients before and after highly active antiretroviral therapy. *Ethnicity and Disease*, Vol. 18, No. 2, (April 2008), pp. (189-194), ISSN 1049-510X

McDonald, D. C., Nelson, M., Bower, M., & Powles, T. (2008). Hepatocellular carcinoma, human immunodeficiency virus and viral hepatitis in the HAART era. *World Journal Gastroenterology*, Vol. 14, No. 11, (March 2008), pp. (1657–1663), ISSN 1007-9327

Miller, Y. E. (2004). Lung cancer and other pulmonary neoplasms, In: *Cecil Textbook of Medicine*, Lee Goldman & Dennis Ausiello, pp. (1201-1207), Saunders, ISBN 978-0721696522, United States

Mitsuyasy, R. T., Reddy, & D., Copper. J. S. (2011). AIDS-Related malignancies, In: *Cancernetwork*, March 25, 2011, Available from: http://www.cancernetwork.com/display/article/10165/1802726

Molpus, K. L., & Jones, H. W. (2004). Gynecologic cancer, In: *Cecil Textbook of Medicine*, Lee Goldman & Dennis Ausiello, pp. (1238-1241), Saunders, ISBN 978-0721696522, United States

National Institutes of Health. (2005). Head and neck cancer: questions and answers, In: *National Cancer Institute*, June 26, 2011, Available from: http://www.cancer.gov/cancertopics/factsheet/Sites-Types/head-and-neck

National Institutes of Health. (n.d.). Anal cancer, In: *National Cancer Institute*, June 22, 2011, Available from: http://www.cancer.gov/cancertopics/types/anal

Newcomb-Fernandez, J. (2003). Cancer in the HIV-infected population, In: *The Body*, June 22, 2011, Available from: http://www.thebody.com/content/art16834.html

Nguyen, M. L., Farrell, K. J., & Gunthel C. J. (2010). Non-AIDS-Defining malignancies in patients with HIV in the HAART era. Current Infectious Disease Reports, Vol.12 (January 2010), pp. (46-55) ISSN 1523-3847

Patel, P., Hanson, D. L., Sullivan, P. S., Novak, R. M., Moorman, A. C., Tong, T. C., Holmberg, S. D., & Brooks, J. T. (2008). Incidence of types of cancers among HIV-infected persons compared with the general population in the United States, 1992-2003. Annals of Internal Medicine, Vol. 148, No. 10, (May 2008), pp. (728-736), ISSN 1539-3704

Portlock, C. S., & Yahalom, J. (2004). Hodgkin's disease, In: Cecil Textbook of Medicine, Lee Goldman & Dennis Ausiello, pp. (1166-1173), Saunders, ISBN 978-0721696522, United States

Posner, M. (2004). Head and neck cancer, In: Cecil Textbook of Medicine, Lee Goldman & Dennis Ausiello, pp. (1195-1200), Saunders, ISBN 978-0721696522, United States

Powrie, R. O., & Cu-Uvin, S. (2007). Women, In: HIV, Howard Libman & Harvey J. Makadon, pp. (295-303), American College of Physicians, ISBN 978-1930513730, United States

Samet, J. H. (2007). Injection-drug users, In: HIV, Howard Libman & Harvey J. Makadon, pp. (317-324), American College of Physicians, ISBN 978-1930513730, United States

Simard, E. P., Pfeiffer, R. M., & Engels, E. A. (2010). Spectrum of cancer risk late after AIDS onset in the United States. Archives of Internal Medicine, Vol. 170, No. 15, (August 2010), pp. (1337-1345), ISSN 0003-9926

9

Clinical Immunosuppression in Solid Organ and Composite Tissue Allotransplantation

Barbara Kern and Robert Sucher
Department of Visceral-, Transplant- and Thoracic Surgery,
Medical University Innsbruck
Austria

1. Introduction

Although organ and tissue transplantation has been a fantasy for centuries, the epidemic of discovery in transplantation has taken place primarily during the past 55 years. In 1954, Dr J. Murray was presented with the unique opportunity to transplant a human kidney between identical twins without facing the challenges of acute or chronic allograft rejection as well as side effects of long-term immunosuppression (1, 2). Adding to scientific knowledge through basic research helped us to perform complex vascularized composite allotransplants (VCA) like the hand and face today and vascularized tissues recovered from a different individual will soon be extended to all reconstructive transplant procedures currently requiring autologous tissues (3-5).

The development of novel surgical techniques and the discovery of potent immunosuppressive drugs in the second half of the 20th century propelled the clinical development of organ transplantation(6). The combination of corticosteroids and azathioprine, which was the primary immunosuppressive regimen, used from the late 1960's until 1980 culminated in one-year survival rates of only 40% - 50%. Most notably, the discovery of cyclosporine A and tacrolimus in the 1970's and 1980's represented another major milestone in solid organ transplantation resulting in excellent short-term and acceptable long-term survival rates. With current immunosuppressive regimens mainly consisting of the triple combination of corticosteroids, mycophenolate mofetil, and tacrolimus the overall graft and patient survival has improved substantially and reached one-year graft survival rates of 80%-95% leading to consider organ and tissue transplantation as treatment modality of choice for patients with end–stage organ failure or severe tissue defects due to trauma or burn. Despite significant improvements in acute rejection rates, long-term solid organ allograft survival remained unchanged for the last 15 years (7). The major causes for late graft loss include chronic allograft rejection and death with a functioning graft (8, 9).

Since the immunologic graft-loss-rate seemed to be highest within the first months after transplantation, it became the rule that heightened immunosuppression is required early, with progressive reduction over time, leading to the definition of three distinct periods of immunosuppression after transplantation: The perioperative "induction period", where immunosuppressants are initially given at high doses, the "early maintenance period", which is characterized by progressive taper of the individual drugs, and the "chronic maintenance period", characterized by the combination of different immunosuppressants used at their lowest effective doses.

At the end of 20th century, vascularized composite allotransplantation (VCA) like the hand and face has been performed in humans with success using the same immunosuppressive medications and therapeutic principles used for solid organ transplantation (10). However, since hand and face transplants must be considered as non life-saving operative procedures, novel immunosuppressive treatment protocols for these types of transplants must be developed not only to minimize graft rejection, but also to avoid complications related to adverse effects. Several challenges seem to impede the pharmaceutical industry in bringing novel immunosuppressive agents to the clinic. However, new powerful immunosuppressants are urgently in demand to enable the transplantation of highly immunogenic tissues like the skin and at the same time reduce the incidence of drug-induced toxicity. This goal can only be achieved by either combining synergistic immunosuppressive medications to maximize efficacy and minimize toxicity or by developing minimization protocols where conventional immunosuppression is tapered or even withdrawn shortly after transplantation.

2. Maintenance immunosuppression regimens

Maintenance immunosuppression remains the mainstay of therapy for successful outcomes after solid organ transplantation. Over the past decades, immunosuppressive regimens tried to target multiple immune pathways aiming to decrease acute and chronic allograft rejection and maintain long–term graft survival. Although current maintenance therapy after solid organ transplantation typically includes calcineurin inhibitors, antimetabolites, and corticosteroids, newer therapeutic options including induction therapy with biological agents, mTOR inhibitors, and cellular based therapies have emerged as alternative immunosuppressive strategies. The following paragraph will discuss immunosuppressants that are currently employed in solid organ transplantation.

2.1 Calcineurin-Inhibitors – Backbone of current immunosuppressive regimens

Cyclosporine A

The discovery of cyclosporine A (CsA) still has to be considered as one of the most important breakthroughs in transplantation medicine. CsA was initially discovered in 1968 as a product of *Tolypocladium inflatum gams* and isolated from the soil of the Norwegian plain of Hardanger Vidda (11, 12). At the same time, it was retrieved from fungi imperfecti native to Wisconsin. Almost a decade later, in 1976, Jean-Francois Borel described the immunosuppressive effects for the first time and hence, the first clinical use in a cadaveric kidney transplantation was reported two years later in 1978. Since then, CsA represents the backbone of a multitude of maintenance immunosuppressive protocols used in solid organ transplantation.

The immunosuppressive effects of CsA are based on the inhibition of proliferating CD4+ T cells by interfering with the IL-2 pathway. In other words, CsA was observed to form a complex with cyclophilin that furthermore engages the calcium/calmodulin dependent protein phosphatase calcineurin, which in a further step activates "the nuclear factor of activated T cells" (NFAT) in cell nucleoli to ultimately upregulate interleukin-2 (IL-2) expression. Based on this IL-2 inhibiton, CsA halts T cell growth and T cell differentiation and thereby acts immunosuppressive (13).

Tacrolimus

Since the early 1990's, tacrolimus (FK 506), a macrolide antibiotic, which has been isolated from *Streptomyces tsukubaensis*, represents a mainstay in immunosuppression. Similar to CsA, tacrolimus blocks T cell activation and proliferation by interfering with the IL-2 pathway. FK 506 has been shown to bind the FK-binding protein 12 (FKBP12), which ultimately results in the inhibition of the calcineurin pathway leading to decreased IL-2 mediated T cell proliferation. The binding potency of FK 506 is 10 to 100 times stronger when compared to CsA, which results in decreased dosage demand by nonetheless retaining it's immunosuppressive capacity (14, 15).

Tacrolimus and cyclosporine A have both similar interactions with other medications, because of their common metabolism occurring in the liver by the cytochrome P–450 family. In addition, they also have a similar side effect profile such as acute and chronic renal insufficiency, dyslipidemia, hypertension, electrolyte disturbances, and post transplant diabetes. Furthermore, tacrolimus is more strongly associated with neurological complications including, seizures, headaches, and tremors.

2.2 Mycophenolate mofetil – A powerful substitute for azathioprine in antiproliferative immunosuppressive therapy

Mycophenolate Mofetil (MMF) is an antimetabolite immunosuppressant whose active component, mycophenolic acid (MPA), inhibits the key enzyme in the purine synthesis pathway, inosine monophosphate dehydrogenase (16). The discovery of this antiproliferative agent dates back to 1896, when it was first isolated from cultures of *Penicillium brevicompactum*. Initial analyses and studies to proof the immunosuppressive competence of MMF were conducted in the early 1980's. MMF has been shown to inhibit B and T cells proliferation, and induce apoptosis of activated T cells. It furthermore limits the expression of adhesion molecules on lymphocytes, which results in a decrease of nitric oxide production and hence, decreases the recruitment of inflammatory cells (17). Nevertheless, it took 15 more years until the Food and Drug Administration (FDA) approved this drug for the prevention of renal allograft rejection in 1995 (18).

Several clinical trials in the recent past pointed out that the combination of MMF with calcineurin inhibitors results in enhanced patient and graft survival and reduces events of acute and chronic rejection (19). MMF furthermore might be an alternative drug for patients developing drug-induced nephrotoxicity due to other immunosuppressive treatment (20). Besides bone marrow suppression and subsequent leucopenia, diarrhea, and GI distress are the most notable side effects of this immunosuppressant. However, recently a new " enteric coated" formulation of MMF has been developed, which has been shown to improve the mycophenolate exposure and hence, decreases GI side effects. In addition, MMF replaced azathioprine after 5 decades of its successful utilization as an antiproliferative immunosuppressive agent in the area of solid organ transplantation.

2.3 Azathioprine

Azathioprine has a long history of use in the field of solid organ transplantation (21). As an antimetabolite, azathioprine exerts its immunosuppressive properties by halting DNA replication of T and B cells, as well as by interfering with costimulatory signals, which ultimately results in lymphocyte depletion (22). Before the discovery of CsA, the combination of azathioprine and steroids represented the standard treatment of choice in solid organ transplantation, however, like most immunosuppressive agents, azathioprine has multiple drug interactions and side effects. If co-administered with allopurinol for the treatment of gout or hyperuricemia due to a decrease in drug metabolism of both agents, azathioprine should only be dosed at 20% to 30% of normal dosage (23). The main toxicity associated with azathioprine is a dose dependent myelosuppression resulting in leucopenia, thrombocytopenia, and macrocytic anemia. Additionally, hepatotoxicity and an increased incidence in malignancies have been reported. Today, azathioprine has widely been replaced by mycophenolate mofetil.

2.4 mTOR-Inhibitors
Another powerful class of immunosuppressive drugs comprises inhibitors of the mammalian target of rapamycin (mTOR), a key signaling kinase that affects broad aspects of cellular function like cell growth, as well as protein synthesis, and transcription (24, 25). The first mTOR inhibiting substance, sirolimus (Rapamycin), was isolated from soil obtained on Easter Island (Rapa Nui) and was initially identified as a potent antifungal metabolite (26).
However, this macrolide produced by *Streptomyces hygroscopicus* also turned out to inhibit cell proliferation and thereby produced antitumor and immunosuppressive activity. Finally, in 1999 sirolimus got its FDA approval for the prevention of kidney allograft rejection. Initially, the implementation of sirolimus was supposed to potentiate the therapy with CsA, but the combination controversially increased nephrotoxicity, hypertension, as well as the incidence of hemolytic-uremic syndrome. Hence, a controlled trial in kidney transplantation confirmed increased nephrotoxicity and hypertension in the treatment group of sirolimus combined with tacrolimus, which has been compared to the combined use of mycophenolate mofetil and tacrolimus.
The synthetic derivate of sirolimus, everolimus, showed an increased bioavailability, but there were no affects in interaction with CsA compared to sirolimus observed. Severe side effects of both lipophilic macrolides have been reported including hyperlipidemia, thrombocytopenia, aggravation of proteinuria, mouth ulcers, skin lesions, as well as pneumonitis, and impaired wound healing (27). Especially in kidney grafts, delayed recovery from acute tubular necrosis was observed.

2.5 Corticosteroids
From the early beginnings of solid organ transplantation, corticosteroids have played a key role in maintenance immunosuppression as well as treatment of acute rejection episodes. Today, most immunosuppressive protocols contain high doses of methylprednisolone perioperatively with a subsequent tapering to approximately 5 to 7.5mg per day over the ensuing months.
Although it has been shown that corticosteroids have anti-inflammatory and immunosuppressive properties due to their suppression of prostaglandin synthesis, their stabilization of lysosomal membranes, and subsequently their reduction of histamine and bradykinin, the exact mechanism of action remains incompletely understood (18). Experimental data provide evidence that a continuous corticosteroid treatment due to the presence of glucocorticoid receptors on T cells, results in steroid mediated T regulatory FOXP3 expression and thus suppressor activity (28, 29).

In addition to their therapeutic immunosuppressive effects, corticosteroids have several severe side effects, especially when administered for a long time, which limit their applicability in post-transplant therapy (30). These sequels include inter alia: diabetes, hypertension, obesity, cushingoid features, osteoporosis, poor wound heeling, and adrenal suppression (31). However, despite many transplant clinicians search out steroid-sparing or even steroid–free regimens due to their deleterious side effects, especially induction therapy regimens still continue to include steroids in their treatment regimens.

3. Induction therapy

Many transplant centers in the United States and Europe are currently preferring to apply intense therapy at the time of transplantation with the goal to deplete the recipient's immune system in the immediate post-transplant period to decrease early deleterious interactions between the recipient's immune system and the donor allograft to ultimately induce a tolerogenic state (32). It has been widely accepted that early alloreactivity not only leads to an increase in acute rejection episodes, but also promotes chronic rejection which ultimately leads to poor long–term graft survival. While current induction immunosuppression agents have reduced the incidence of acute rejection, the goal of transplant tolerance has not been realized.

3.1 Antibodies

OKT3

Antibody mediated immunosuppressants have been used as induction therapy to suppress the recipient's immune system immediately after transplantation. There are both, polyclonal as well as monoclonal, antibodies available. OKT3 is a murine monoclonal antibody, which targets the T cell receptor CD3 complex resulting in a decrease of T cell activation (33). As a side effect OKT3 treatment commonly causes a "cytokine release syndrom" with fevers, chills, headaches and myalgias. As a consequence, patients are premedicated with steroids, acetaminophen, and diphenhydramine as a prophylaxis against this inflammatory response. Other less frequent side effects include pulmonary edema, seizures, aseptic meningitis, and renal insufficiency (34).

Basiliximab (Simulect)

Basiliximab is another antibody, commonly used as an induction agent, which interferes with the alpha subunit (CD25) of the IL-2 receptor (35). This monoclonal antibody of chimeric human-murine origin formidably decreases T cell proliferation and differentiation without T cell depletion. It is preferentially used in patients with the risk of low to moderate rejection episodes and it's currently approved for dosing 20mg on the first and fourth day after transplant (36). Being humanized, there were only minimal toxic effects reported, although basiliximab has been associated with pulmonary edema and ARDS-like symptoms (37).

Alemtuzumab (Campath)

Alemtuzumab is a humanized-rat monoclonal antibody directed against CD52, which is present on the surface of mature lymphocytes (38). Originally prescribed in lymphocytic leukemia and lymphoma, alemtuzumab is currently also used as a potent induction agent in solid organ and vascularized composite allografts. Although the function of CD52 remains incompletely understood, it is present on the cell surface of B and T cells, as well as macrophages, and NK cells which get depleted upon binding of alemtuzumab. Although alemtuzumab has a half-life of about 2 weeks, different cells have different rates of recovery after therapy. Additionally, alemtuzumab has been shown to deplete T cells inhomogenously, with a relative sparing of memory T cells and T regulatory cells. In terms of side effects, alemtuzumab has been associated with neutropenia, anemia, pancytopenia, first-dose reactions, and autoimmunity (37).

Antithymocyte Globulin

Anthithymocyte globulin (ATG) is a polyclonal antibody derived from animals that have been immunized with human lymphocytes. As a result, ATG is nonspecifically directed against human lymphocytes, which upon treatment get depleted through multiple mechanisms including complement-mediated lysis and opsonisation. In addition, ATG might induce alloantigen specific immunological tolerance as ATG binds lymphocyte costimulatory molecules and similar to OKT3 and alemtuzumab expands T regulatory cells *in vitro and in vivo* (39). Polyclonal antithymocyte globulin is preferrably used as an agent in steroid-free regimes due to its positive effects in the treatment of steroid-resistant rejection episodes. However, ATG treatment frequently induces an acute reaction to initial administration consisting of fever, rigors and anaphylaxis with some patients developing leucopenia and thrombocytopenia.

3.2 Fusion proteins

CTLA4-Ig (Abatacept, Belatacept)

Full T cell activation depends on two signals. The first signal is generated upon MHC-antigen - T cell receptor (TCR) interaction. The costimulation pathway, or signal two, is activated when accessory molecules bind to their ligands. Specifically the CD28/B7 pathway (CD80 and CD86) has proven itself to be relevant for sustained naïve T cell activation. Interfering with these pathways has been one of the most intensively investigated areas in immunology, particularly when considering therapeutic interventions.

After 25 years of research, the fusion receptor protein CTLA4-Ig (abatacept), a competitive antagonist for CD80/CD86 binding, was finally approved for the therapy of rheumatoid arthritis. For the specific use in solid organ transplantation, where an even more robust immunosuppression is required, a second-generation fusion protein called belatacept was developed. Belatacept has proven efficient in prolonging renal allograft survival alone or in combination therapies with basiliximab or MMF and prednisone (40).

3.3 Immunosuppression in Vascularized Composite Allotransplantation

Immunosuppression in vascularized composite allotransplantation (VCA) remains a difficult issue, since the treatment with conventional immunosuppression used in solid organ transplantation is associated with life–threatening infectious complications (41) and metabolic side effects, which seem to be intolerable for non life-saving procedures like hand and face transplantation (42, 43). As a consequence, reconstructive surgeons and immunologists more than ever seek to establish stable donor antigen specific immunological tolerance to vascularized composite allografts, a state that impairs the immune system not to mount responses against a specific allograft, but at the same time facilitates natural defenses

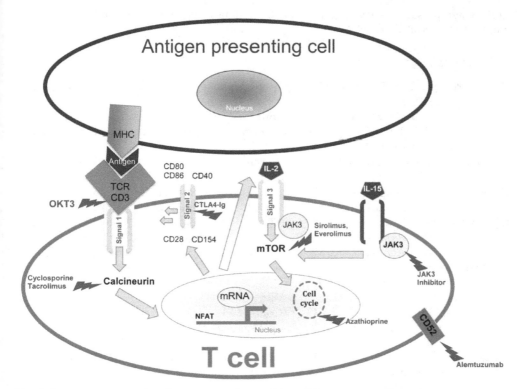

Fig. 1. Immunosuppressive drugs currently used in solid organ transplantation

against viral and bacterial infections. However, in the early days of reconstructive transplantation, immunosuppressive regimens consisted of initial high–dose induction therapy, mainly ATG, or alemtuzumab, which in most cases was followed by a conventional triple combination of corticosteroids, calcineurin inhibitors, and mycophenolate mofetil (44). Exceptions to this conventional immunosuppressive treatment include some recent cases in hand transplantation, where patients received induction therapy with alemtuzumab followed by maintenance immunosuppression with tacrolimus and mycophenolate mofetil (Louisville) or tacrolimus and prednisone (Innsbruck). More recently, the "Pittsburgh Protocol" consisting of an induction therapy with alemtuzumab and a donor specific bonemarrow cell transfusion within 2 weeks after transplantation proofed that maintenance immunosuppression with tacrolimus alone can successfully be achieved in VCA. The idea of donor cell infusion for either the induction of chimerism or the intensification of clonal exhaustion or deletion of alloreactive T cells is appealing, however, the combination of such a concept with high–dose multi drug immunosuppression might be counterproductive, because such phenomena may require the persistence of a certain degree of immune response to be effective. Recent innovative immunosuppressive protocols proofed to be effective in weaning patients off immunosuppression or at least in allowing a reduction of immunosuppression to a minimum level (45, 46). Nevertheless, from the current clinical point of view in reconstructive transplantation, it is difficult to conclude the superiority from one immunosuppressive regimen over another and it seems mandatory to pursue multicenter prospective trials despite the limited number of patients that are currently eligible to be enrolled in such trials.

4. References

[1] Murray JE. The first successful organ transplants in man. J Am Coll Surg. 2005 Jan;200(1):5-9.

[2] Murray JE. The Nobel Lectures in Immunology. The Nobel Prize for Physiology or Medicine, 1990. The first successful organ transplants in man. Scand J Immunol. 1994 Jan;39(1):1-11.

[3] Dubernard JM, Owen E, Herzberg G, Lanzetta M, Martin X, Kapila H, et al. Human hand allograft: report on first 6 months. Lancet. 1999 Apr 17;353(9161):1315-20.

[4] Devauchelle B, Badet L, Lengele B, Morelon E, Testelin S, Michallet M, et al. First human face allograft: early report. Lancet. 2006 Jul 15;368(9531):203-9.

[5] Schneeberger S, Ninkovic M, Gabl M, Hussl H, Rieger M, Loescher W, et al. First forearm transplantation: outcome at 3 years. Am J Transplant. 2007 Jul;7(7):1753-62.

[6] Vincenti F, Kirk AD. What's next in the pipeline. Am J Transplant. 2008 Oct;8(10):1972-81.

[7] Meier-Kriesche HU, Schold JD, Srinivas TR, Kaplan B. Lack of improvement in renal allograft survival despite a marked decrease in acute rejection rates over the most recent era. Am J Transplant. 2004 Mar;4(3):378-83.

[8] Nankivell BJ, Borrows RJ, Fung CL, O'Connell PJ, Allen RD, Chapman JR. The natural history of chronic allograft nephropathy. N Engl J Med. 2003 Dec 11;349(24):2326-33.

[9] Gaston RS, Cecka JM, Kasiske BL, Fieberg AM, Leduc R, Cosio FC, et al. Evidence for antibody-mediated injury as a major determinant of late kidney allograft failure. Transplantation. Jul 15;90(1):68-74.

[10] Sucher R, Hautz T, Brandacher G, Lee WP, Margreiter R, Schneeberger S. [Immunosuppression in hand transplantation: state of the art and future perspectives]. Handchir Mikrochir Plast Chir. 2009 Aug;41(4):217-23.

[11] Kahan BD. The era of cyclosporine: twenty years forward, twenty years back. Transplant Proc. 2004 Mar;36(2 Suppl):5S-6S.

[12] Kostakis A. Early experience with cyclosporine: a historic perspective. Transplant Proc. 2004 Mar;36(2 Suppl):22S-4S.

[13] Morris PJ. Cyclosporine, FK-506 and other drugs in organ transplantation. Curr Opin Immunol. 1991 Oct;3(5):748-51.

[14] Reichenspurner H. Overview of tacrolimus-based immunosuppression after heart or lung transplantation. J Heart Lung Transplant. 2005 Feb;24(2):119-30.

[15] Sigal NH, Dumont FJ. Cyclosporin A, FK-506, and rapamycin: pharmacologic probes of lymphocyte signal transduction. Annu Rev Immunol. 1992;10:519-60.

[16] Allison AC, Eugui EM. Mechanisms of action of mycophenolate mofetil in preventing acute and chronic allograft rejection. Transplantation. 2005 Oct 15;80(2 Suppl):S181-90.

[17] Allison AC, Eugui EM. Mycophenolate mofetil and its mechanisms of action. Immunopharmacology. 2000 May;47(2-3):85-118.

[18] Bhorade SM, Stern E. Immunosuppression for lung transplantation. Proc Am Thorac Soc. 2009 Jan 15;6(1):47-53.

[19] Sollinger HW. Mycophenolates in transplantation. Clin Transplant. 2004 Oct;18(5):485-92.

[20] Hirose R, Vincenti F. Immunosuppression: today, tomorrow, and withdrawal. Semin Liver Dis. 2006 Aug;26(3):201-10.

[21] Taylor AL, Watson CJ, Bradley JA. Immunosuppressive agents in solid organ transplantation: Mechanisms of action and therapeutic efficacy. Crit Rev Oncol Hematol. 2005 Oct;56(1):23-46.

[22] Maltzman JS, Koretzky GA. Azathioprine: old drug, new actions. J Clin Invest. 2003 Apr;111(8):1122-4.

[23] Brooks RJ, Dorr RT, Durie BG. Interaction of allopurinol with 6-mercaptopurine and azathioprine. Biomed Pharmacother. 1982;36(4):217-22.

[24] Brown EJ, Albers MW, Shin TB, Ichikawa K, Keith CT, Lane WS, et al. A mammalian protein targeted by G1-arresting rapamycin-receptor complex. Nature. 1994 Jun 30;369(6483):756-8.

[25] Hay N, Sonenberg N. Upstream and downstream of mTOR. Genes Dev. 2004 Aug 15;18(16):1926-45.

[26] Saunders RN, Metcalfe MS, Nicholson ML. Rapamycin in transplantation: a review of the evidence. Kidney Int. 2001 Jan;59(1):3-16.

[27] Chhajed PN, Dickenmann M, Bubendorf L, Mayr M, Steiger J, Tamm M. Patterns of pulmonary complications associated with sirolimus. Respiration. 2006;73(3):367-74.

[28] Chen X, Murakami T, Oppenheim JJ, Howard OM. Differential response of murine CD4+CD25+ and CD4+CD25- T cells to dexamethasone-induced cell death. Eur J Immunol. 2004 Mar;34(3):859-69.

[29] Demirkiran A, Hendrikx TK, Baan CC, van der Laan LJ. Impact of immunosuppressive drugs on CD4+CD25+FOXP3+ regulatory T cells: does in vitro evidence translate to the clinical setting? Transplantation. 2008 Mar 27;85(6):783-9.

[30] Bodziak KA, Hricik DE. New-onset diabetes mellitus after solid organ transplantation. Transpl Int. 2009 May;22(5):519-30.

[31] Compston JE. Osteoporosis after liver transplantation. Liver Transpl. 2003 Apr;9(4):321-30.

[32] Krischock L, Marks SD. Induction therapy: why, when, and which agent? Pediatr Transplant. May;14(3):298-313.

[33] Chatenoud L, Bluestone JA. CD3-specific antibodies: a portal to the treatment of autoimmunity. Nat Rev Immunol. 2007 Aug;7(8):622-32.

[34] Hong JC, Kahan BD. Immunosuppressive agents in organ transplantation: past, present, and future. Semin Nephrol. 2000 Mar;20(2):108-25.

[35] Gabardi S, Martin ST, Roberts KL, Grafals M. Induction immunosuppressive therapies in renal transplantation. Am J Health Syst Pharm. Feb 1;68(3):211-8.

[36] Delgado JF, Vaqueriza D, Sanchez V, Escribano P, Ruiz-Cano MJ, Renes E, et al. Induction treatment with monoclonal antibodies for heart transplantation. Transplant Rev (Orlando). Jan;25(1):21-6.

[37] Tang IY, Meier-Kriesche HU, Kaplan B. Immunosuppressive strategies to improve outcomes of kidney transplantation. Semin Nephrol. 2007 Jul;27(4):377-92.

[38] Weaver TA, Kirk AD. Alemtuzumab. Transplantation. 2007 Dec 27;84(12):1545-7.

[39] Merion RM, Howell T, Bromberg JS. Partial T-cell activation and anergy induction by polyclonal antithymocyte globulin. Transplantation. 1998 Jun 15;65(11):1481-9.

[40] Larsen CP, Pearson TC, Adams AB, Tso P, Shirasugi N, Strobert E, et al. Rational development of LEA29Y (belatacept), a high-affinity variant of CTLA4-Ig with potent immunosuppressive properties. Am J Transplant. 2005 Mar;5(3):443-53.

[41] Schneeberger S, Lucchina S, Lanzetta M, Brandacher G, Bosmuller C, Steurer W, et al. Cytomegalovirus-related complications in human hand transplantation. Transplantation. 2005 Aug 27;80(4):441-7.

[42] Bonatti H, Brandacher G, Margreiter R, Schneeberger S. Infectious complications in three double hand recipients: experience from a single center. Transplant Proc. 2009 Mar;41(2):517-20.

[43] Schneeberger S, Kreczy A, Brandacher G, Steurer W, Margreiter R. Steroid- and ATG-resistant rejection after double forearm transplantation responds to Campath-1H. Am J Transplant. 2004 Aug;4(8):1372-4.

[44] Schneeberger S, Landin L, Kaufmann C, Gorantla VS, Brandacher G, Cavadas P, et al. Alemtuzumab: key for minimization of maintenance immunosuppression in reconstructive transplantation? Transplant Proc. 2009 Mar;41(2):499-502.

[45] Kirk AD, Mannon RB, Swanson SJ, Hale DA. Strategies for minimizing immunosuppression in kidney transplantation. Transpl Int. 2005 Jan;18(1):2-14.

[46] Schneeberger S, Landin L, Jableki J, Butler P, Hoehnke C, Brandacher G, et al. Achievements and challenges in composite tissue allotransplantation. Transpl Int. Aug;24(8):760-9.

10

E-Health 2.0 Developments in Treatment and Research in Multiple Sclerosis

Peter Joseph Jongen
The MS4 Research Institute (MS4RI)
The Netherlands

1. Introduction

The treatment of multiple sclerosis (MS) is entering a new era, characterized by the availability of a broad range of disease modifying drugs (DMDs) for patients in the relapsing-remitting (RR) phase of the disease. Through interference with immune-mediated inflammatory processes the DMDs reduce the number and severity of relapses and the increase in relapse-related disability. Each DMD is characterized by a unique combination of mode of action, route of administration, degree of efficacy and potential side effects. In the past two decades the injectable drugs interferon beta-1a (INFb-1a), INFb-1b and glatiramer acetate (GA) have been proven to be safe first-line treatments. In more recent years, the intravenously administered monoclonal antibody natalizumab and the oral drugs fingolimod and cladribine have been demonstrated to be efficacious in RRMS. These DMDs are more potent, but also potentially more hazardous, which by and large restricts their use to patients who have very active disease or are refractory to first-line treatment. Lately, phase II/III studies showed beneficial effects of the oral drugs teriflunomide, laquinimod and BG-12, and the monoclonal antibodies rituximab and alemtuzumab in RRMS.

The advent of the new treatments coincides with the Web 2.0 evolution of the internet technology. Web 2.0 offers patients, doctors, and nurses unforeseen possibilities to fundamentally change, and hopefully improve, the ways in which care is delivered and clinical, patient-centered research is performed. The term Web 2.0 is associated with web applications that facilitate participatory information sharing, inter-operability, user-centered design and collaboration on the World Wide Web [1]. A Web 2.0 site allows users to interact and collaborate with each other, e.g. as creators of user-generated content in a virtual community, in contrast to websites where users are limited to the passive viewing of content that was created for them [2].

Basically, e-health 2.0 can be defined as the merging of the Web 2.0 phenomenon within health care [3]. However, e-health 2.0 goes beyond the social networking technology to include a reformative or even revolutionary change in the fields of health care and clinical research [3]. According to O'Grady the main point of e-health 2.0 is the use of social software and its ability to promote collaboration between patients, their caregivers, and medical professionals [3]. Thus, using the web to exchange information with others substantially relates to learning and education about an illness, what treatment options are available, how to make decisions, and for support [3]. In a broad sense, it can be conceived that Web 2.0 technologies enable and facilitate social networking, participation, openness, and collaboration, within and between health care consumers, caregivers, patients, health professionals, and biomedical researchers [4].

This chapter highlights actual developments at the crossroads of MS treatment and research and interactive applications of the internet, thereby focusing on online self-assessment, interactive web-based care and interactive phase IV research, and their potential for patient empowerment.

2. Multiple sclerosis

2.1 Disease characteristics

MS is a chronic disease of the central nervous system (CNS) that is pathologically characterized by multiple areas of inflammation, demyelination, axonal loss and gliosis, predominantly but not exclusively in the white matter. Compared to other chronic CNS disorders MS is distinguished by a wide range of symptoms and a highly variable course. Typical clinical features are optic neuritis, paresis, diplopia, paresthesias, incoordination, bladder and bowel disturbances, cognitive dysfunction, anxiety, depression and fatigue [5].

In most patients the onset of disease is between 20 and 40 years of age. In 80% to 85% of the patients the initial phase is characterized by relapses and remissions: RRMS. Relapse / remission episodes are alternated by relatively stable periods of months to years. During a relapse symptoms typically evolve over days to weeks, and after a plateau phase often spontaneously improve, completely or incompletely. The total duration of a relapse / remission episode, from initial symptom to final recovery, varies from less than a week to more than half a year.

To explain the etiology of MS it is thought that myelin-specific auto-reactive lymphocytes are primed in the periphery by unknown factors, after which they migrate to the CNS, leading to inflammatory demyelination and axonal loss [6]. Recent studies have suggested that the innate immune system also plays a role both in the initiation and progression of MS [6]. Inflammation composed of mononuclear cells, breakdown of the blood brain barrier, focal plaques of demyelination and axonal damage characterize the acute MS lesions and underlie relapses [7]. Importantly, the frequency and severity of the immune-mediated changes can be reduced by DMDs.

As the disease duration increases the tendency of relapses to recover diminishes, which results in a higher risk of relapse-related deficits and a step-wise accrual of disability. Eventually, after a period of 10 to 20 years, most RRMS patients transgress to the secondary progressive phase (SPMS), characterized by a relentless continuous progression of disability. In about 15% of the MS patients symptoms start insidiously and continue to slowly progress without relapses, the primary progressive course (PPMS). In both SPMS and PPMS clinical deficits mainly result from axonal degeneration, whereas inflammation plays only a minor role. Accordingly, DMDs are not efficacious in SPMS and PPMS.

2.2 Diagnosis

In the last two decades the sensitivity and specificity of the MS diagnosis has considerably improved due to two developments. Firstly, the wide-spread use of the magnetic resonance imaging (MRI) technique for detection of lesions in brain and spinal cord, and secondly, new diagnostic criteria proposed by McDonald et al.. The improved diagnosis in combination with the availability of DMDs has increased doctors' awareness of MS as a possible cause of an episode of CNS disturbances in young adults. In such patients ancillary MRI and cerebrospinal fluid (CSF) analyses may yield abnormal findings that, in combination with the clinical features, justify the diagnosis possible or definite RRMS according to the revised McDonald criteria [8]. Patients who do not fulfill these criteria and in whom other disorders have been adequately excluded are diagnosed as having a so-called clinically isolated syndrome (CIS) suggestive of MS, briefly CIS [8]. A CIS may be monofocal – when clinical abnormalities relate to a single CNS lesion – or multifocal, and often involve the optic nerve, brainstem, cerebellum, spinal cord, or cerebral hemispheres [8].

On T2-weighed brain MRI the great majority of MS patients show multiple hyper-intense lesions. These are typically ovoid shaped with the longitudinal axis perpendicular to the ventricles, of varying hyper-intensity, and located peri-ventricular, juxta-cortical or infra-tentorial in an asymmetric bilateral pattern [8]. In most MS patients MRI of the spinal cord also shows T2 hyper-intense abnormalities, and the absence of spinal lesions on a technically adequate MRI scan is considered a red flag.

2.3 Assessment and treatment of major symptoms

Fatigue

Fatigue is reported by over 80% of MS patients [9] and often interferes with family life, work or social activities [10]. It is a major determinant of impaired health-related quality of life (HRQoL) in MS [11]. Psychometrically validated questionnaires for measuring MS-related fatigue are the Fatigue Impact Scale (FIS), the Modified Fatigue Impact Scale (MFIS), and the Fatigue Severity Scale (FSS). Treatment options include a management program for a more efficient use of energy, progressive resistance training, cognitive behavioral therapy, and pharmacotherapy. Drugs that are believed to potentially improve MS-related fatigue are amantadine, 4-aminopyridine, 3,4-diaminopyridine, and modafinil. When 6 to 8 weeks after start of a drug treatment the patient has not experienced a relevant decrease in fatigue, the treatment is discontinued and a different drug is considered.

Bladder dysfunction

Symptoms of bladder dysfunction are uncommon at presentation but frequently develop in the course of the disease, and are often associated with spastic paraparesis and sexual problems [5]. The increased urge and voiding frequency result from detrusor muscle over-activity and detrusor-sphincter dyssynergia. Urinary tract infections, resulting from incomplete bladder emptying, are a frequent complication and may lead to worsening of MS symptoms. A 3-day Voiding Diary, the Urinary Distress Inventory (UDI-6) and the Incontinence Impact Questionnaire (IIQ-7) are validated tools to comprehensively assess bladder dysfunction in MS. Pharmacotherapeutic options include anticholinergics, cannabinoids and botulinum toxin.

Anxiety and depression

Anxiety and depression are increasingly being recognized as frequent symptoms in MS and as a major determinant of worsened HRQoL [11]. The Hospital Anxiety and Depression Scale (HADS) questionnaire is a validated assessment tool. In daily practice anxiety disorders, and to a lesser degree depression, are often under-diagnosed in MS patients. As a consequence, patients are deprived of psychological and pharmacological treatments that might be effective in reducing symptoms and disease burden.

Cognitive impairment

Cognitive disturbances are a prominent feature of MS, occurring in about half of all patients [12] and in one third of patients with early RRMS [13]. The most frequently impaired domains are complex attention, information processing speed, and memory and executive functions. MS patients with problems in cognitive performance have increased odds of becoming unemployed [12]. Importantly, cognitive symptoms in early RRMS are predictive of disability several years later [14], and in benign RRMS failure on neuropsychological tests predicts clinical worsening over a 3-year period [15].

The detection of cognitive impairment in a RRMS patient is a reason to evaluate the current policy. Routine evaluation of cognition is useful for helping patients to address ensuing problems and to detect cognitive decline as a sign of disease progression or treatment failure [16]. Two neuropsychological test batteries have been developed for use in MS patients, the Brief Repeatable Neuropsychological Battery (BRNB) and the Minimal Assessment of Cognitive Functioning in Multiple Sclerosis (MACFIMS) [for brief descriptions see reference 17]. The high rater and patient burden (the MACFIMS taking around 90 minutes to administer) and the high degree of expertise needed to administer, seriously limit the utility of BRNB and MACFIMS in patient care and clinical trials [17]. A recent study reported the preliminary validation of a brief computerized cognitive battery in RRMS [17]. Previous data supported the reliability of the Symbol Digit Modalities Test (SDMT) and the Multiple Sclerosis Neuropsychological Questionnaire (MSNQ) as potential tools for screening and monitoring of cognition in MS [18]. Studies investigating the utility of the SDMT as an online test are ongoing. Neuropsychological (memory) training, aiming to improve or stabilize cognitive performance, and adjustment of coping strategies are management options. Drugs for treatment of cognitive symptoms are under study, although presently no pharmacotherapy is available [17].

2.4 Disease modifying drugs

The DMDs exert their effect by modifying immune mechanisms related to the inflammatory disease process, and thus prevent demyelination and axonal damage. The first-line DMDs INFb and GA combine a moderate efficacy with proven safety, in both the short and the long term. In contrast, the highly efficacious DMDs natalizumab, fingolimod and cladribine are more likely to have potentially serious side effects on the short term, whereas their long term safety still has to be established. The ongoing debate on the optimal use of the DMDs in RRMS patients directly relates to their perceived benefits and risks.

In the escalating treatment approach naïve patients are first prescribed a moderately efficacious DMD, and in case of an insufficient response the drug is discontinued and a more potent DMD is started. This step-wise regimen is deemed appropriate in patients with low disability and a favorable prognosis. The alternative induction regimen is considered in treatment-naïve patients who, in spite of a short disease duration, already have acquired permanent neurological deficits due to frequent or severe relapses, and with a poor prognosis. The aim is to induce a substantial and long-lasting reduction in disease activity, in order that future relapses can be prevented by a moderately efficacious DMD. The inductive effects of the immunosuppressive agents mitoxantrone and cyclophosphamide have been studied in clinical trials. Natalizumab is, strictly speaking, not an inductive agent, as it's discontinuation is followed by a reappearance of disease activity.

In either scenario, escalation or induction, there is a need to closely monitor disease activity, in order to prevent further increase in disability (escalation regimen) or unnecessary risk of serious side effects (induction regimen).

2.5 Concept of (very) early treatment

Pathological findings indicate that inflammation occurring early in the disease leads to axonal damage and permanent tissue loss. These histological changes are in due course mirrored by the appearance of permanent T1-weighed hypo-intense lesions, and brain and spinal cord atrophy on MRI. Recent epidemiological data indicate that as soon as a disability level of Expanded Disability Status Score (EDSS) 3 or 4 has been reached, the increase in disability during the further course of the disease no longer relates to relapses or treatment with DMDs. Interestingly, observational data indicate that start of DMD treatment within 24 months of disease onset, and even more so in the first 12 months, is associated with less long-term disability, later transgression to SPMS and a slower progression during SPMS. The concept of (very) early DMD treatment is based on these and related studies and proposes to start treatment after the first episode, including CIS, or at least in the first 12 to 24 months. However, the disease course and accrual of disability is highly variable between patients. So, in order not to unnecessarily treat patients who would have a benign course without treatment, the (very) early use of DMDs is restricted to those patients in whom prognostic features are unfavorable.

2.6 Prognostic features

There is a body of evidence suggesting that to a certain degree the short-term disease course can be predicted from the presence or absence of specific clinical, MRI and CSF findings. However, the methodological limitations of the investigations on the predictive value of parameters with respect to the long-term disability make that in individual patients a formal prognosis cannot be established. Yet, a comprehensive appraisal of the available patient data might justify an 'educated guess' on a patient's prospects, especially for the short term.

The following clinical characteristics of a first RRMS episode or of CIS are considered prognostically unfavorable: multifocal symptoms, pyramidal, cerebellar, or sphincter symptoms, need of steroid treatment, and incomplete recovery. In patients with two or more relapses a short interval between the first and the second attack is unfavorable, as is the occurrence of three or more relapses in the first three years. Some abnormalities suggestive of MS on diagnostic MRI also have a prognostic relevance: the occurrence of three or more T2-weighed hyper-intense lesions, two or more infra-tentorial lesions, corpus callosum lesions, cortical lesions, diffuse lesions in the cervical spinal cord, cerebral or cervical spinal cord atrophy, T1-weighed hypo-intense lesions, and one or more gadolinium-enhancing lesions. Finally, the presence of immunoglobuline G oligoclonal bands (IgG-OCB), intrathecal immunoglobulin M (IgM) synthesis, and a high concentration of light chain neurofilament on CSF analyses have also been associated with a less favorable course.

2.7 Therapeutic goals

Conventional clinical measures of the effectiveness of DMD treatment include the number and severity of relapses, need of steroid-treatment for relapses, and EDSS or Multiple

Sclerosis Functional Composite (MSFC) score (disability). In clinically stable patients new or enlarged T2-weighed hyper-intense lesions, new or enlarged T1-weighed hypo-intense lesions or gadolinium-enhanced T1- weighed MRI lesions, and (increase of) cerebral or spinal cord atrophy all reflect subclinical disease activity. Clinical and MRI parameters may be combined into a composite measure of disease activity or disease free status. Thus, in a recent study sustained freedom of disease activity was defined as the patient having no relapse, no 3-month sustained increase in EDSS, and no new MRI lesions (no T1 gadolinium-enhancing or new/enlarged T2 lesions) over a specified period [19].

The ultimate goal of DMD treatment is not only to prevent clinical and MRI disease activity, but also the transgression to SPMS. For DMDs to have a maximum chance to obtain this long-term goal, treatment should not only be started timely but also managed in such a way that EDSS 3 to 4 is not reached. To this end the following short-term clinical and MRI measures of disease activity may be monitored: occurrence of a relapse, change in disability (EDSS), new or enlarging T2-weighed hyper-intense or T1-weighed hypo-intense lesions, gadolinium-enhancing lesions, and (increase of) brain and spinal cord atrophy. It was recently found that early EDSS change and medication possession ratio are moderate predictors of long-term disability [20] [21]. A higher medication possession ratio predicted better long-term clinical outcomes, while greater early increase in EDSS score predicted worse outcomes. In contrast, change in MRI parameters were only weakly associated with long-term outcome [20]. So, it seems that short-term clinical changes and adherence to DMD treatment have a higher prognostic value than MRI measures. The added value of composite measures remains to be established.

3. E-health 2.0 in multiple sclerosis treatment

The availability of a broad range of DMDs for the treatment of RRMS, the prognostic relevance of early disease activity in CIS and RRMS, the prognostic relevance of early disease activity after start of treatment, the importance of the timing of treatment initiation, the potentially serious side effects of the newer drugs and our ignorance of their long-term risks, implicate that in the coming years MS treatment is increasingly being characterized by both complexity and personalization. In this context, the use of Web 2.0 techniques for interactive online monitoring and care might make a crucial contribution to the management of MS patients. Interactive online monitoring and care are believed to enhance the chances that the potential benefits of the DMDs are realized and that treatment goals are achieved.

3.1 Monitoring

Aspects of monitoring

Monitoring may be defined as repeated testing aimed at guiding and adjusting the management of a chronic or recurrent condition [22]. Minimum criteria for monitoring are that clinically significant changes in the condition or effect of treatment occur over time, that there is an available monitoring test that reliably detects clinically significant changes when they occur, and that cost-effective action can be taken on the basis of the test result [22]. As monitoring involves a series of tests over time a monitoring strategy needs to consider frequency and timing of tests in the context of a series of sequential results [22]. It should address the following questions: Who should be monitored? What outcome should be monitored? What test should be used? When, and at what interval? Who should do the monitoring? What action to take on the monitoring result? [23]. Only since the occurrence in 2005 of progressive multifocal leukencelopathy, a potentially lethal CNS disorder, as a rare side effect of natalizumab has monitoring become a topic in MS neurology. As monitoring of disease activity and adverse events in DMD-treated patients is a rather recent development, most of the fundamental questions regarding the optimal monitoring strategies still have to be answered.

Monitoring in multiple sclerosis

In view of the nature of the parameters for current or future disease activity mentioned above, the conventional monitoring of CIS and RRMS patients focuses on doctor-centered clinical and MRI outcomes. In fact, in daily clinical practice the natural course of the disease as well as the course after start of DMD treatment is monitored by means of assessments during the patients' regular visits to the out-patient department, with intervals that usually vary from 3 to 12 months. Doctors and nurses ask about relevant changes in symptoms, notably those suggestive of a relapse or progression, and ideally disability is measured using a validated clinical scale, e.g. the EDSS or MSFC. However, in general neurological practices the regular and standardized quantification of disability is probably an exception, rather than the rule. Moreover, it is doubtful whether CIS and RRMS patients have a T2-weighed and gadolinium-enhanced T1-weighed brain and spinal MRI scan performed on a sufficiently regular basis, given the costs of scanning time and of gadolinium. Importantly, practical circumstances, like travel distances and expenses, scarcity of qualified medical personnel, and restricted availability of MRI machines, often prevent the conventional monitoring process from being optimal, both in terms of the selection of patients, the tests used, and the frequency of assessments.

Monitoring by online self-assessment

Compared to doctor-centered or technical measures patient-reported outcomes have various advantages. Firstly, they have an intrinsic clinical relevance; secondly, data are less expensive to acquire; and thirdly, the assessment schedule is more flexible and can easily be adjusted to changing circumstances or unexpected outcomes. For example, the frequency of assessments can be increased if there is a narrow time window regarding the start of DMD treatment, or if a dose increase is associated with a risk of serious side effects. Traditionally, patient-reported outcomes are obtained via questionnaires on site, per postal questionnaire or per telephone. Prospective well-designed studies in MS patients using patient-reported outcomes via the internet are scarce. Yet, especially the web-based applications of accepted and validated measures have obvious advantages compared to doctor-centered outcomes obtained on site. Online questionnaires and diaries can be completed at home at time points convenient to patients; errors and missing data are minimized by instantaneous checks of completeness and consistency; and electronic data capture into a database prevents transmission errors. Moreover, as online questionnaires are ready available, assessment intervals can be short and flexible, and monitoring schedules can easily be tailored to individual needs, e.g. for detection of early changes. Finally, patient-centered data may provide information that complements or partially substitutes doctor-reported data, rendering monitoring less time-consuming for neurologists and MS nurses.

We investigated in an exploratory manner whether monitoring by online self-assessments with monthly intervals is feasible and informative in RRMS patients starting a DMD [24].

We included 167 RRMS patients in a 12-month observational study during which patients were asked to complete two short questionnaires, on HRQoL and fatigue, at monthly intervals. 73.7% completed both questionnaires at all 13 time points, whereas 85.1% of the patients completed both questionnaires in at least 7 of the 13 time points. For both questionnaires the mean changes between baseline and month 12 were similar to those found in studies using paper questionnaires completed on site or at home with 6-month intervals. These data indicate the feasibility and potential usefulness of monitoring by monthly online self-assessment. Intensive online monitoring appears to be an informative and patient-friendly tool for assessing short-term effectiveness. It can be argued that the full advantages of monitoring by online self-assessment are only realized in the context of an interactive care setting.

3.2 Treatment and care

In the past two decades the expanding knowledge on the inflammatory mechanisms leading to tissue damage in MS and the pathophysiological changes underlying the major symptoms have initiated a plethora of therapeutic studies, varying from placebo-controlled randomized trials to observational studies and anecdotal reports. Study data have given neurologists and MS-nurses ample opportunities to substantially lessen the disease burden in their patients. However, it is recognized that as yet most patients insufficiently benefit from the insights and therapeutic potential generated by research data [25]. The unmet needs in MS patients relate to the fact that the implementation of treatment options is hampered by limited resources and organizational insufficiencies and inefficiencies. One of the measures to improve both effectiveness and efficiency of MS care may be the introduction of Web 2.0 applications in the care process.

Interactive online care

To outline the potential advantages of interactive online care in MS patients a typical example, the MSmonitor project, is described here. This project aims to improve MS care in the Netherlands by interactive use of the internet on the basis of patient-reported outcomes, obtained via online self-assessment. MSmonitor started in 2010 and at present 12 MS centers and neurological practices participate. Basically, every six months patients complete the Multiple Sclerosis Impact Profile (MSIP) and the Multiple Sclerosis Quality of Life-54 (MSQoL-54) or the Leeds Multiple Sclerosis Quality of Life (LMSQoL) scale online 1 to 2 weeks before their regular out-patient visit.

The MSIP is a psychometrically validated outcome measure for disability and disability perception in MS patients [26]. The scale is based on the International Classification of Functioning, Disability and Health (ICF) of the World Health Organization (WHO). The MSIP disability data are complementary to the doctor-centered EDSS. In those neurological practices where the EDSS cannot be assessed (time constraints, lack of qualified personnel) the MSIP disability data may provide a validated patient-reported alternative. In addition, the disability perception part of the MSIP informs on the subjective dimension of symptoms and signs and provides a systematic, complete, detailed, and quantitative overview of experienced burden of disease. In the online application of the MSIP answers that represent a worsening compared to the previous assessment are automatically highlighted. Thus, the online MSIP gives a quick screen of both the current condition and of recent changes. The individual data are made available on the secured project website to treating MS-nurse and neurologist, and helps them to prepare the on site consultation. In fact, the MSIP overview may guide the conversation between patient and MS-nurse or neurologist, by focusing on changes with high disability perception. The inventory of symptoms according to relevance and the preview opportunity for caregivers are thought to enhance effectiveness and efficiency of outpatient visits.

The MSQoL-54 and the LMSQoL measure HRQoL. HRQoL is a multidimensional concept related to a person's perception of well-being and the level of role fulfillment across a range of dimensions, including physical, psychosocial, social and symptom-related dimensions [27]. It is a term that refers to an individual's assessment of how a health problem as well as its treatment affect his/her ability to perform activities and roles that he/she values [28]. A critical element of HRQoL is that it reflects the patient's assessment of the impact of his/her illness, not the physician's perspective, as most physiologically oriented measures and traditional clinical scales do [29]. As HRQoL comprises not only perceptions of physical functioning and general health, but also perceived psychological functioning and social/role functioning [30], its assessment is thought to provide a comprehensive evaluation of an individual's health [31]. Using the MSIP it was demonstrated that HRQoL impairment in MS patients was most related to emotional problems, cognitive dysfunction, and sleep disturbances [26]. In DMD-treated patients the HRQoL data help to assess the treatment's overall effectiveness from the patient's perspective [32] [33].

In addition to the 6-monthly assessments, MS-nurse and neurologist may in selected patients activate these scales at additional time points or activate symptom-related questionnaires for in-depth assessment of specific symptoms, e.g. when a subjective worsening has been reported by e-mail or by phone; or to obtain valid pre-treatment values by repeated measurements; or to closely follow initial changes after start of treatment; or to evaluate specific treatment effects. An example: the beneficial effect of symptomatic drug treatment of MS-related fatigue usually manifests itself within 6 to 8 weeks. The low chance of a relevant change in fatigue and the possibility of side effects urge a timely evaluation. The repeated online use of the MFIS informs on the baseline condition and the degree of short-term change in MS-related fatigue. Other symptoms can also be quantified online by symptom-specific validated questionnaires, such as depression and anxiety by the HADS, bladder symptoms by a Voiding Diary, and comorbidity by the Self-Report Comorbidity Questionnaire for Multiple Sclerosis (SRCQ-MS). The SDMT may be included for assessment of cognition, as soon as preliminary data on an the validity of the online version have been confirmed.

The combination of the instantaneous availability of patient-reported outcomes on disability, disability perception and symptoms prior to and during out-patient visits, the possibility of repeated assessments and of symptom-related in–depth measurements, the online evaluation by caregivers via the secured website, and the flexible feedback by short-message service (SMS) or e-mail has the potential to improve effectiveness and efficiency of MS treatment and care. Moreover, an outcome value that represents a clinically minimally important change may be set as an alert level. As soon as the outcome variable reaches the predefined limit an alert pops up on the screen, a message is sent by e-mail to the neurologist or MS-nurse, or appears on their screen after log in, whatever is decided. E.g. patients with a tendency to depressive symptoms who start INFb treatment may use the online HADS for monitoring mood with a predefined alert set-point. Preliminary data from the MSmonitor project indicate that the use of Web 2.0 technology in MS care benefits both patient and caregiver in terms of flexibility and efficiency, as self-assessment, evaluation, and feedback do not depend on consulting hours or simultaneous availability of patient and caregiver. A next step will be the development of an interactive education program for patients and caregivers.

4. E-health 2.0 in multiple sclerosis research

4.1 Web-based phase IV research

Randomized placebo-controlled phase II/III trials provide data on a DMD's efficacy to reduce in the short term the frequency and severity of the clinical manifestations of inflammation (relapses) and of surrogate parameters (MRI lesions). Such trials do not inform on the long-term efficacy, in terms of preventing disability increase or conversion to SPMS, or slowing progression during SPMS; nor on long-term side effects. It is also of note that in fact the phase II/III results do not pertain to patients treated in real life, as data are typically obtained from selected patients, treated in dedicated MS centers in large, often academic hospitals.

Data on the long-term effectiveness and safety in patients treated in daily practice can be acquired in observational phase IV studies, and the internet enables virtually every MS patient to participate in such studies. Within the framework of a prospective observational study every patient who starts a treatment can be asked to regularly complete online a set of standard questions concerning aspects of effectiveness and side effects. In a web-based study a patient's participation does not depend on his/her geographic location or distance to out-patient clinic, and therefore an online study may include large cohorts in whole regions or even countries. Methodologically, the representative character of the online acquired data enables the external validation of the phase III data. As to drug safety, an online observational study covering a whole population or region with virtually no restrictive selection criteria yields an almost complete picture of adverse events in real life.

4.2 Interactive observational research

An important aspect of web-based phase IV research is that study data on effectiveness and safety from individual patients can be made available to treating MS-nurse or neurologist for monitoring purposes. We started in the Netherlands the Dutch MS Study, a prospective, online, patient-centred study of long-term disability, disability perception and HRQoL in patients with MS or CIS. Every 6 months patients complete the MSIP (disability and disability perception) and the MSQoL-54 (HRQoL). Disease characteristics and demographic, diagnostic and medication data are recorded online at the start of a patient's participation, and thereafter relapses and medication use can be updated every month. A patient may consent to give his/her MS-nurse or neurologist access to the study data for evaluation of treatment or the natural course of the disease. Actually, as the information provided by the study data may lead to an adjustment of the disease management, e.g. discontinuation or change of medication, we have created a setting in which there is an interaction between observation and daily practice. As a result, the study data may give insight not only into factors that relate to changes in the disease course, but also in those that drive the decisions regarding treatment and care processes.

The study's inclusion criteria are: having the diagnosis MS or CIS, and being willing and able to participate in the investigations. The latter criterion implies the availability of a computer for online access. In fact, as almost every patient with MS or CIS is eligible the Dutch MS study is developing into an interactive Dutch MS registry.

4.3 Adherence and adherence research

The effectiveness of DMD treatment depends on adequate adherence and implies year-long continued drug administration with a minimum of missed doses. The two aspects of inadequate adherence are: 1) missing doses, and 2) early discontinuation for other reason than insufficient response, serious side effects or persistent moderate side effects. Patients treated with the injectable first-line DMDs miss 30% of the doses [34], and the 6-month discontinuation rate may be as high as 27% [35]. It has been known that DMD discontinuation for more than three months is associated with a increased risk of relapses. Recent data show that in RRMS patients the degree of disability eight years after start of INFb-1a treatment is related to the medication possession ratio [21] Adherence is influenced by the socio-economic situation, health care and caregivers, disease, treatment and patient characteristics. In MS patients self-efficacy expectations are thought to be related to adherence, as are patient education and optimal support. A detailed knowledge of those aspects of care that significantly relate to adherence may lead to adherence-improving measures. Moreover, the identification of patients at high risk of inadequate adherence could lead to more efficient care.

The CAIR (Correlative analyses of Adherence In Relapsing remitting multiple sclerosis) study investigates in GA-treated RRMS patients the relationship between drug adherence and multidisciplinary care, as well as factors associated with adherence [36]. The study is a prospective, web-based, patient-centered, nation-wide, observational cohort study in the Netherlands. The primary objective is to investigate whether adherence is associated with specific disciplines of care or quantities of specific care. The secondary objective is to investigate whether adherence is associated with specific aspects of the socio-economic situation, health care and caregivers, disease, treatment or patient characteristics.

All data are acquired online via a study website (www.cairstudie.nl) and all RRMS patients in the Netherlands starting GA treatment were eligible. At pre-defined and random time-points patients are requested to complete a short questionnaire on missed doses and eventual discontinuation. Every two weeks patients record the care they received (discipline, frequency, duration). The Dutch Adherence Questionnaire-90 (DAQ-90), a 90-item questionnaire based on the World Health Organization (WHO) 2003 report on adherence, comprehensively assesses the five domains of evidence-based determinants of adherence: socio-economic, health care and caregivers, disease, treatment, and patient-related factors. Self-efficacy is assessed by the Multiple Sclerosis Self-Efficacy Scale (MSSES), and mood and HRQoL by the MSQoL-54.

Importantly, adherence data from online self-assessment can be used in an interactive web-based care setting, like the MSmonitor project. Access to individual data enables neurologist and MS-nurse to monitor adherence, whereas the regular completion of a short questionnaire may per se be an adherence promoting activity. Based on the online data caregivers will be able to give feedback to patients with inadequate adherence, whereas the choice of adherence improving measures can be guided by the pre-treatment online inventory of risk factors (DAQ-90). It is expected that in the near future online monitoring of adherence and interactive web-based care, tailored to the individual risk factors, may help to improve adherence and thus the effectiveness of DMD treatments.

4.4 Patient empowerment

The interactive use of the internet for monitoring and care purposes enables patients to better understand and evaluate their own conditions. As a result, patients become educated partners in the relation with caregivers and may take initiatives as to how their MS should be managed. Interactive programs that inform and educate on treatment options, e.g. using evidence-based algorithms, will help patients to position themselves as independent actors in the process of benefit-to-risk evaluation and shared decision making. As the Web 2.0 technology is likely to increase knowledge and awareness in many individual patients, it may thus collectively transform web-based patient communities into grassroots movements that initiate and drive research projects on topics that are relevant to patients but do not appeal to pharmaceutical companies and academia.

5. Conclusion

Current developments suggest that in the coming years Web 2.0 technologies will be integrated in the treatment and care of MS patients and in MS research. Monitoring of effectiveness, safety and adherence by online self-assessment is the basis of interactive online care and (interactive) observational phase IV research. E-health 2.0 developments are likely to increase patients' empowerment and will favor patient-driven decision making and research. In the context of ever diminishing health care resources and an increasing likelihood of drastic changes in the health care system, for MS patients e-health 2.0 could make the difference between, on the one hand, an ongoing suboptimal use of ever more efficacious drugs with persistence of unmet needs, and, on the other hand, personalized, more effective and safe treatments that may prevent long-term disability.

6. References

[1] http://www.techpluto.com/web-20-services.
[2] http://en.wikipedia.org/wiki/Web_2.0.
[3] http://health20.org/wiki/Health_2.0_Definition.
[4] Eysenbach G. Medicine 2.0: Social Networking, Collaboration, Participation, Apomediation, and Openness. J Med Internet Res 2008;10(3):e22; doi:10.2196/jmir.1030.
[5] Multiple Sclerosis. Clinical and pathogenetic basis. CS Raine, HF McFairland, WW Tourtelotte (eds). London, Chapman & Hall Medical, London, 1997.
[6] Gandhi R, Laroni A, Weiner HL. Role of the innate immune system in the pathogenesis of multiple sclerosis. Review. J Neuroimmunol 2010;221(1-2):7-14.
[7] Nessler S, Brück W. Advances in multiple sclerosis research in 2009. J Neurol 2010; 257(9):1590-1593.
[8] Polman CH, Reingold SC, Banwell B,Clanet M, Cohen JA, Filippi M, et al. Diagnostic criteria for multiple sclerosis: 2010 revisions to the McDonald criteria. Ann Neurol 2011;69(2):292-302. doi: 10.1002/ana.22366.
[9] Krupp LB. Mechanisms, measurement, and management of fatigue in multiple sclerosis. In Multiple sclerosis: clinical challenges and controversies. AJ Thompson, C Polman, R Hohlfeld (eds). London, Martin Dunitz, 1997: pp 283-294.
[10] Fisk JD, Pontefract A, Ritvo PG, Archibald CJ, Murray TJ: The impact of fatigue on patients with multiple sclerosis. Can J Neurol Sci 1994; 21:9-14.

[11] Ziemssen T. Multiple sclerosis beyond EDSS: depression and fatigue. J Neurol Sci 2009;277(Suppl 1):S37-41.

[12] Strober L, Englert J, Munschauer F, Weinstock-Guttman B, Rao S, Benedict RH. Sensitivity of conventional memory tests in multiple sclerosis: comparing the Rao Brief Repeatable Neuropsychological Battery and the Minimal Assessment of Cognitive Function in MS. Mult Scler 2009;15:1077-1084.

[13] Amato MP, Zipoli V, Portaccio E: Cognitive changes in multiple sclerosis. Expert Rev Neurother 2008;8:1585-1596.

[14] Deloire M, Ruet A, Hamel D, Bonnet M, Brochet B. Early cognitive impairment in multiple sclerosis predicts disability outcome several years later. Mult Scler;16:581-587.

[15] Portaccio E, Stromillo ML, Goretti B, Zipoli V, Siracusa G, Battaglini M, et al. Neuropsychological and MRI measures predict short-term evolution in benign multiple sclerosis. Neurology 2009;73:498-503.

[16] Benedict RH, Zivadinov R. Risk factors for and management of cognitive dysfunction in multiple sclerosis. Nat Rev Neurol 2011; 7(6):332-342. doi: 10.1038/nrneurol.2011.61.

[17] Edgar C, Jongen PJ, Sanders E, Sindic C, Goffette S, Dupuis M, et al. Cognitive performance in relapsing remitting multiple sclerosis: A longitudinal study in daily practice using a brief computerized cognitive battery. BMC Neurol 2011;11:68.

[18] Morrow SA, O'Connor PW, Polman CH, Goodman AD, Kappos L, Lublin FD, et al. Evaluation of the symbol digit modalities test (SDMT) and MS neuropsychological screening questionnaire (MSNQ) in natalizumab-treated MS patients over 48 weeks. Mult Scler 2010;16(11):1385-1392.

[19] Giovannoni G, Cook S, Rammohan K, Rieckmann P, Sorensen PS, Vermersch P, et al. Sustained disease-activity-free status in patients with relapsing-remitting multiple sclerosis treated with cladribine tablets in the CLARITY study: a post-hoc and subgroup analysis. The Lancet Neurology 2011;10(4); 329–337.

[20] Traboulsee A, Uitdehaag BMJ, Kappos L, Sandberg-Wollheim M, Li D, Jongen PJ, et al. Clinical and Magnetic Resonance Imaging Predictors of Long-Term Outcomes in Patients with Relapsing–Remitting Multiple Sclerosis: Additional Analyses. 63rd Annual Meeting of the American Academy of Neurology, Honolulu, Hawaii; 9–16 April 2011.

[21] Uitdehaag B, Constantinescu C, Cornelisse P, Jeffery D, Kappos L, Li D. Impact of exposure to interferon beta-1a on outcomes in patients with relapsing-remitting multiple sclerosis: exploratory analyses from the PRISMS long-term follow-up study. Ther Adv Neurol Disord 2011;4(1):3-14.

[22] Glasziou PP, Aronson JK. An introduction to monitoring therapeutic interventions in clinical practice. In Glasziou PP, Irwig L, Aronson JK (eds). Evidence-based medical monitoring. From principles to practice. Oxford, Blackwell Publishing 2008, pp. 3-14.

[23] Mant D. An introduction to monitoring therapeutic interventions in clinical practice. In Glasziou PP, Irwig L, Aronson JK (eds). Evidence-based medical monitoring. From principles to practice. Oxford, Blackwell Publishing 2008, pp. 15-30.

[24] Jongen PJ, Sanders E, Visser L, Zwanikken C, van Noort E, Koopmans P, et al. Automated on-line monitoring of health-related quality of life and fatigue in

relapsing remitting MS patients treated with glatiramer acetate. 1st International Congress on Clinical Neurology & Epidemiology, Munich, August 27-30, 2009.

[25] Bates D. Unmet Needs for People with Multiple Sclerosis. European Neurological Review. Touch Briefings 2008. http://www.touchbriefings.com/pdf/3248/bates.pdf European Neurology - Volume 3 Issue 2.

[26] Wynia K, Middel B, van Dijk JP, De Keyser JH, Reijneveld SA. The impact of disabilities on quality of life in people with multiple sclerosis. Mult Scler 2008;14:972–980.

[27] Zwibel H. Health and quality of life in patients with relapsing multiple sclerosis. J Neurol Sci 2009;287 S1:S11-S16

[28] Schipper H, Clinch JJ, Olweny CLM. Quality of life studies: de®nitions and conceptual issues. In Spilker B. (ed). Quality of life and pharmacoeconomics in clinical trials. 2nd ed. Philadelphia, Lippincott-Raven 1996, pp. 11-23.

[29] Hobart JC. Measuring health outcomes in multiple sclerosis: why, which, and how? In Thompson AJ, Polman C, Hohlfeld R, (eds). Multiple sclerosis: clinical challenges and controversies. London, Martin Dunitz 1997, pp. 211-225.

[30] Fischer JS, LaRocca NG, Miller DM, Ritvo PG, Andrews H, Paty D. Recent developments in the assessment of quality of life in multiple sclerosis (MS). Mult Scler 1999;5(4):251-259.

[31] Hopman WM, Coo H, Edgar CM, McBride EV, Day AG, Brunet DG. Factors associated with health-related quality of life in multiple sclerosis. Can J Neurol Sci 2007; 34(2):160-166.

[32] Jongen PJ, Sindic C, Carton H, Zwanikken C, Lemmens W, Borm G. Functional composite and quality of Life in Avonex-treated Relapsing multiple sclerosis patients study group. Improvement of health-related quality of life in relapsing remitting multiple sclerosis patients after 2 years of treatment with intramuscular interferon-beta-1a. J Neurol 2010;257(4):584-589.

[33] Jongen PJ, Lehnick D, Sanders E, Seeldrayers P, Fredrikson S, Andersson M, et al. Health-related quality of life in relapsing remitting multiple sclerosis patients during treatment with glatiramer acetate: a prospective, observational, international, multi-centre study. Health Qual Life Outcomes 2010;8:133.

[34] Lafata JE, Cerghet M, Dobie E, Schulz L, Tunceli K, Reuther J, Elias S. Measuring adherence and persistence to disease modifying agents among patients with relapsing remitting multiple sclerosis. J Am Pharm Assoc 2008;48:752-757.

[35] Tremlett HL, Oger J: Interrupted therapy: stopping and switching of the beta-interferons prescribed for MS. Neurology 2003;61:551-554.

[36] Jongen PJ, Hengstman G, Hupperts R, Schrijver H, Gilhuis J, Vliegen JH, et al. Drug adherence and multidisciplinary care in patients with multiple sclerosis: protocol of a prospective, web-based, patient-centred, nation-wide, Dutch cohort study in glatiramer acetate treated patients (CAIR study). BMC Neurol 2011;11:40.

Permissions

The contributors of this book come from diverse backgrounds, making this book a truly international effort. This book will bring forth new frontiers with its revolutionizing research information and detailed analysis of the nascent developments around the world.

We would like to thank Suman Kapur, for lending her expertise to make the book truly unique. She has played a crucial role in the development of this book. Without her invaluable contribution this book wouldn't have been possible. She has made vital efforts to compile up to date information on the varied aspects of this subject to make this book a valuable addition to the collection of many professionals and students.

This book was conceptualized with the vision of imparting up-to-date information and advanced data in this field. To ensure the same, a matchless editorial board was set up. Every individual on the board went through rigorous rounds of assessment to prove their worth. After which they invested a large part of their time researching and compiling the most relevant data for our readers. Conferences and sessions were held from time to time between the editorial board and the contributing authors to present the data in the most comprehensible form. The editorial team has worked tirelessly to provide valuable and valid information to help people across the globe.

Every chapter published in this book has been scrutinized by our experts. Their significance has been extensively debated. The topics covered herein carry significant findings which will fuel the growth of the discipline. They may even be implemented as practical applications or may be referred to as a beginning point for another development. Chapters in this book were first published by InTech; hereby published with permission under the Creative Commons Attribution License or equivalent.

The editorial board has been involved in producing this book since its inception. They have spent rigorous hours researching and exploring the diverse topics which have resulted in the successful publishing of this book. They have passed on their knowledge of decades through this book. To expedite this challenging task, the publisher supported the team at every step. A small team of assistant editors was also appointed to further simplify the editing procedure and attain best results for the readers.

Our editorial team has been hand-picked from every corner of the world. Their multi-ethnicity adds dynamic inputs to the discussions which result in innovative outcomes. These outcomes are then further discussed with the researchers and contributors who give their valuable feedback and opinion regarding the same. The feedback is then collaborated with the researches and they are edited in a comprehensive manner to aid the understanding of the subject.

Apart from the editorial board, the designing team has also invested a significant amount of their time in understanding the subject and creating the most relevant covers. They scrutinized every image to scout for the most suitable representation of the subject and create an appropriate cover for the book.

The publishing team has been involved in this book since its early stages. They were actively engaged in every process, be it collecting the data, connecting with the contributors or procuring relevant information. The team has been an ardent support to the editorial, designing and production team. Their endless efforts to recruit the best for this project, has resulted in the accomplishment of this book. They are a veteran in the field of academics and their pool of knowledge is as vast as their experience in printing. Their expertise and guidance has proved useful at every step. Their uncompromising quality standards have made this book an exceptional effort. Their encouragement from time to time has been an inspiration for everyone.

The publisher and the editorial board hope that this book will prove to be a valuable piece of knowledge for researchers, students, practitioners and scholars across the globe.

List of Contributors

Nathalie Cools, Viggo F. I. Van Tendeloo and Zwi N. Berneman
Laboratory of Experimental Hematology, Vaccine & Infectious Disease Institute, University of Antwerp, Belgium

Raffaele Girlanda, Cal S. Matsumoto, Keith J. Melancon and Thomas M. Fishbein
Transplant Institute, Georgetown University Hospital, Washington DC, USA

Stephen P. McAdoo and Frederick W. K. Tam
Imperial College Kidney and Transplant Institute, London, United Kingdom

L. De Filippis and L. Rota Nodari
Department of Biotechnologies and Biosciences, Università Milano Bicocca, Milan, Italy

Maurizio Gelati
Laboratorio Cellule Staminali, Cell Factory e Biobanca, Azienda Ospedaliera "Santa Maria", Terni, Italy

Rosangela Correa Villar
Department of Radiation Oncology, University of Sao Paulo, Medicine School, Brasil

Cheguevara Afaneh, Meredith J. Aull, Sandip Kapur and David B. Leeser
Department of Surgery, Division of Transplant Surgery, New York-Presbyterian Hospital-Weill Cornell Medical College, New York, NY, USA

Artur Pupka and Tomasz Płonek
Wroclaw Medical University, Poland

Angel Mayor, Yelitza Ruiz, Diana Fernández and Robert Hunter-Mellado
Retrovirus Research Center, Universidad Central del Caribe School of Medicine, Bayamón, Puerto Rico

Barbara Kern and Robert Sucher
Department of Visceral, Transplant and Thoracic Surgery, Medical University Innsbruck, Austria

Peter Joseph Jongen
The MS4 Research Institute (MS4RI), The Netherlands

Printed in the USA
CPSIA information can be obtained
at www.ICGtesting.com
JSHW011402221024
72173JS00003B/385

9 781632 422415

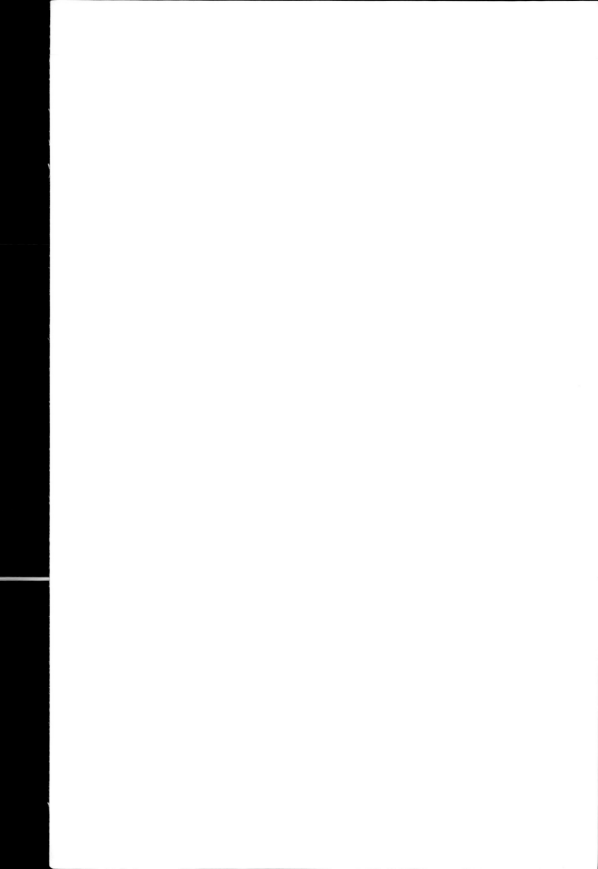